Peripheral Nerve Surgery - A Compendium

Katharina Hobitsch

Peripheral Nerve Surgery - A Compendium

Anatomy, Diagnostics, Pathologies and Surgical Approaches

Springer

Katharina Hobitsch
Department of Neurosurgery and Neurorestauration
Klinikum Klagenfurt am Wörthersee
Klagenfurt, Austria

ISBN 978-3-032-03408-3 ISBN 978-3-032-03409-0 (eBook)
https://doi.org/10.1007/978-3-032-03409-0

This Springer imprint is published by the registered company Springer Nature Switzerland AG
The registered company address is: Gewerbestrasse 11, 6330 Cham, Switzerland

Foreword

It is an honor to write the foreword to Periph*eral Nerve Surgery: A Compendium*, published by Springer and authored by Dr. Katharina Hobitsch. This handbook compiles clinically relevant information on peripheral nerve surgery and presents it in useful context and perspective, with dedicated sections on anatomy, diagnostics, pathologies, and surgical approaches.

Dr. Hobitsch is from Carinthia, Austria. She attended medical school from 2012 to 2018 in Timişoara, Romania, learning Romanian for that purpose. She returned to Austria for postgraduate training at the University of Innsbruck from 2019 to 2020 and then began her neurosurgical residency in March 2020 in Klagenfurt, Austria, near her home. She completed her neurosurgical board examination early and prepared this book during her six years of residency. In 2026, she will join the team in Klagenfurt and continue her work in complex nerve surgery, where she is currently documenting and registering nerve and tumor patients.

From early on, Dr. Hobitsch developed a keen interest in peripheral nerve surgery and strived to gain additional exposure and knowledge. She was influenced by her department chair, Thomas Kretschmer, MD, PhD, who, in addition to his broad training and expertise across various neurosurgical subspecialties, has maintained a major interest in and focus on peripheral nerve surgery. Under his guidance and encouragement, she spent three months in 2023 with Mariano Socolovsky, MD, PhD, in Buenos Aires, Argentina, for an embedded nerve fellowship supported by a grant from the Carinthian Medical Science Society—learning Spanish to do so. Her notes, based on these experiences, have been transformed into this book.

This handbook will become a treasured resource not only for those seeking to learn peripheral nerve surgery but also for those motivated to advance it. It blends facts and clinical pearls in a readable format and style, consolidating concepts and contributions made over generations. This book is well-illustrated and referenced and is appropriately sized. It continues a long thread of history, passing the baton of knowledge from mentor to mentee across generations, disciplines, and international borders. This book celebrates innovative international neurosurgeons and their threads: Thomas, mentored by Hans-Peter Richter and David Kline; Mariano, by Hector Giocoli (trained by Hanno Millesi) and Mario Siqueira. The book is also time-efficient and timely. It will fill a void and complement Stephen Russell's "Examination of Peripheral Nerve Injuries: An Anatomical Approach," first written in 2006 and updated in 2015, directly based on his postgraduate clinical training with David Kline.

A foreword is meant to provide perspective on the past, present, and future. This compendium will carry us forward. I commend the author on her perseverance and her mentors for their inspiration, dedication, and pursuit of excellence: the common ingredient being a passion for peripheral nerve surgery sustained through friendship and legacy.

Mayo Clinic
Rochester, MN, USA
November 2025

Robert J. Spinner, MD

Foreword

Peripheral Nerve Surgery: A Compendium is a beautiful piece of work from our resident and now faculty Katharina Hobitsch. In a nutshell, this is a structured compilation of knowledge, facts, and tips, up to mnemonics, which are supposed to be a real aid for nerve learners, who want to dive deeper into this beautiful field. Dr. Hobitsch structured her work in eight chapters: in Chaps. 1, 2, and 3, Anatomy; Chap. 4, clinical examination; Chap. 5, diagnostic tools; Chap. 6, surgery, including techniques, remarks on spasticity and neuroplasticity; Chap. 7, Pathology; and finally in Chap. 8, things good to know for nerve compression, tumor, and trauma. This clever chapter organization enabled her to organize numerous notes of her day-to-day learner's experience in a digestible plus easily retrievable format. Each chapter entails beautiful drawings made by Dr. Hobitsch's sister, a nurse at our department, and photographs from the operation room (Buenos Aires and Klagenfurt). The examination photos feature her brother as "the patient." This outline already points to the rather unusual approach of the compendium. Dr. Hobitsch has an interest in nerve from the beginning of her residency. She easily accumulated knowledge, fast and continuously, asked the right questions, and simply had joy to treat these patients. To broaden her horizon, she went on a three-month clinical fellowship in 2023 to visit Professor Socolowsky's nerve surgery team at Buenos Aires on a study grant from the Carinthian Medico-Scientific Society. She returned as a nerve enthusiast full of ideas; many thanks to the Buenos Aires team and the Society!

The structured learner that she is, she immediately started a note file there, which after her return transformed into the idea of a book supposed to be for her and other scholars of nerve. This is not, and never intended to be, a comprehensive textbook on nerve. It is a condensed compilation of facts and knowledge for the beginning and advanced "scholar of nerve" who is eager to start building and brushing up his knowledge-web with key facts chosen from a learner's perspective. From this perspective, chosen content and prioritization is different and that is crucial.

The European Association of Neurosurgical Societies (EANS) has been excellent to support the peripheral nerve subdiscipline and the international teaching efforts of the peripheral nerve family. I am confident that the compendium will also be used as a study resource for its annual nerve courses.

I am very proud of Dr. Hobitsch and her project, which in a way also was a family endeavor of its own kind. The way and time frame she handled this task is very remarkable, and the result is astounding and excellent.

So, I hope this work finds the distribution that it deserves and is an aid and starting point for future nerve experts.

I congratulate Dr. Hobitsch for her work and her perseverance!

Thomas Kretschmer, MD, PhD

Neurosurgeon, Klinikum Klagenfurt
Department of Neurosurgery
and Neurorestoration
Klagenfurt, Austria
November 2025

Preface

The present volume is addressed to young doctors who are interested in peripheral nerve surgery as a structured and coherent framework offering a fundamental knowledge, intended to serve as a basis for further study and clinical experience.

The material presented herein is derived from authoritative monographs, current literature, and—most importantly—on information I received from numerous outstanding peripheral nerve surgeons, whose willingness to share their expertise has been invaluable. It should serve as a straightforward introduction to the subspecialty of peripheral nerve surgery.

The structure of the book is designed to facilitate a progressive learning trajectory starting from the anatomy of a nerve, proceeds through methods of clinical examination and diagnostics, and culminates with an overview of the most relevant pathologies. In addition, current therapeutic guidelines are incorporated to align the content with contemporary standards of care.

Recognizing the pivotal role of clinical examination in guiding surgical decision-making, special emphasis has been placed on this chapter.

Another notable part in this book is dedicated to clinical and intraoperative considerations and advices with the intention to facilitate the complexity that young surgeons may face in the beginning of their "peripheral nerve surgery career."

The didactic value of the text is further enhanced by numerous illustrations and clinical photographs—many of which are unique—to give the book a more vivid character and facilitate comprehension and retention.

Due to its well-organized and condensed structure, it aids in fast finding, thereby serving as a useful reference for specific nerve knowledge prior to surgical intervention.

My goal gues embarking upon a career in peripheral nerve surgery by providing an extended overview of peripheral nerves without being overloaded, and at the same time informative and compact. Having one book instead of multiple sources simplifies the learning process.

Klagenfurt, Austria — Katharina Hobitsch

Acknowledgments

The idea for *Peripheral Nerve Surgery: A Compendium* arose from my growing dedication to peripheral nerves since I had the chance to get deeper into this field four years ago.

During my fellowship in Buenos Aires, I was privileged to observe numerous surgeries performed by Prof. Dr. Mariano Socolovsky—an internationally respected neurosurgeon in the field of peripheral nerve surgery—and his accomplished team. As I was a young resident at that time, I had plenty of questions, all of which Prof. Socolovsky answered with remarkable patience and generosity.

After two months devoted exclusively to peripheral nerve surgeries, I had filled a notebook with valuable information and remarks, which I wished to put together in a structured form for myself and for my colleagues at my hospital in Austria.

It was during this process when Prof. Socolovsky encouraged me to transform these notes into a proper book.

And this was the beginning; in April 2023, I started to convert my notes into book form.

Initially, my plan was to produce a concise pocket guide in PDF format for a limited circle of colleagues. However, when my Chief, Prof. Dr. Thomas Kretschmer, got to know about my project, he saw the potential for publishing the book in a bigger format accessible to a wider readership.

His continuous support made it possible to bring this book to completion. Throughout my residency, Prof. Dr. Kretschmer allowed me to participate in his nerve surgeries, generously shared his knowledge and operative techniques. Beyond his clinical guidance, he provided invaluable advice on the process of writing a book, shared his personal experiences, and introduced me to many distinguished surgeons in this field.

An essential part of this book—the illustrations—would not have been possible without the support of my family and friends.

My sister Viktoria, whose artistic talent is extraordinary, created all of the anatomical drawings. Despite her professional responsibilities and the demands of raising her daughter, she consistently found time to complete the illustrations with great dedication, thereby being an absolute perfectionist.

My brother and brother-in-law assisted with the photographs included in the clinical examination chapter.

I am also grateful to two colleagues for the valuable contributions: Dr. Daniela Binaghi, a radiologist from Buenos Aires and now living in

Quakenbrück, who provided the radiological images; and Dr. Johannes Troger, my colleague from the Department of Neurology in Klagenfurt, who supplied the electrophysiological illustrations.

I wish to express my sincere gratitude to all who have supported me throughout this endeavor. It is my earnest hope that this book will not only reflect the enrichment of my own professional development but will also serve as a useful resource for others pursuing the fascinating field of peripheral nerve surgery.

Contents

Abbreviations

ADUT	Anterior division of the upper trunk
ADP	Adductor pollicis muscle
AIN	Anterior interosseous nerve
AMS	Active move scale
BMI	Body mass index
BP	Brachial plexus
BPA	Brachial plexus avulsion
BPI	Brachial plexus injury
CC7	Contralateral C7
CFNG	Cross-facial nerve grafting
CIPD	Chronic inflammatory demyelinating polyneuropathy
CMP	Compound muscle action potential
CN	Cranial nerve
CNS	Central nervous system
CRPS	Complex regional pain syndrome
CSA	Cross-sectional area
CT	Computed tomography
CV	Conduction velocity
DBRN	Deep branch of the radial nerve
DIP	Distal interphalangeal joint
DREZ	Dorsal root entry zone
EMG	Electromyography
ENoG	Electroneurography
FDI	First dorsal interossei muscles
FCU	Flexor carpi ulnaris
GON	Greater occipital nerve
ILP	Isolated limb perfusion
IP	Interphalangeal joints
LFCN	Lateral femoral cutaneous nerve
LON	Lesser occipital nerve
LPI	Lumbar plexus injury
HB	House-Brackmann
HGC	Hourglass-like constriction
MCP	Metacarpophalangeal joint
MEP	Motor evoked potential
MCN	Musculocutaneous nerve
MMNST	Melanotic malignant peripheral nerve sheath tumor

MNT	Masseteric-to-facial nerve transposition
MPNST	Malignant peripheral nerve sheath tumor
MRC	Medical Research Council
MRI	Magnetic resonance imaging
MRN	Magnetic resonance neurography
MUAP	Motor units action potential
NAP	Nerve action potential
NF	Neurofibromatosis
NSM	Nerve sheath myxoma
OBPP	Obstetric brachial plexus palsy
PDUT	Posterior division of the upper trunk
PET	Positron emission tomography
PIN	Posterior interosseous nerve
PIP	Proximal interphalangeal joint
PNP	Polyneuropathy
PNS	Peripheral nervous system
PNST	Peripheral nerve sheath tumor
QSS	Quadrilateral space syndrome
ROM	Range of motion
SBRN	Superficial branch of the radial nerve
SCS	Spinal cord stimulation
SEP, SSEP	Somatosensory evoked potential
SNAP	Sensitive nerve action potential
SNES	Suprascapular nerve entrapment syndrome
T-SPOTT	Total split posterior tibial tendon transfer
Th7	Seventh thoracic vertebra
TIVA	Total intravenous anesthesia
TON	Third occipital nerve
TOS	Thoracic outlet syndrome
US	Ultrasound

Anatomy of the Nerve

1

The anatomy of peripheral nerves is defined by a clear structural organization crucial for their function and resilience. The nerve is encapsulated by the ***epineurium****, a fibrous and vascularized external layer allowing mobility of the nerve within its surrounding tissues and stretching to a certain degree without lesioning. Internally, the* ***perineurium*** *forms a protective barrier around the nerve fascicles which contain the nerve fibers called axons, while the* ***endoneurium*** *encases individual myelinated axons. Axons represent the smallest functional unit of a nerve and are classified by their size and conduction velocity into myelinated (Groups A and B) and unmyelinated (Group C), with the Schwann cells playing a key role in insulation and signal conduction.*

Nerve vascularization involves an extensive network extending from the mesoneurium to the endoneurial vessels.

Injury to peripheral nerves can be classified by ***Seddon*** *into neurapraxia, axonotmesis, and neurotmesis, and by the* ***Sunderland's*** *five-grade systems, according to the extent of axonal and connective tissue disruption.*

Regeneration *depends on the injury type and hinges on the integrity of the Schwann cells and their guidance structures, such as Büngner bands, with varying axonal regrowth rates. Functional recovery is influenced by various factor including the lesion site, the degree of injury, and—in cases of surgery—time to surgical intervention as well as the right method of surgery.*

Besides loss of nerve function, irreversible muscle atrophy and fibrosis may ensue if reinnervation fails within a critical period, underlining the need for timely and targeted nerve repair strategies.

1.1 Structural Units

The *epineurium* represents the external layer covering the whole nerve. It contains small vessels (intrinsic and extrinsic) and fatty tissue, and consists of an outer layer which is composed of collagen type I/III and elastin, as well as an inner layer which encloses the fascicles. Due to this composition, stretching of the nerve less than 12% of its length can be tolerated [1]. Stretching of the nerve at approximately 16% can lead to ischemia [2], while a continuous stretching of up to 1 mm per day is possible without lesioning the nerve [3].

The nerve is not fixed, but embedded in a vascularized *paraneurium (=mesoneurium)* allowing a smooth gliding within the tissue, which is important for movements especially in the extremities and joints.

Epithelioid myofibroblasts form the *perineurium* and create concentric layers in a lamellar configuration. The cells of the perineurium have gap junctions and tight junctions thereby forming a mechanical barrier towards the entering chemical substances from the blood.

K. Hobitsch, *Peripheral Nerve Surgery - A Compendium*,
https://doi.org/10.1007/978-3-032-03409-0_1

Injury to the perineurium—as it is seen in trauma—can lead to demyelination of the nerve and subsequent compromised neural transmission.

Another layer, called the *endoneurium* can be found surrounding each myelinated nerve fiber. This layer—formed of collagen type I and III as well as fibroblasts and macrophages—is rich of glycoproteins situated in an endoneurial fluid which is equivalent to the cerebral spinal fluid of the central nerve system (CNS), and may probably be involved in the regeneration of the nerve by sending out signals for the axons to grow.

Fascicles contain nerve fibers—called *axons*—representing the smallest functional unit of a nerve. The axon constitutes the elongated part of the nerve between the soma and the dendrites transmitting the electrical impulses from one neuron to another via synapses located at the dendrites, or to their end-targets (e.g. muscle fibers). They vary in length and diameter, factors that influence conduction velocity and are further dependent on the presence of myelin sheath. These properties are aligned with their specific function, with the sciatic nerve containing the longest axon.

Some axons may have bifurcations—so-called branches—that can modulate the direction of firing (Fig. 1.2).

Axons bigger than 1 μm in diameter are sheathed by *Schwann cells* [7]. Their degree of myelinization depends on the growth factor neuroregulin-1 and the proportion is approximately 1:1 [8]. They

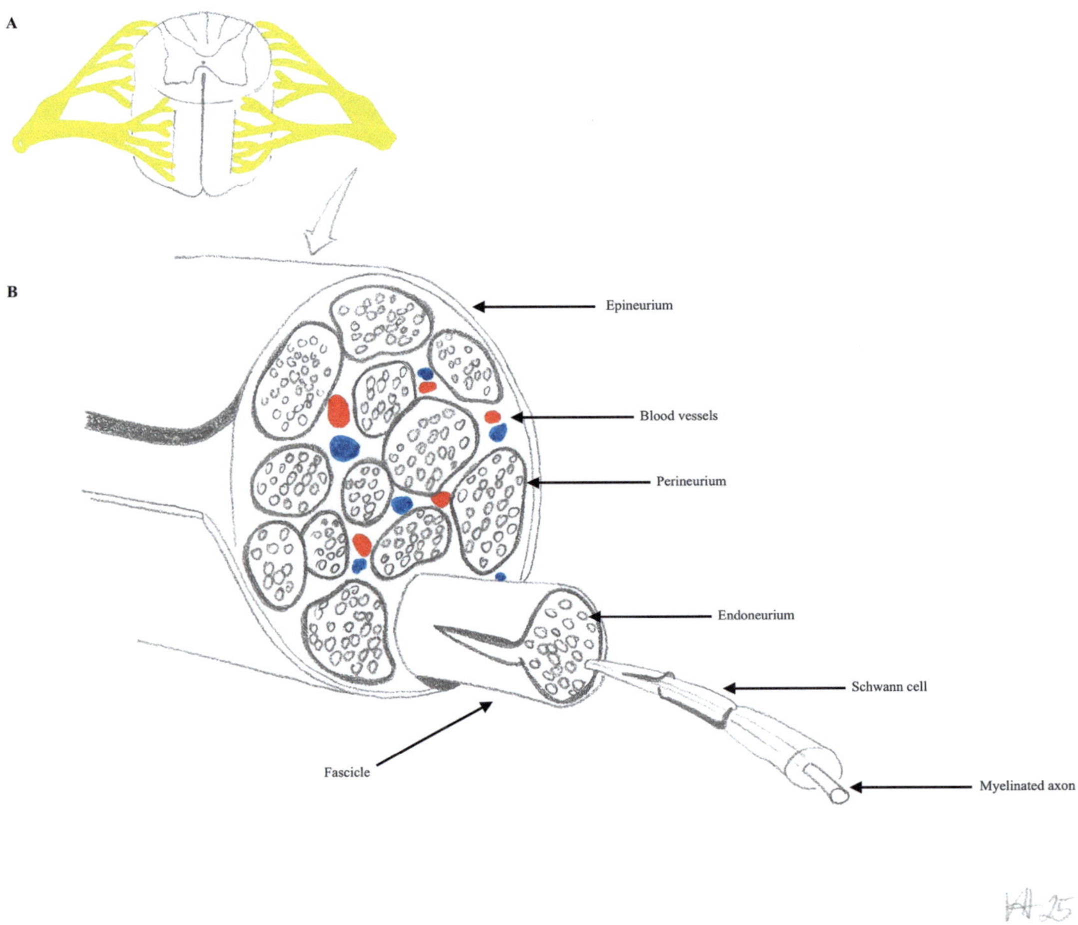

Fig. 1.1 (**a**) Ventral and dorsal ramus forming the spinal nerve. (**b**) Transverse section of a spinal nerve

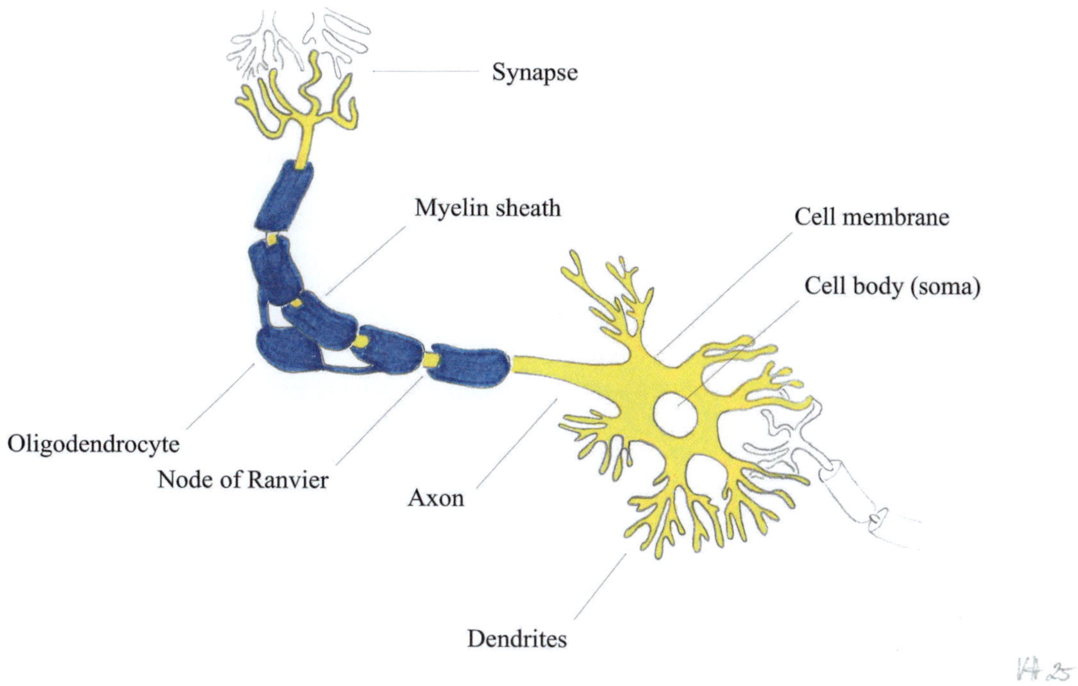

Fig. 1.2 Anatomy of an axon

are represented by motor and sensory axons and are usually of large diameter.

On the other hand, axons smaller than 1 μm in diameter are also coated by the Schwann cells but no myelinization takes place. Examples for those axons are nociceptive nerves or axons of the autonomic nervous system.

Remak bundles are unmyelinated axons (C-fibers) sheathed together by Schwann cells unlike being individually surrounded by them.

Wrapping of the Schwann cells provides insulation, thus increasing the velocity of the electrical signal.

Small unmyelinated gaps with a high number of ion channels along the axons are called nodes of Ranvier and enable an even faster "saltatory" electrical conduction.

Based on their size and conduction velocity, nerve fibers can be classified into three groups (Erlanger and Gasser 1924):

- *Group A* are fibers with the thickest myelinization—thus being fibers with the fastest rate of transmission—and can be further subdivided into alpha Aα, beta Aβ, gamma Aγ, and delta Aδ; according to their amount of myelin sheath. Their conduction velocity can reach up to 120 m/s (Aδ fibers).
- *Group B* have a moderate amount of myelinization with a conduction velocity of 3–15 m/s. They are predominantly located within the autonomic nervous system.
- *Group C* represent the smaller, unmyelinated fibers serving as the sensory afferent nerve fibers (e.g. nociceptive or tactile fibers). Their conduction velocity accounts 0.25–1.5 m/s.

Within mixed sensorimotor nerves, the fascicles are interconnected in a plexus-like manner. Axons may alter their trajectory by passing from one fascicle to another, a phenomenon that occurs predominantly in the proximal portion of the nerve and decreases distally.

Regarding the vascularization of a nerve, vessels are found in the mesoneurium; their branches run laterally from the epineurium to the perineurium where they form a longitudinally orientated plexus. They further cross the perineurium and join the central artery to form the endoneural microvessels.

1.2 Degeneration

According to literature, 2.8% of trauma patients are suffering from a peripheral nerve injury [14].

Lesion to the nerve can be divided in either three or five groups according to Seddon or Sunderland classification, respectively [16].

Seddon

1. **Neurapraxia** results from transient stress or injury to a peripheral nerve, commonly due to blunt trauma, compression, or local ischemia. The pathological hallmark is focal segmental demyelination without lesion of the axon itself. This may cause a partial or complete block of the conduction velocity and decreased amplitude of the action potential. Prognosis is favorable, as spontaneous recovery is typically observed once remyelination occurs.
2. **Axonotmesis** is most frequently encountered in nerve entrapment or contusion injuries associated with prolonged compression. In this injury pattern, the axon is disrupted, while the surrounding endoneurium remains intact. Electromyography (EMG) typically demonstrates abnormal spontaneous activity. Although axonal regeneration is required, functional recovery is often possible without surgical intervention.
3. **Neurotmesis** represents the most severe form of peripheral nerve injury and is characterized by complete disruption of the axon, Schwann cells, and the surrounding connective tissue layers (endoneurium, perineurium and epineurium). Spontaneous recovery is not possible, and surgical reconstruction is required to restore continuity. Neuroma formation may develop at the proximal stump of the transected nerve.

   Neuromas do not form at the distal nerve stumps of a transected nerve.

   A neuroma presents an undirected, failed attempt of regeneration in which the axons are not able to reach the distal stump of the transected nerve.

Sunderland

Sunderland subdivides axonotmesis into three subgroups (grade II–IV, as grade I and V represent neurapraxia and neurotmesis respectively) according to their degree of damage of the outer layers:

- **Grade II**: Damaged axon with intact endoneurium
- **Grade III**: Damaged axon and endoneurium with intact perineurium
- **Grade IV**: Damaged axon as well as endoneurium and perineurium but with the epineurium being intact (Fig. 1.3, Table 1.1)

In the absence of neural input, targeted muscles undergoe progressive atrophy. This process remains potentially reversible if timely reinnervation occurs, either through spontaneous axonal recovery or surgical intervention.

Once denervation persists, myofiber apoptosis begins approximately 7 days after loss of innervation. Subsequently, muscle tissue undergoes irreversible replacement by fibrous and fatty connective tissue [19]. This degenerative transformation typically evolves over a period of 3–12 months.

Even in cases where axonal regeneration is achieved at a later stage, the affected muscle fibers may not longer be excitable, and functional recovery is significantly compromised.

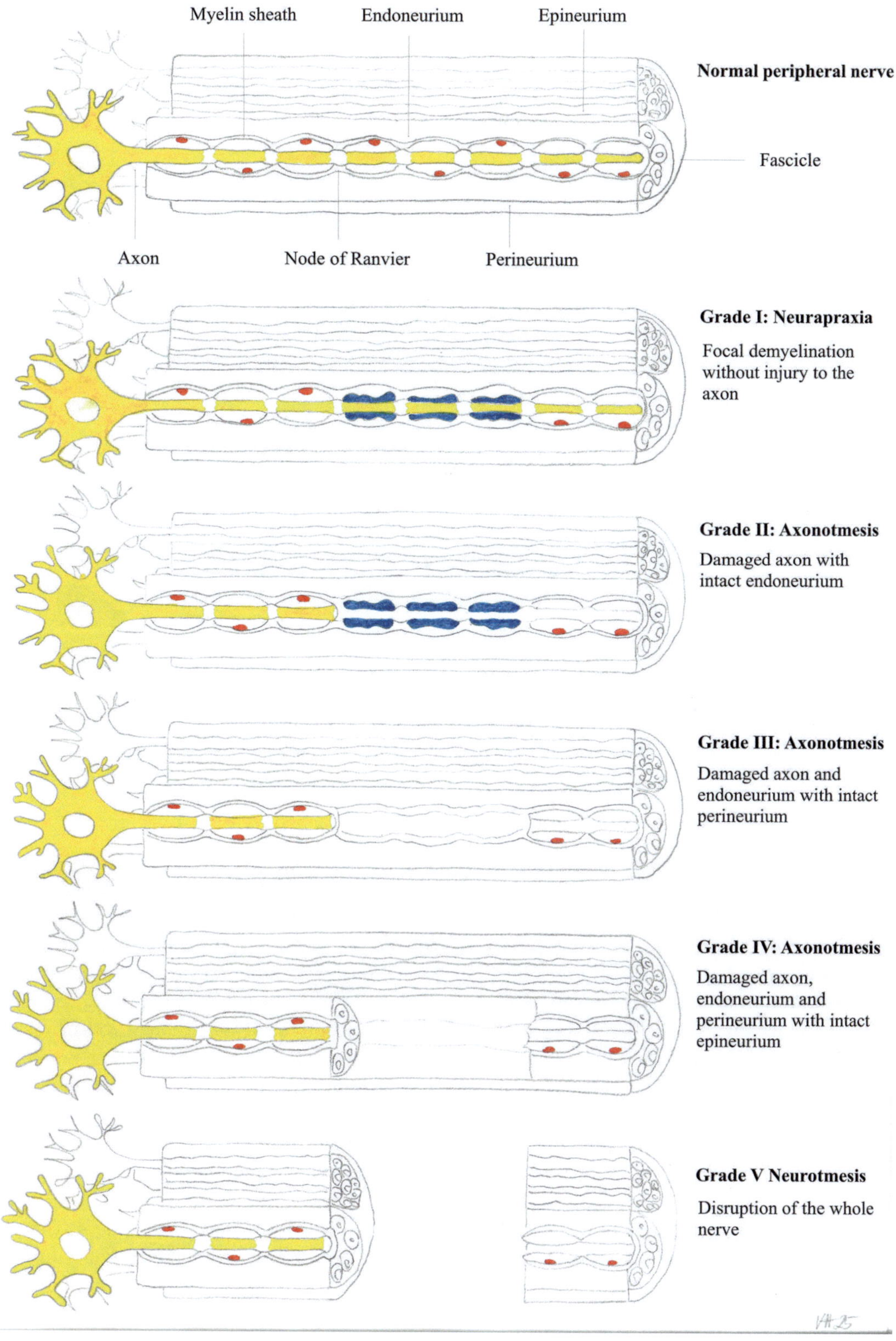

Fig. 1.3 Schematic diagram illustrating a normal peripheral nerve and the different grades of nerve injury according to the Sunderland classification

Table 1.1 Sunderland and Seddon classification showing the degree of peripheral nerve injury

Sunderland (1951) [16]	I	II	III	IV	V
Seddon (1942)	Neurapraxia (Transient block)	Axonotmesis (Injury in continuity)			Neurotmesis (Discontinuity of the nerve)

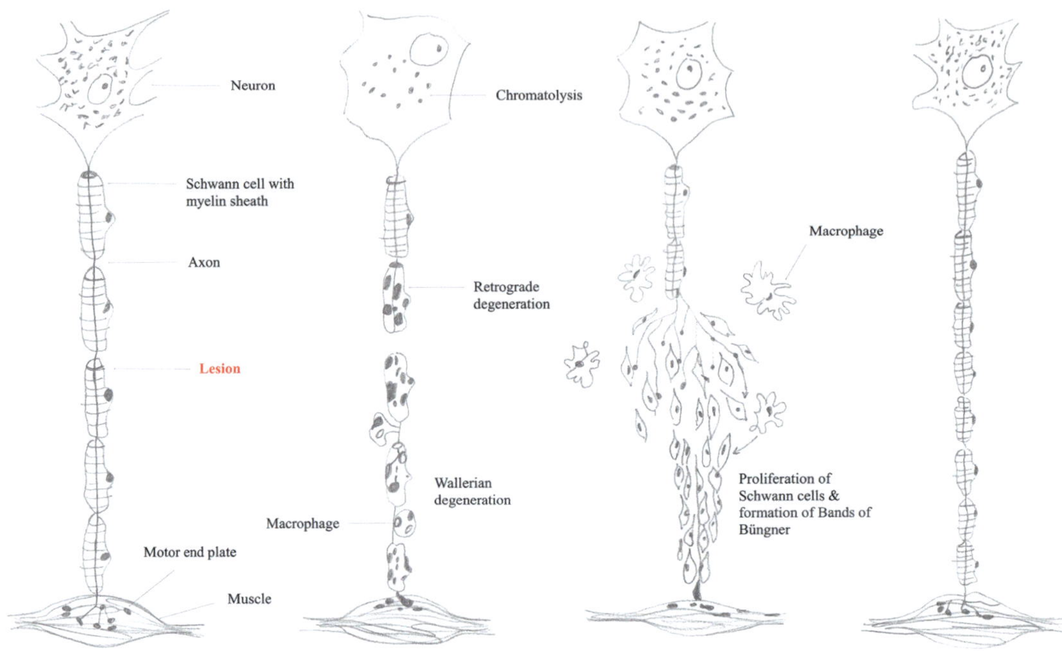

Fig. 1.4 Diagram illustrating nerve degeneration and regeneration. The first section shows a healthy neuron with labeled parts: neuron, Schwann cells with myelin sheath, axon, lesion, motor end plate, and muscle. The second section depicts chromatolysis and retrograde degeneration with macrophages. The third section shows Wallerian degeneration and macrophage activity. The final section illustrates the proliferation of Schwann cells and formation of Bands of Büngner

1.3 Regeneration

Following axonal transection, Schwann cells proliferate and extend longitudinally, forming the so-called bands of Büngner. These structures act as "guiding pathways" within the basal lamina, directing the regrowth of regenerating axons toward their distal targets.

The rate of regeneration depends on the severity of nerve injury: In cases of axonotmesis, regeneration typically progresses at approximately 3–4 mm/day. In contrast, following neurotmesis, regenration is slower, averaging 2–3 mm/day, owing to the necessity of surgical repair [21] (Fig. 1.4).

If axonal regeneration fails and the regenrating axons do not reach their distal targets, the muscular motor end plates degenerate, leading to progressive fibrosis of the denervated muscle and dedifferentiation of the Schwann cells.

The survival of neurons with transected axons depends largely on the location of injury within the peripheral nervous system (PNS). Lesions occurring distal to the neuronal soma are generally associated with a favorable prognosis. In contrast, lesions proximal to the soma – such as root avulsion in brachial plexus injuries – are associated with a poor prognosis, with motor unit survival rates as low as 10–20% [23].

For sensory neurons, approximately 40% undergo apoptosis following injury [24].

Importantly, early surgical intervention can reduce neuronal death in both motor and sensory neurons.

Overall, prognosis is dependent on both the site of injury and the time interval between trauma and surgical repair.

Another critical prognostic factor is the degree of vascularization achieved after nerve grafting. Thin grafts allow for revascularization through the surrounding capillary network. By contrast, large caliber grafts may undergo ischemic cell death before sufficient revascularization is established (e.g. peroneal versus sural nerve grafts). Notably, fat tissue and synovium provide a favorable biological environment for nerve regeneration.

Further Reading

1. Dahlin LB. Aspects on pathophysiology of nerve entrapments and nerve compression injuries. Neurosurg Clin N Am. 1991;2(1):21–9.
2. Ogata K, Naito M. Blood flow of peripheral nerve effects of dissection, stretching and compression. J Hand Surg Br. 1986;11(1):10–4. https://doi.org/10.1016/0266-7681(86)90003-3.
3. Vekris MD, Bates M, Terzis JK. Optimal time for distraction osteogenesis in limbs with nerve repairs: experimental study in the rat. J Reconstr Microsurg. 1999;15(3):191–201. https://doi.org/10.1055/s-2007-1000091.
4. Stewart JD. Peripheral nerve fascicles: anatomy and clinical relevance. Muscle Nerve. 2003;28(5):525–41. https://doi.org/10.1002/mus.10454.
5. Kretschmer T, editor. Nervenchirurgie: trauma, tumor, kompression. Berlin: Springer; 2014.
6. Standring S, Borley NR, Gray H. Gray's anatomy: the anatomical basis of clinical practice. 40th ed., anniversary ed. London: Churchill Livingstone/Elsevier; 2008.
7. Salzer JL. Schwann cell myelination. Cold Spring Harb Perspect Biol. 2015;7(8):a020529. https://doi.org/10.1101/cshperspect.a020529.
8. Jessen KR, Mirsky R. The origin and development of glial cells in peripheral nerves. Nat Rev Neurosci. 2005;6(9):671–82. https://doi.org/10.1038/nrn1746.
9. Topp KS, Boyd BS. Peripheral nerve: from the microscopic functional unit of the axon to the biomechanically loaded macroscopic structure. J Hand Ther. 2012;25(2):142–52. https://doi.org/10.1016/j.jht.2011.09.002.
10. ResearchGate. Pain: physiologic background and therapeutic consequences – types of nerve fibres (Erlanger-Gasser definition) [Figure]. n.d. Retrieved 14 May 2025, from https://www.researchgate.net/figure/Types-of-nerve-fibres-Erlanger-Gasser-definition_tbl1_339381885.
11. Whitwam JG. Classification of peripheral nerve fibres. An historical perspective. Anaesthesia. 1976;31(4):494–503. https://doi.org/10.1111/j.1365-2044.1976.tb12354.x. PMID: 779513.
12. Sunderland S. Nerve and nerve injuries. 2nd ed. Edinburgh: Churchill Livingstone; 1978.
13. Muangsanit P, Shipley RJ, Phillips JB. Vascularization strategies for peripheral nerve tissue engineering. Anat Rec (Hoboken). 2018;301(10):1657–67. https://doi.org/10.1002/ar.23919.
14. Walsh S, Midha R. Practical considerations concerning the use of stem cells for peripheral nerve repair. Neurosurg Focus. 2009;26(2):E2. https://doi.org/10.3171/FOC.2009.26.2.E2.
15. Houschyar KS, Momeni A, Pyles MN, Cha JY, Maan ZN, Duscher D, Jew OS, Siemers F, van Schoonhoven J. The role of current techniques and concepts in peripheral nerve repair. Plast Surg Int. 2016;2016:4175293. https://doi.org/10.1155/2016/4175293.
16. Sunderland S. A classification of peripheral nerve injuries producing loss of function. Brain J Neurol. 1951;74(4):491–516. https://doi.org/10.1093/brain/74.4.491.
17. Biso GMNR, Munakomi S. Neuroanatomy, neurapraxia. In: StatPearls [Internet]. StatPearls Publishing; 2022. https://www.ncbi.nlm.nih.gov/books/NBK557746/figure/article-25766.image.f1/.
18. Cisterna BA, Cardozo C, Sáez JC. Neuronal involvement in muscular atrophy. Front Cell Neurosci. 2014;8:405. https://doi.org/10.3389/fncel.2014.00405.
19. Wu P, Chawla A, Spinner RJ, Yu C, Yaszemski MJ, Windebank AJ, Wang H. Key changes in denervated muscles and their impact on regeneration and reinnervation. Neural Regen Res. 2014;9(20):1796–809. https://doi.org/10.4103/1673-5374.143424.
20. Terenghi G. Peripheral nerve regeneration and neurotrophic factors. J Anat. 1999;194 (Pt 1)(Pt 1):1–14. https://doi.org/10.1046/j.1469-7580.1999.19410001.x.
21. Stoll G, Müller HW. Nerve injury, axonal degeneration and neural regeneration: basic insights. Brain Pathol. 1999;9(2):313–25. https://doi.org/10.1111/j.1750-3639.1999.tb00229.x.
22. Gordon T. Peripheral nerve regeneration and muscle reinnervation. Int J Mol Sci. 2020;21(22):8652. https://doi.org/10.3390/ijms21228652.
23. Novikov L, Novikova L, Kellerth JO. Brain-derived neurotrophic factor promotes axonal regeneration and long-term survival of adult rat spinal motoneurons in vivo. Neuroscience. 1997;79(3):765–74. https://doi.org/10.1016/s0306-4522(96)00665-3.
24. Oliveira AL. Apoptosis of sensory neurons and satellite cells after sciatic nerve transection in C57BL/6J mice. Braz J Med Biol Res. 2001;34(3):375–80. https://doi.org/10.1590/s0100-879x2001000300012.
25. Ma J, Novikov LN, Kellerth JO, Wiberg M. Early nerve repair after injury to the postganglionic plexus: an experimental study of sensory and motor neuronal survival in adult rats. Scand J Plast Reconstr Surg Hand Surg. 2003;37(1):1–9. https://doi.org/10.1080/alp.37.1.1.9.

2 Anatomy of the Brachial Plexus and Its Terminal Branches

The brachial plexus (BP) represents a complex network of nerves originating from spinal roots C5 to T1, with potential contributions from C4 or T2 in prefixed or postfixed variations, respectively. Its main function is the motor and sensory innervation of the upper limb. At the intervertebral foramen, motor and sensory roots unite to form spinal nerves, which contribute to the formation of the brachial plexus. It further organizes into roots, trunks (superior, middle, inferior), divisions (anterior, posterior), and cords (lateral, medial, posterior), to finally end into terminal branches. At each level, several motor and sensory nerves branch to innervate specific muscles.

The lateral cord gives off the musculocutaneous and contributes to the median nerve; the posterior cord—formed by the posterior divisions of all three trunks—bifurcates into the axillary and radial nerves; and the medial cord gives rise to the ulnar nerve and also contributes to the formation of the median nerve. The median nerve is unique as it receives fibers from both the lateral and medial cords. Each terminal nerve has a defined course and function, with multiple points of potential entrapment or injury.

Finally, the cervical plexus (C1–C4) contributes motor and sensory innervation to the neck and shoulder and communicates with cranial and sympathetic nerves.

This detailed anatomical understanding is essential for diagnosing nerve lesions, planning surgical interventions, and interpreting electrophysiological studies.

2.1 Brachial Plexus

At the level of the intervertebral foramen, motor and sensory roots merge to form a spinal nerve. They further unite with the sympathetic ganglia.

The **brachial plexus (BP)** in turn is formed by spinal nerves C5–T1. Anatomical variations exist in which C4 or T2 may also contribute to the formation of the BP—this is called prefixed or postfixed, respectively [1].

The only bony attachment of the spinal nerves is at the transverse process, which provides partial protection against avulsion from the spinal cord. However, this attachment is structurally weaker at the level of the C8–T1 spinal nerves compared to C5–C7, rendering the lower roots more susceptible to traction injuries and avulsion [2].

> It is important to note that the sympathetic fibers innervating the face (via the trigeminal nerve) originate from the **thoracic spinal cord**, traversing the **T1 and T2 spinal nerves**. Consequently, injury at these levels may disrupt the sympathetic pathway and result in **Horner syndrome**.

K. Hobitsch, *Peripheral Nerve Surgery - A Compendium*,
https://doi.org/10.1007/978-3-032-03409-0_2

Prior to joining the brachial plexus, the spinal nerves are referred to as "***roots***". Each brachial plexus root corresponds to a specific **sensory dermatome** and an associated **myotome**, reflecting its cutaneous and motor distribution.

C5 myotome ➔ Abduction and external rotation of the shoulder
C6 myotome ➔ Elbow flexion
C7 myotome ➔ Elbow extension
C8 myotome ➔ Flexion of the fingers
T1 myotome ➔ Abduction of the fingers

After formation of the BP, the spinal nerve roots converge to form ***trunks:*** the superior *(C5, C6)*, ***middle*** *(C7)*, and ***inferior*** *(C8, T1)* trunk.

At the level of the trunks, the *suprascapular nerve* arises as a branch of the superior trunk. This nerve courses posteriorly, passing between the omohyoid and trapezius muscles, and traverses the suprascapular notch to supply the supraspinatus and infraspinatus muscles.

A second branch of the superior trunk is the *nerve to the subclavius*, which innervates the subclavius muscle. Situated beneath the clavicle, this muscle functions to stabilize the bone during movements of the shoulder girdle. Its function cannot be assessed either clinically or electrophysiologically [7].

Before contributing to the superior trunk, the **C5 root** gives rise to three important nerves:

The *phrenic nerve* (C3–C5) courses ventrally to the anterior scalene muscle and descends to innervate the diaphragm. Injury to the C5 root may cause an ipsilateral paralysis of the diaphragm.

> "C3, 4 and 5 keeps the human alive"

The *long thoracic nerve* (C5–C7) travels in a caudal direction posteriorly to the brachial plexus to supply the serratus anterior muscle which stabilizes the scapula. Injury produces scapular winging and shoulder pain.

The *dorsal scapular nerve* (C5) passes posterior to the brachial plexus, perforates the middle scalene muscle, and courses beneath the levator scapulae supply to the rhomboid major and minor muscles, which anchor the scapula to the spine and act antagonistically to the serratus anterior muscle. It may also provide partial innervation to the levator scapulae muscle.

Lesion to the dorsal scapular nerve may also result in scapular winging, typically presenting with lateral displacement.

The brachial plexus trunks emerge between the anterior and middle scalene muscles, accompanied by the subclavian artery. Each trunk further divides into an ***anterior division*** (primarily supplying flexor musculature) and a ***posterior division*** (primarily supplying extensor musculature).

Distally, these divisions recombine to form three ***cords,*** named according to their relation to the axillary artery beneath the pectoral minor muscle:

Lateral Cord

- From the anterior divisions of the superior and middle trunk.
- Has a branch to the lateral pectoral nerve which innervates the clavicular head of the pectoralis major muscle.

> Frequently communicates with the medial pectoral nerve

- Terminal branches are the *musculocutaneous* and the *median nerve*.

Posterior Cord

- Formed by the posterior divisions of all trunks.
- Receives contributions from all roots of the BP.
- Has branches to the upper subscapular nerve—a short nerve innervating the subscapular muscle—to the lower subscapular nerve, which innervates the lower part of the subscapular and the teres major muscle; and to the thoracodorsal nerve which arises between the upper and the lower subscapular nerves and innervates the latissimus dorsi muscle.

> Branches from the posterior cord innervate the adductors and internal rotators of the arm

- Terminal branches are the *axillary* and the *radial nerve*.

> The radial nerve represents the largest terminal nerve

Medial Cord

- Arises from the anterior division of the inferior trunk.
- Has a branch to the median pectoral nerve which innervates the pectoralis minor and the sternal head of pectoralis major muscle, the medial brachial cutaneous, and the medial antebrachial cutaneous nerve.
- Terminal branches are the *median* and the *ulnar nerve*.

It is important to note that the median nerve is the only terminal branch of the brachial plexus that does not represent a direct continuation of a single cord. Instead, it is formed by contributions from the lateral cord and the medial cord. The fibers from the lateral cord are primarily sensory, whereas the fibers from the medial cord carry the motor component. The union of these two roots occurs anterior to the axillary artery, creating an anatomical configuration that resembles the shape of an "M" (Fig. 2.1 and 2.2).

2.1.1 Overview of the Brachial Plexus Anatomy

- Spinal nerves C5–T1 ➔ Brachial plexus
- Supraclavicular, in the area of the scalenus aperture:
  - C5 + C6 ➔ **Superior trunk**
  - C7 ➔ **Middle trunk**
  - C8 + T1 ➔ **Inferior trunk**
- The trunks bifurcate each in an anterior and a posterior division
- Formation of the cords at the infra-/retroclavicular level:
  - All three posterior divisions ➔ **Posterior cord**
  - Anterior division of superior and middle trunk ➔ **Lateral cord**
  - Anterior division of inferior trunk ➔ **Medial cord**
- The cords are named based on their positional relation to the subclavian/axillary artery
- Terminal branches at the infraclavicular level:
  - Posterior cord ➔ **Radial and axillary nerve**
  - Lateral cord ➔ **Median and musculocutaneous nerve**
  - Medial cord ➔ **Median and ulnar nerve**

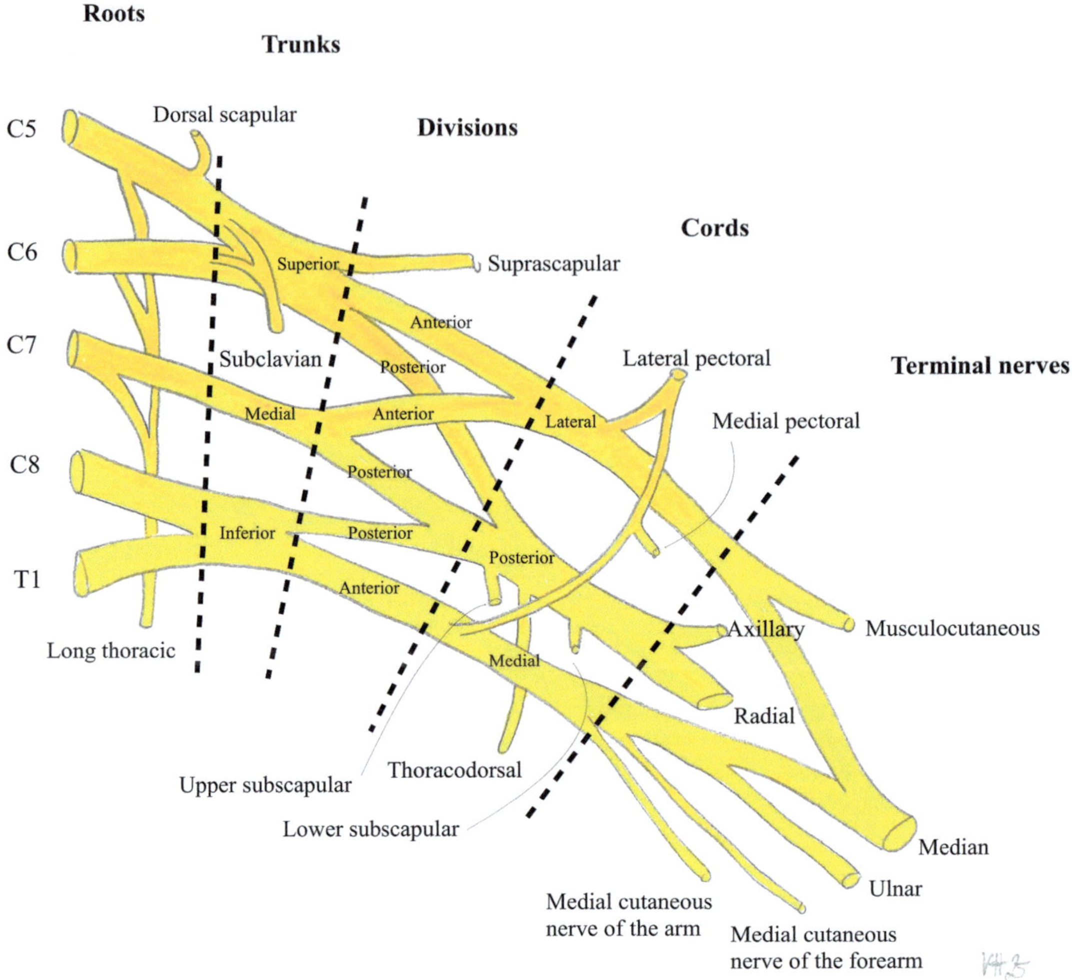

Fig. 2.1 Schematic representation of the brachial plexus, illustrating the nerves originating from spinal roots C5 to T1. The image shows the progression from roots to trunks, divisions, cords, and terminal nerves

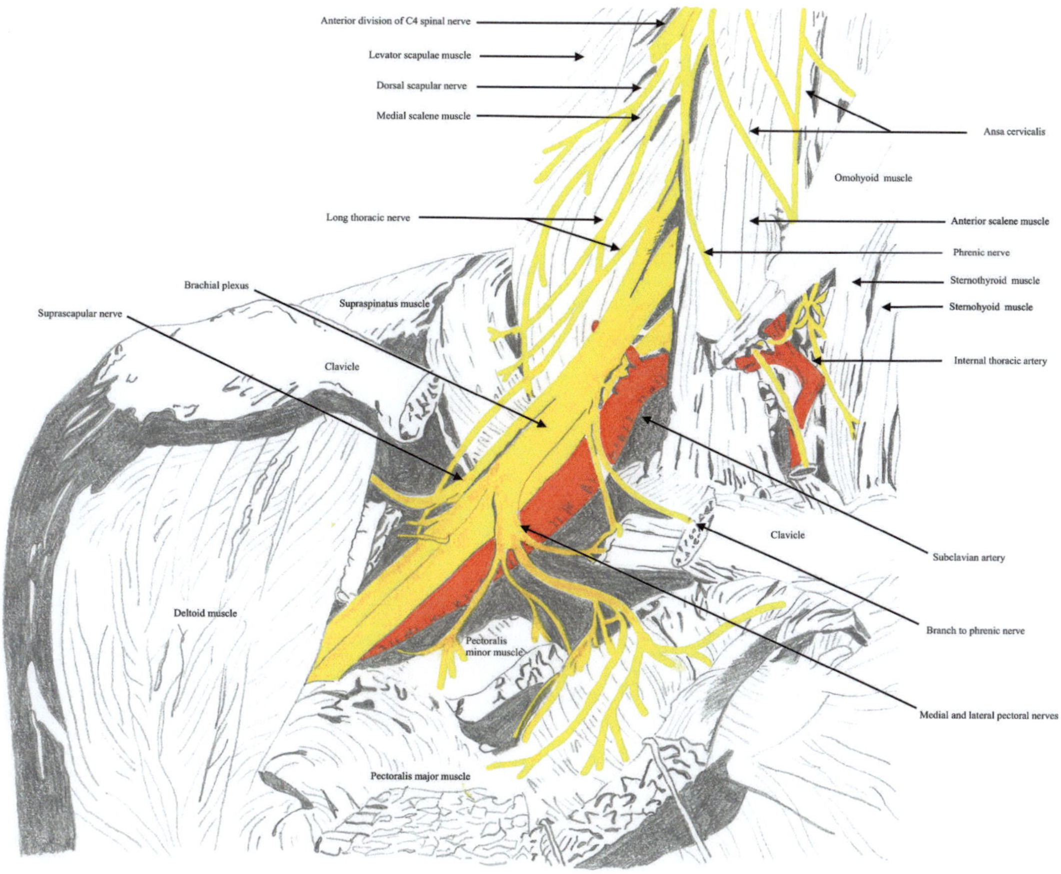

Fig. 2.2 Anatomy of the brachial plexus

2.2 Terminal Branches

2.2.1 Musculocutaneous Nerve (C5–C6)

At the level of the axilla, the **musculocutaneous nerve** courses along the lateral aspect of the arm, piercing the coracobrachialis muscle—which it innervates—before continuing between the brachialis and the biceps brachii muscles with the brachialis lying deep to the nerve and the biceps brachii positioned superficially (= flexor compartment). Several branches exit at that level to innervate the two above mentioned muscles.

As it travels more distally, the musculocutaneous nerve enters the antecubital fossa, further pierces the fascia lateral to the biceps brachii and proceeds into the forearm. At that level, the nerve is named *lateral antebrachial cutaneous nerve*, having an anterior and posterior division, where it innervates the lateral half of the forearm (Fig. 2.3).

Motor Innervation

Muscular branches ➔

Coracobrachialis muscle
Biceps brachii muscle
Brachialis muscle

Sensory Innervation

Lateral antebrachial cutaneous nerve ➔

Lateral half of forearm

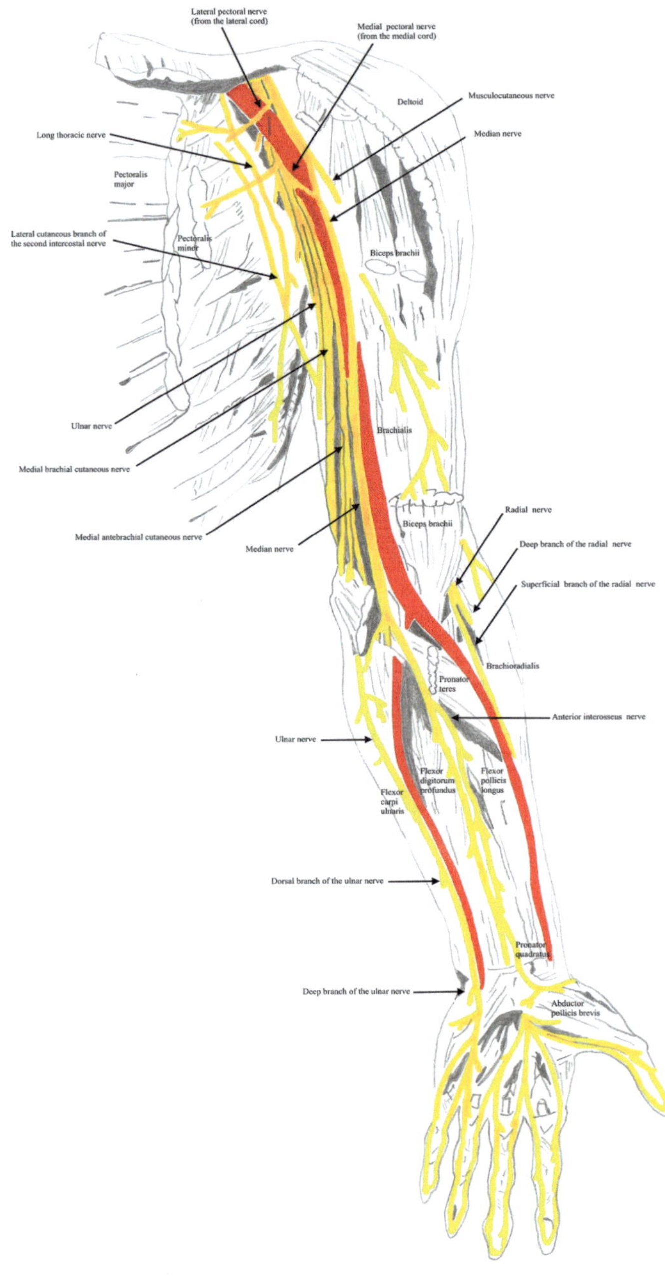

Fig. 2.3 Anatomical diagram of the human arm, illustrating the nerve pathways. The image highlights various nerves, including the median and ulnar nerves, with labels pointing to each

2.2.2 Median Nerve (C6–T1)

As mentioned above, the **median nerve** receives its fibers from the lateral (sensory axons C6–C7) and the medial cord (motor axons C8–T1).

After the formation of the median "M" superficial to the brachial artery, the median nerve descends anterolaterally to the brachial artery and parallel to the intermuscular septum, which is separating the triceps muscle from the biceps and the brachialis muscles.

Rarely, at the medial aspect of the distal humerus, a fibrous band may be present—called the *Struthers' ligament*—extending from the supracondylar process to the medial epicondyle. If present, it may compress the median nerve and the brachial artery as these structures are running beneath the Struthers' ligament [15].

The median nerve further crosses to the medial side of the brachial artery and descends under a bicipital aponeurosis, called the lacertus fibrosus, to reach the forearm.

As it descends, the median nerve passes beneath the humeral head of the pronator teres muscle—crosses at that point the ulnar artery—and continues deep to a third structure—the two heads of flexor digitorum superficialis muscle. The fibrous ridge between the two heads is called sublimis ridge and plays a role in entrapment syndromes of the median nerve.

The median nerve continues its course distally between the flexor digitorum superficialis and the flexor digitorum profundus muscle.

The *anterior interosseus nerve* branches after one third of its way and terminates at the distal forearm deep to the pronator quadratus.

Approximately 5 cm before reaching the wrist, the median nerve becomes more superficial and courses medial to the tendon of the flexor carpi radialis muscle [18]. Before finally entering the hand under the transverse carpal ligament, another branch exits named the *palmar cutaneous branch*, which runs superficially to the carpal tunnel.

After passing through the carpal tunnel, a third branch—the *recurrent branch* (*thenar motor branch*) exits.

Finally, in the deep palm of the hand, the median nerve terminates by dividing into two rami running deep to the superficial palmar arterial arch: the radial division, which in turn branches into the *common digital nerve* (thumb) and the *proper digital nerve* (radial half of index finger); and the ulnar division branching into the common digital nerve, which ultimately splits into the *proper digital nerves*.

Anatomical Variations

Martin-Gruber-Anastomosis: It is present in approximately 15% of the population and represents an anastomosis located in the median third of the forearm. It involves the nerve fibers of the median nerve—a branching to the recurrent motor ramus which innervates the muscles of the thenar—and the ulnar nerve. Those fibers are entering the palm of the hand with the deep branch of the ulnar nerve. They may then travel back to the recurrent motor branch to innervate the intended muscles (Fig. 2.4).
A lesion of the median nerve distally to this anastomosis may thus preserve the function of the thenar muscles.
Note, that the electrophysiological results may also differ.

Marinacci-Anastomosis: Also named "Reversed Martin-Gruber Anastomosis" is a very rare anatomical variation of ulnar nerve fibers joining the median nerve in the area of the distal forearm, thus the name reversed Martin-

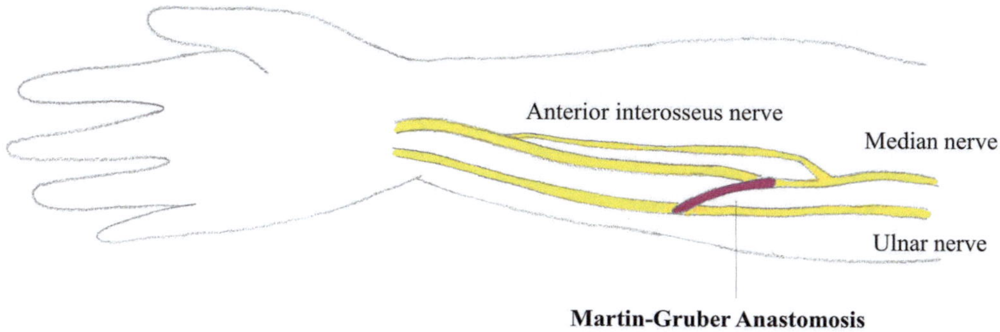

Fig. 2.4 Schematic representation of the Martin-Gruber-Anastomosis

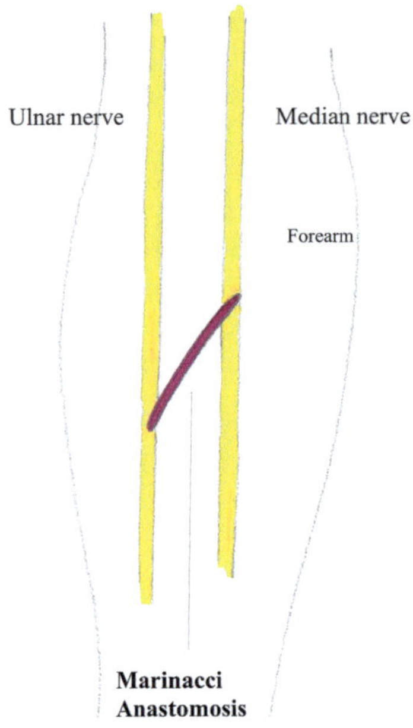

Fig. 2.5 Schematic representation of the Marinacci-Anastomosis

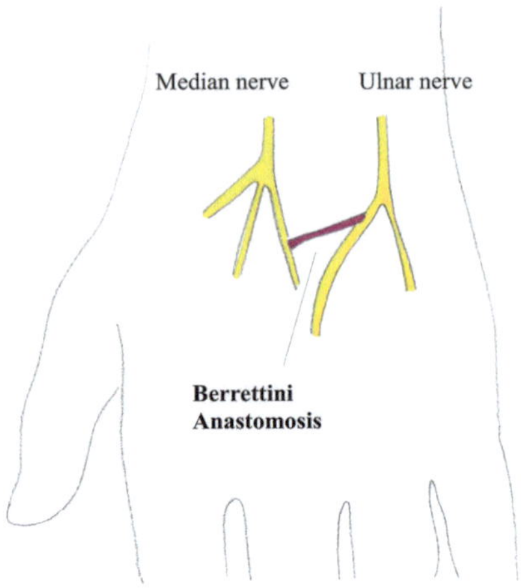

Fig. 2.6 Schematic representation of the Berrettini-Anastomosis

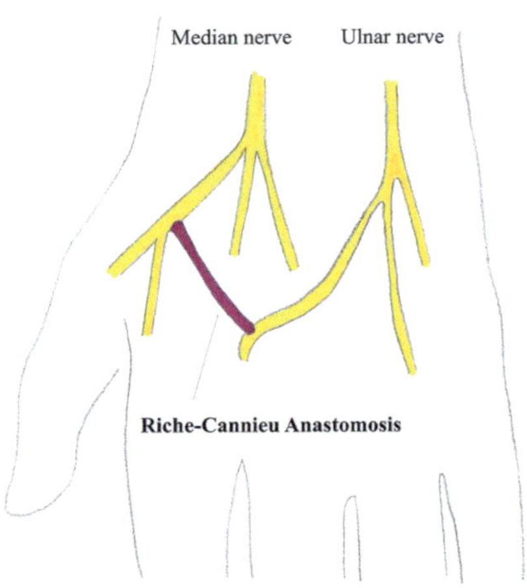

Fig. 2.7 Schematic representation of the Cannieu-Riche-Anastomosis

Gruber Anastomosis. It has no clinical relevance (Fig. 2.5).

Berrettini-Anastomosis: The Berrettini-Anastomosis is the most frequent anastomosis and represents a communication between the common palmar digital nerve III and the common palmar digital nerve IV of the ulnar and median nerves, respectively. This anastomosis is assumed to be purely sensitive. It is commonly seen in both hands (Fig. 2.6).

Cannieu-Riche-Anastomosis: This anastomosis represents a connection—located in the palm of the hand—between the recurrent motor branch of the median nerve and the deep ulnar branch (Fig. 2.7).

A median nerve injury distally to this communication may preserve the function of the addressed muscle, namely, the flexor pollicis brevis [22].

Motor Innervation

No branches in the upper arm.

Muscular branches ➔

Superficial flexors of the forearm:

- Pronator teres muscle
- Flexor carpi radialis muscle
- Palmaris longus muscle
- Flexor digitorum superficialis muscle

Anterior interosseus nerve ➔

Deep flexors of the forearm:

- Flexor digitorum profundus muscle
- Flexor pollicis longus muscle
- Pronator quadratus muscle

Recurrent (thenar) motor branch ➔
Thenar group:
Abductor pollicis brevis muscle
Flexor pollicis brevis muscle
Opponens pollicis muscles
Radial and ulnar divisions ➔
Terminal group: First and second lumbrical muscles

<u>Sensory Innervation</u>
Palmar cutaneous nerve ➔
Proximal palmar hand
Radial division ➔
Thenar (palmar surface)
Ulnar division ➔
Radial half of the index finger (palmar surface)
Proper palmar digital nerves of the median nerve (3 nerves) ➔
2 nerves innervate the sides of the thumb
1 nerve innervates the radial digit II
Common palmar digital nerves (2 nerves) ➔
Sides of digit II + IV

2.2.3 Ulnar Nerve (C8–T1)

The **ulnar nerve** is primarily formed by fibers from the medial cord of the inferior trunk, with occasional contributions from C7 root.

Prior to the formation of the ulnar nerve, the medial cord gives rise to two important sensitive branches—the *medial brachial cutaneous nerve* and *the medial antebrachial cutaneous nerve* (which further divides into anterior and posterior branches). These nerves provide sensory innervation in the skin of the medial half of the arm and forearm, respectively. Clinical signs of hypoesthesia in these regions suggest a lesion proximal to the ulnar nerve. It is important to note that anatomical variations exist, and in some cases, these cutaneous branches may arise directly from the ulnar nerve itself.

As it descends, the ulnar nerve is accompanied anteromedially by the brachial artery, adjacent to the intermuscular septum that separates the flexor from the extensor compartment. At approximately the midpoint of the arm, it pierces the septum and continues its descend medially, together with the superior ulnar collateral artery— a branch of the brachial artery—toward the head of the triceps muscle.

In approximately 86.7% [26] of the population, the intermuscular septum is thickened forming an arch or arcade, known as the arcade of Struthers.

The **arcade of Struthers** should not be confused with the **Struther's ligament.** These are distinct anatomical structures: the arcade of Struthers is a fascial-muscular band that can compress the **ulnar nerve** in the arm, whereas the Struther's ligament is a fibrous band extending from the supracondylar process of the humerus to the medial epicondyle, which may cause entrapment of the **median nerve**.

The incidence of the arcade of Struthers varies considerably in anatomical studies, with some authors reporting its presence in approximately 13.5% of individuals [29]. This structure is located proximal to the medial epicondyle and may be clinically relevant in cases of ulnar nerve compression.

After passing beneath the arcade of Struthers, the ulnar nerve enters the posteromedial cubital fossa accompanied by the ulnar artery, a branch of the brachial artery.

In the cubital region, the ulnar nerve courses dorsally around the medial epicondyle within the post-condylar groove, which represents its most vulnerable site for traumatic injury.

Distally, the ulnar nerve passes beneath the flexor carpi ulnaris muscle which consists of the humeral and the ulnar head. The aponeurosis connecting these heads may be thickened in about 75% of the population, being called the Osborne band [3, 30]. Compression of the nerve is likely to happen here, especially during elbow and wrist flexion, which leads to contraction of the flexor carpi ulnaris muscle.

In some individuals, absence of this aponeurosis can result in ulnar subluxation or "snapping" over the medial epicondyle.

A rare anatomical variant, the anconeus epitrochlearis muscle, extends from the medial epicondyle to the olecranon, and occurs in about about 3–34% of the population; it may also contribute to ulnar nerve irritation [33, 34].

Typically, only a *single branch* of the ulnar nerve innervates the flexor digitorum profundus muscle.

As the ulnar nerve continues its course beneath the flexor carpi ulnaris toward the pisiform bone of the wrist, it becomes uncovered by muscle at the distal third of the forearm, where the tendon of the flexor carpi ulnaris lies laterally and the flexor digitorum superficialis medially to the nerve.

At this level, two sensory branches exit about 5–10 cm proximal to the wrist—the *dorsal ulnar cutaneous nerve* and the *palmar ulnar cutaneous nerve* (at the volar-lateral side).

The ulnar nerve then enters—together with the ulnar artery being located lateral to the nerve—the Guyon canal to ultimately reach the palm.

The Guyon canal has one entrance but two exits and its boundaries are the following:

Ulnar ➔ Pisiform bone
Distal radial ➔ Hook of the hamate bone
Dorsal ➔ Transverse carpal ligament
Palmar ➔ Superficial palmar carpal ligament and palmaris brevis muscle

Prior to entering the canal, the ulnar nerve gives off a branch to innervate the hypothenar muscles. Within the Guyon canal, the ulnar nerve bifurcates into a *deep motor branch* and a *superficial sensory branch*, with the accompanying ulnar artery dividing into corresponding deep and superficial palmar branches.

Motor Innervation

Motor branch ➔
- Forearm group:
  - Flexor carpi ulnaris muscle
  - Flexor digitorum profundus muscle IV–V

Superficial branch ➔
- Hypothenar group:
  - Palmaris brevis muscle

Deep branch ➔
- Hypothenar group:
  - Abductor digiti minimi muscle
  - Flexor digiti minimi muscle
  - Opponens digiti minimi muscle
- Thenar group:
  - Adductor pollicis muscle
  - Flexor pollicis brevis muscle
- Intrinsic group:
  - Palmar and dorsal interossei muscles
  - Lumbrical muscles digits III + IV

Sensory Innervation

Medial brachial and antebrachial cutaneous nerve (from the medial cord) **➔**
- Medial half of arm and forearm

Articular branch ➔
- Elbow

Dorsal ulnar cutaneous branch ➔
- Skin of the median dorsal hand, hypothenar, and half of digit IV

Palmar ulnar cutaneous branch ➔
- Skin of the median palmar hand

Superficial sensory division ➔
- Anterior aspect of hypothenar and half of digit IV

Proper palmar digital nerve ➔
- Medial digit V

Common palmar digital nerve ➔
- Ulnar side of digit IV and V

2.2.4 Axillary Nerve (C5–C6)

The **axillary nerve** originates from the posterior cord of the brachial plexus. It emerges deep to the axillary artery and courses alongside the posterior humeral circumflex artery toward the surgical neck of the humerus, passing through the quadrangular (or quadrilateral) space. This space is anatomically defined by the teres minor muscle superiorly, the humeral neck laterally, the teres major muscle inferiorly, and the long head of the triceps muscle medially. Within this confined space, the axillary nerve exhibits limited mobility, rendering it susceptible to stretch injuries.

Upon exiting the quadrangular space, the axillary nerve bifurcates into anterior and posterior divisions. The *anterior division* courses beneath the deltoid to provide motor innervation to the deltoid.

The *posterior division* supplies a branch to the teres minor muscle before piercing the fascia of the brachialis to continue as the *superior lateral cutaneous nerve*, providing sensory innervation to the upper lateral aspect of the arm.

In rare cases, the quadrangular space may serve as a site for axillary nerve compression, a condition termed quadrangular space syndrome .

Additionally, the axillary nerve contributes sensory fibers to the shoulder joint via its *articular branch*.

Axillary nerve lesions most commonly result from shoulder trauma, such as dislocations or proximal humeral fractures. In cases of isolated axillary nerve injury versus partial damage of the posterior division of the brachial plexus, the muscles innervated by the radial nerve are preserved (Fig. 2.8).

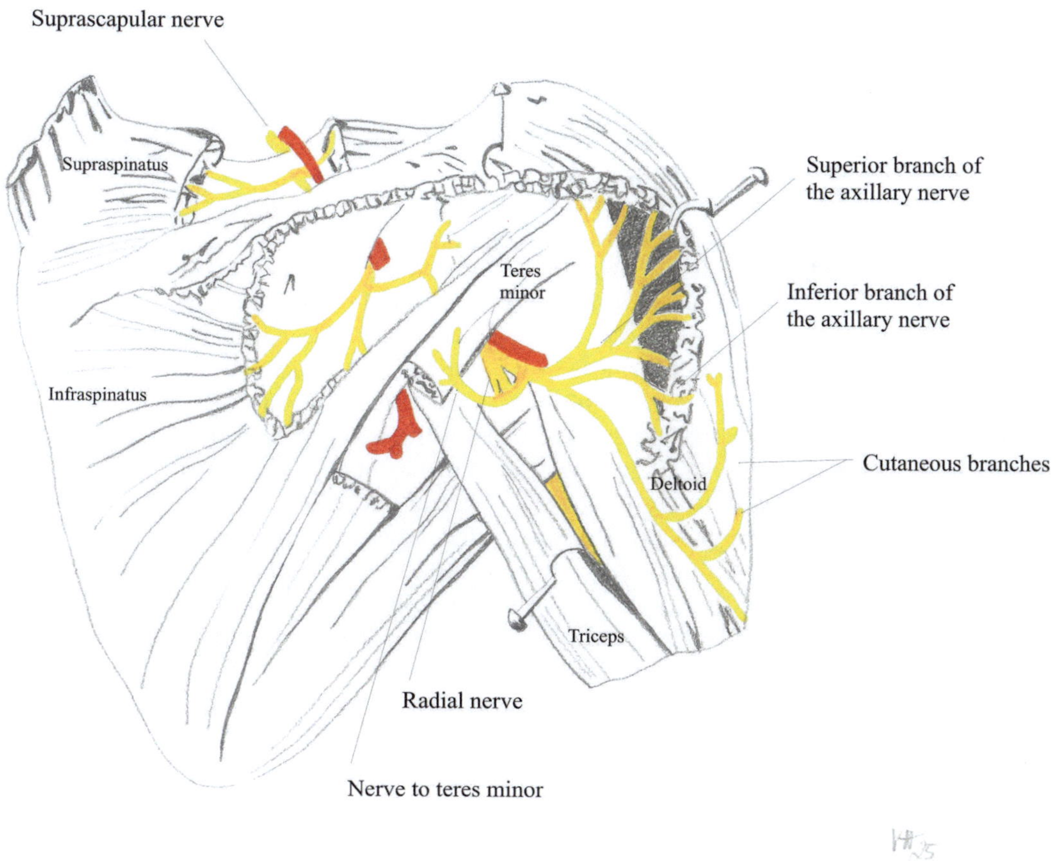

Fig. 2.8 An anatomical diagram of the shoulder region, highlighting the anatomical course of the axillary nerve

Motor Innervation

Anterior division →

Deltoid muscle

Posterior division →

Teres minor muscle

Posterior part of deltoid muscle

Long head of triceps brachii muscle

Sensory Innervation

Upper lateral cutaneous nerve →

Upper lateral arm

Articular branch →

Glenohumeral joint

2.2.5 Radial Nerve (C5–C8)

The **radial nerve** is a continuation of the posterior cord of the brachial plexus and receives additional fibers from T1 spinal nerve.

Initially located posterior to the brachial artery, it courses laterally between the medial and the lateral head of the triceps muscle, giving off branches to the *long and lateral heads.* It then passes toward the dorsal aspect of the humeral bone where it lies superficial to the subscapular, latissimus dorsi, and the teres major muscles.

The radial nerve proceeds then alongside with the profunda brachii artery (deep brachial artery) in the spiral groove, anterior to the long head of the triceps, in direct contact with the humeral shaft. At this level, the *posterior cutaneous antebrachii branch* and *branches to the medial head of the triceps muscle* emerge.

As it continues distally, the radial nerve pierces the lateral intermuscular septum approximately 10 cm proximal to the lateral epicondyle—a site of vulnerability due to limited mobility.

It then reaches the cubital fossa, coursing anteroinferiorly between the brachialis and the brachioradialis muscles.

At the radial head, the nerve bifurcates into the purely sensitive *superficial branch* and the *posterior interosseus nerve*—being a motor. The posterior interosseus nerve proceeds—together with the recurrent radial artery—through a pocket formed by the two heads of the supinator muscle and continues along the radial bone between the extensor digitorum communis and the abductor pollicis longus muscles to ramify into *multiple muscular branches* called the "cauda equina of the forearm" [43]. The above-mentioned pocket may have a fibrous edge, named the arcade of Frohse, which represents a common site of compression [44].

Another potential entrapment site is the leash of Henry, where branches of the recurrent artery cross the posterior interosseus nerve immediately distal to its bifurcation from the superficial branch.

Terminal branches of the posterior interosseus nerve supply the radial-innervated muscles of the thumb, lying deep to the interosseous membrane in the distal forearm.

The superficial branch of the radial nerve continues along the extensor carpi radialis longus muscle, becoming superficial in the distal third of the forearm, and terminates by dividing into four or more *sensory rami* at the dorsolateral wrist (Fig. 2.9).

Motor Innervation

Motor branch of the triceps group →

Long head of the triceps muscle (close to the axillobrachial junction)

Medial and lateral head of triceps muscle (proximal to entering in spiral groove)

Motor branch of the lateral epicondyle group →

Brachioradialis muscle C5, C6 (proximal to lateral epicondyle)

Extensor carpi radialis longus muscle C6, C7 (distal to the lateral epicondyle)

Extensor carpi radialis brevis muscle C7, C8 (distal to the lateral epicondyle)

Supinator muscle C6, C7 (proximal forearm)

Posterior interosseus group →

Superficial group (C7, C8):

Extensor carpi ulnaris muscle

Extensor digitorum communis muscle

Extensor digiti minimi muscles

Deep group (C7, C8):

Abductor pollicis longus muscle

Extensor pollicis longus muscle

Extensor pollicis brevis muscle

Extensor indicis muscles

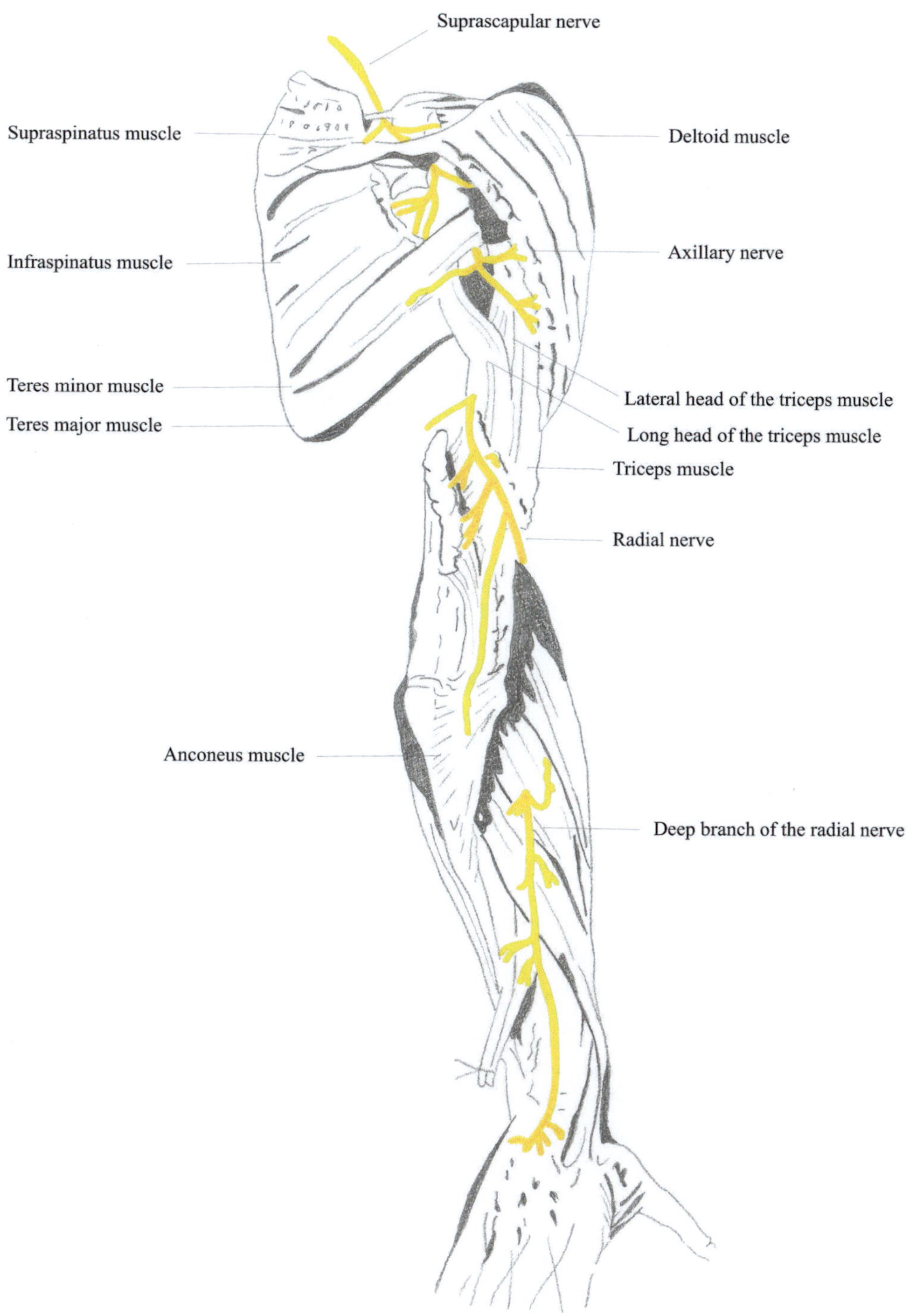

Fig. 2.9 Diagram of the human arm showing the anatomy and course of the radial nerve

The brachial muscle may receive accessory innervation from the radial nerve; however, this contribution is typically insufficient to produce significant elbow flexion.

The *Froment-Rauber nerve* is a rare anatomical variant arising from a terminal branch that communicates with the deep motor branch of the ulnar nerve, innervating intrinsic hand muscles, particularly the first dorsal interosseous and occasionally the second and third interossei.

Sensory Innervation

Posterior cutaneous nerve ➔
Upper dorsal area of the upper arm till the olecranon

Clinical presentation: Hypoesthesia due to injury of the posterior cutaneous nerve suggests a lesion proximal to the spinal groove

Inferior lateral cutaneous nerve ➔
Lower dorsal and lateral aspect of the upper arm (has branches in the spiral groove)

Posterior cutaneous antebrachial nerve➔
Dorsolateral part of the forearm (divides from the radial nerve at the brachial-axillary angle)

Overlapping of this area by the ulnar cutaneous nerve and the lateral antebrachial cutaneous nerve makes it a good donor for grafts. It is called "the sural nerve of the arm".

Superficial sensory radial nerve ➔
Dorsolateral half of hand and proximal two-thirds of digits I–IV

Terminal branch of posterior interosseus nerve ➔
Dorsal wrist capsule (proprioception but no pain)

Dorsal digital nerves ➔
Dorsal side of proximal and middle phalanx of the thumb

2.3 Cervical Plexus

Another plexus of the neck represents the **cervical plexus** which arises from the ventral rami of C1–C4. Each of these rami bifurcates into a superficial sensory branch and a deep motor branch—with the exception of the C1 root (Figs. 2.10 and 2.11)

In some references, the C5 spinal root is considered part of the cervical plexus due to its contribution to the phrenic nerve.

Anatomically, the cervical plexus is located deep to the sternocleidomastoid muscle and the jugular vein, and anterolateral to the levator scapulae muscle.

Prior to bifurcation, cervical nerves communicate with their superior and inferior neighbors, thus anastomosing with the sympathetic fibers of the CNS.

Moreover, the nerves of the cervical plexus communicate with the hypoglossal (CN XII) and the spinal accessory (CN XI) nerves.

The *superficial branches* provide cutaneous innervation to the neck, shoulder, and upper chest.

These four sensory branches emerging from the cervical plexus are named *lesser occipital* (originating from the dorsal ramus of C2), *greater auricular, transverse cervical,* and the *supraclavicular nerves*.

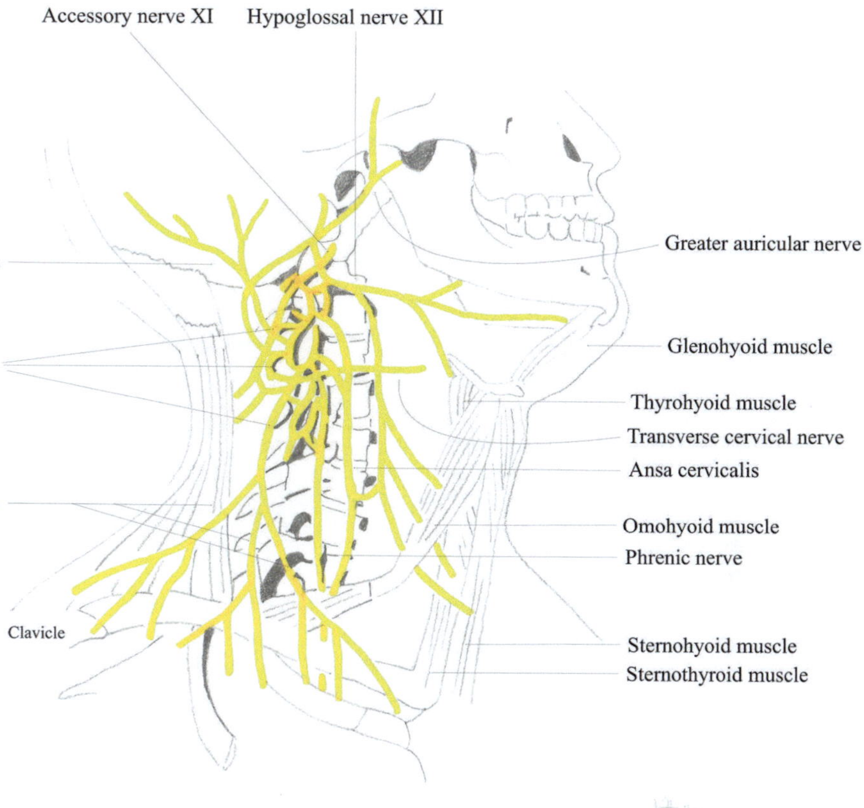

Fig. 2.10 Anatomical drawing of the cervical plexus and its branches

The C1 root does not contribute to cutaneous sensation.

The lesser occipital and greater auricular nerves are following an ascending course, whereas the transverse cervical nerve courses horizontally across the sternocleidomastoid muscle.

The supraclavicular nerves descend posterior to the sternocleidomastoid, dividing at the level of the clavicle to supply their sensory territory.

By acting as the motor part of the cervical plexus, the *deep branches* mainly innervate the muscles of the neck. They are formed by the ansa cervicalis (C1–C3), the phrenic nerve, and some smaller branches.

Motor Innervation

Ansa cervicalis, C1 branch (hypoglossal nerve) ➔
Geniohyoid muscle

Ansa cervicalis, C1-C3 branch ➔
Sternohyoidmuscle
Sternothyroid muscle
Omohyoid muscle
Thyrohyoid muscle (hypoglossal nerve)

➔ Mnemonic: **S**usan **S**aw **G**ame **O**f **T**hrones

The infrahyoid muscles (sternohyoid, sternothyroid, omohyoid and thyrohyoid) are four paired muscles located in the anterior region of the neck. They are responsible for movement of the hyoid bone and the larynx during swallowing and speech.

Phrenic nerve (C3–C5) ➔

Diaphragm and pericardium

Note that the phrenic nerve does also have sensory and sympathetic fibers to the diaphragm. It can be identified as it passes anteriorly to the subclavian artery.

Muscular branches ➔

Prevertebral muscles: longus capiti, longus colli, rectus capitis anterior, and lateralis muscles (ventral flexion of the head)

Scalene muscle (movement of the neck)

Sternocleidomastoid muscle (rotation of the head)

Levator scapulae (elevates the scapula)

> The levator capulae muscle is also innervated by the dorsal scapular nerve of the brachial plexus

<ins>Sensory Innervation</ins>

Lesser occipital nerve (C2) ➔

Upper neck and scalp

Great auricular nerve (C2, C3) ➔

Region of the parotid gland and anterior area of the ear as well as the external auricular meatus

Transverse cervical nerve (C2, C3) ➔

Anterior triangle of the neck

Supraclavicular nerve (C3, C4) ➔

Shoulder and upper chest

> ➔ Mnemonic for the sensory branches: **L**et's **G**o **T**o **S**leep

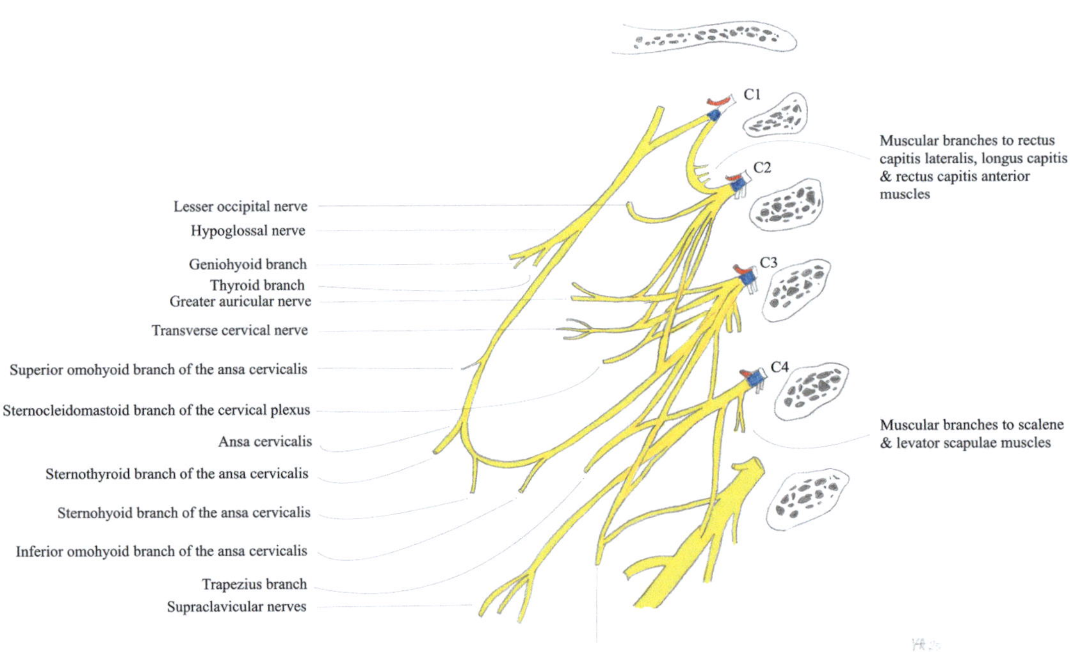

Fig. 2.11 Schematic representation of the cervical plexus

2.3.1 Spinal Accessory Nerve (CN XI)

The spinal accessory nerve is not part of the brachial plexus; however, as it plays an important role regarding neurotization in peripheral nerve surgery it deserves mention.

The nerve exits the jugular foramen having a dual origin: one from the medulla oblongata and another from a spinal contribution (C1–C4). The spinal fibers ascend intramedullary to join the cranial fibers and form the spinal accessory nerve.

On its course inferiorly the spinal accessory nerve bifurcates into an *internal branch,* which contains the cranial fibers, and thereby forms an anastomosis with the vagus nerve to contribute to pharyngeal and laryngeal innervation.

The *external branch*—originating from the spinal fibers—innervates the sternocleidomastoid and the trapezius muscle.

Injury to the spinal accessory nerve typically causes weakness of the trapezius muscle, leading to compromised function of the shoulder girdle. Patients often experience severe shoulder pain, which arises both from injury to the sensory fibers of the spinal accessory nerve and from secondary subacromial impingement [59]. Arm abduction above the head may be restricted but is usually still possible due to compensatory muscle activity, which can sometimes mask a spinal accessory nerve lesion.

The pain often results from overuse and stress of compensating muscles and ligaments in the absence of trapezius function. Mild scapular winging may also be observed.

Weakness of the sternocleidomastoid muscle is typically absent as this muscle also receives innervation from the cervical plexus.

Spinal accessory nerve palsy is mainly of iatrogenic cause, occcurring during cervical lymph node biopsy or dissection.

Moreover, the Vernet Syndrome represents a neuropathic pathology involving cranial nerves IX, X, and XI at the level of the jugular foramen causing injury to them. The etiology is various, including local compression from metastasis or schwannomas, as well as trauma, vascular lesions, or following infections.

Further Reading

1. Johnson EO, Vekris M, Demesticha T, Soucacos PN. Neuroanatomy of the brachial plexus: normal and variant anatomy of its formation. Surg Radiol Anat. 2010;32(3):291–7. https://doi.org/10.1007/s00276-010-0646-0.
2. Herzberg G, Narakas A, Comtet JJ, Bouchet A, Carret JP. Microsurgical relations of the roots of the brachial plexus. Practical applications. Ann Chir Main. 1985;4(2):120–33. https://doi.org/10.1016/s0753-9053(85)80122-8.
3. Russell SM. Examination of peripheral nerve injuries: an anatomical approach. 2nd ed. Thieme; 2015a.
4. Kaiser JT, Lugo-Pico JG. Neuroanatomy, spinal nerves. In: StatPearls [Internet]. StatPearls Publishing; 2023. Available from https://www.ncbi.nlm.nih.gov/books/NBK542218/.
5. Myotomes. Physiopedia. 2025. Retrieved 12:18, May 14, 2025 from https://www.physio-pedia.com/index.php?title=Myotomes&oldid=367775.
6. Blumenfeld H. Neuroanatomy through clinical cases. Sinauer Associates; 2010.
7. Sendić G, Vasković J. Brachial plexus. Kenhub; 2023. https://www.kenhub.com/en/library/anatomy/brachial-plexus
8. Leinberry CF, Wehbé MA. Brachial plexus anatomy. Hand Clin. 2004;20(1):1–5. https://doi.org/10.1016/s0749-0712(03)00088-x.
9. Bayot ML, Nassereddin A, Varacallo M. Anatomy, shoulder and upper limb, brachial plexus. In: StatPearls [Internet]. StatPearls Publishing; 2023. Available from https://www.ncbi.nlm.nih.gov/pubmed/29763192.
10. Oliver KA, Ashurst JV. Anatomy, thorax, phrenic nerves. In: StatPearls [Internet]. StatPearls Publishing; 2023. Available from https://www.ncbi.nlm.nih.gov/books/NBK513325/.
11. Lung K, Lui F. Anatomy, thorax, long thoracic nerve. In: StatPearls [Internet]. StatPearls Publishing; 2023. Available from https://www.ncbi.nlm.nih.gov/books/NBK535396/.
12. Bishop KN, Varacallo MA. Anatomy, shoulder and upper limb, dorsal scapular nerve. In: StatPearls [Internet]. StatPearls Publishing; 2023. Available from https://www.ncbi.nlm.nih.gov/books/NBK459343/.

13. Desai SS, Arbor TC, Varacallo MA. Anatomy, shoulder and upper limb, musculocutaneous nerve. In: StatPearls [Internet]. StatPearls Publishing; 2023. Available from https://www.ncbi.nlm.nih.gov/books/NBK534199/.
14. Pantekidis I, Piagkou M, Koutserimpas C, Samolis A, Tsakotos G, Kostares M, Troupis T. A review of the typical course of the musculocutaneous nerve into the coracobrachialis muscle: its variability and possible clinical implications. Acta Medica Acad. 2023;52(2):95–104. https://doi.org/10.5644/ama2006-124.409.
15. Caetano EB, Sabongi Neto JJ, Vieira LA, Caetano MF. The arcade of Struthers: an anatomical study and clinical implications. Rev Bras Ortop. 2017;52(3):331–6. https://doi.org/10.1016/j.rboe.2016.07.006.
16. Bains KNS, Lappin SL. Anatomy, shoulder and upper limb, elbow cubital fossa. In: StatPearls [Internet]. StatPearls Publishing; 2023. Available from https://www.ncbi.nlm.nih.gov/books/NBK459250/.
17. Wertheimer A, Kiel J. Anatomy, shoulder and upper limb, forearm anterior interosseous nerve. In: StatPearls [Internet]. StatPearls Publishing; 2023. Available from https://www.ncbi.nlm.nih.gov/books/NBK532280/.
18. Murphy KA, Morrisonponce D. Anatomy, shoulder and upper limb, median nerve. In: StatPearls [Internet]. StatPearls Publishing; 2023. Available from https://www.ncbi.nlm.nih.gov/books/NBK448084/.
19. Smith JL, Siddiqui SA, Ebraheim NA. Comprehensive summary of anastomoses between the median and ulnar nerves in the forearm and hand. J Hand Microsurg. 2019;11(1):1–5. https://doi.org/10.1055/s-0038-1672335.
20. Nakashima T. An anatomic study on the Martin-Gruber anastomosis. Surg Radiol Anat. 1993;15(3):193–5. https://doi.org/10.1007/BF01627703.
21. Mendoza M, Sarpong A, Bennett D, Ayala M, Tran P, Sadacharan C, Tippen SP. The Berrettini anastomosis' morphology and "probable zone": a cadaveric study. Cureus. 2025;17(2):e78967. https://doi.org/10.7759/cureus.78967.
22. Ahadi T, Raissi GR, Yavari M, Majidi L. Prevalence of ulnar-to-median nerve motor fiber anastomosis (Riché-Cannieu communicating branch) in hand: an electrophysiological study. Med J Islam Repub Iran. 2016;30:324.
23. Tokmakov M, Markov D, Markov G, Tokmakova K, Poriazova E. Review of the anatomical variations of the median nerve in the carpal tunnel: a concise overview of literature. ResearchGate; 2024.
24. Becker RE, Manna B. Anatomy, shoulder and upper limb, ulnar nerve. In: StatPearls [Internet]. StatPearls Publishing; 2023. Available from https://www.ncbi.nlm.nih.gov/books/NBK499892/.
25. Polatsch DB, Melone CP Jr, Beldner S, Incorvaia A. Ulnar nerve anatomy. Hand Clin. 2007;23(3):283–v. https://doi.org/10.1016/j.hcl.2007.05.001.
26. Tubbs RS, Deep A, Shoja MM, Mortazavi MM, Loukas M, Cohen-Gadol AA. The arcade of Struthers: an anatomical study with potential neurosurgical significance. Surg Neurol Int. 2011;2:184. https://doi.org/10.4103/2152-7806.91139.
27. Natroshvili T, Meene MV, Szweryn WJ, Kemler MA. The controversy surrounding the arcade of Struthers: a systematic review of literature. Indian J Plast Surg. 2024;58(1):11–7. https://doi.org/10.1055/s-0044-1793948.
28. De Jesus R, Dellon AL. Historic origin of the "arcade of Struthers". J Hand Surg Am. 2003;28(3):528–31. https://doi.org/10.1053/jhsu.2003.50071.
29. Siqueira MG, Martins RS. The controversial arcade of Struthers. Surg Neurol. 2005;64(Suppl 1):20–1. https://doi.org/10.1016/j.surneu.2005.04.017.
30. Russell S, editor. Examination of peripheral nerve injuries: an anatomical approach. 2nd ed. Georg Thieme Verlag KG; 2015b. https://doi.org/10.1055/b-003-120831.
31. Range TL, Samra NS. Anatomy, shoulder and upper limb, Osborne band. In: StatPearls [Internet]. StatPearls Publishing; 2023. Available from https://www.ncbi.nlm.nih.gov/books/NBK536999/.
32. Granger A, Sardi JP, Iwanaga J, Wilson TJ, Yang L, Loukas M, Oskouian RJ, Tubbs RS. Osborne's ligament: a review of its history, anatomy, and surgical importance. Cureus. 2017;9(3):e1080. https://doi.org/10.7759/cureus.1080.
33. Massrey C, Iwanaga J, Ishak B, Oskouian RJ, Loukas M, Tubbs RS. Variant of the anconeus epitrochlearis muscle: a case report. Cureus. 2018;10(8):e3201. https://doi.org/10.7759/cureus.3201.
34. Nascimento SRR, Ruiz CR. A study on the prevalence of the anconeus epitrochlearis muscle by magnetic resonance imaging. Rev Bras Ortop. 2018;53(3):373–7. https://doi.org/10.1016/j.rboe.2018.03.015.
35. Depukat P, Henry BM, Popieluszko P, Roy J, Mizia E, Konopka T, Tomaszewski KA, Walocha JA. Anatomical variability and histological structure of the ulnar nerve in Guyon's canal. Arch Orthop Trauma Surg. 2017;137(2):277–83. https://doi.org/10.1007/s00402-016-2616-4.
36. Niitsu M, Kokubo N, Nojima S. Variations of the ulnar nerve in Guyon's canal: in vivo demonstration using ultrasound and 3 T MRI. Acta Radiol. 2010;51(8):939–46. https://doi.org/10.3109/02841851.2010.503193.
37. Okwumabua E, Thompson JH. Anatomy, shoulder and upper limb, axillary nerve. In: StatPearls [Internet].

StatPearls Publishing; 2023. Available from https://www.ncbi.nlm.nih.gov/books/NBK493212/.

38. Gurushantappa PK, Kuppasad S. Anatomy of axillary nerve and its clinical importance: a cadaveric study. J Clin Diagn Res. 2015;9(3):AC13-AC17. https://doi.org/10.7860/JCDR/2015/12349.5680.
39. Tessler J, Talati R. Axillary nerve injury. In: StatPearls [Internet]. StatPearls Publishing; 2023. Available from https://www.ncbi.nlm.nih.gov/books/NBK539895/.
40. Palastanga NP, Soames RW, Palastanga N. Anatomy and human movement: structure and function. 6th ed. Churchill Livingstone; 2011.
41. Glover NM, Black AC, Murphy PB. Anatomy, shoulder and upper limb, radial nerve [updated 2023 Nov 5]. In: StatPearls [Internet]. Treasure Island: StatPearls Publishing; 2024. Available from https://www.ncbi.nlm.nih.gov/books/NBK534840/.
42. Cho H, Lee HY, Gil YC, Choi YR, Yang HJ. Topographical anatomy of the radial nerve and its muscular branches related to surface landmarks. Clin Anat. 2013;26(7):862–9. https://doi.org/10.1002/ca.22115.
43. Kesserwani H. The "Texas longhorn" syndrome: a case of posterior interosseous nerve palsy with noteworthy observations. Cureus. 2021;13(1):e12760. https://doi.org/10.7759/cureus.12760.
44. Debouck C, Rooze M. The arcade of Fröhse: an anatomic study. Surg Radiol Anat. 1995;17(3):245–8. https://doi.org/10.1007/BF01795057.
45. Benes M, Kachlik D, Kunc V, Kunc V. The arcade of Frohse: a systematic review and meta-analysis. Surg Radiol Anat. 2021;43(5):703–11. https://doi.org/10.1007/s00276-021-02718-5.
46. Riffaud L, Morandi X, Godey B, Brassier G, Guegan Y, Darnault P, Scarabin JM. Anatomic bases for the compression and neurolysis of the deep branch of the radial nerve in the radial tunnel. Surg Radiol Anat. 1999;21(4):229–33. https://doi.org/10.1007/BF01631390.
47. Loizides A, Peer S, Ostermann S, Henninger B, Stampfer-Kountchev M, Gruber H. Unusual functional compression of the deep branch of the radial nerve by a vascular branch (leash of Henry): ultrasonographic appearance. Rofo. 2011;183(2):163–6. https://doi.org/10.1055/s-0029-1245738. Epub 2010 Oct 11. PMID: 20938884.
48. Hackl M, Wegmann K, Lappen S, Helf C, Burkhart KJ, Müller LP. The course of the posterior interosseous nerve in relation to the proximal radius: is there a reliable landmark? Injury. 2015;46(4):687–92. https://doi.org/10.1016/j.injury.2015.01.028. Epub 2015 Jan 24. PMID: 25677826.
49. Prasartritha T, Liupolvanish P, Rojanakit A. A study of the posterior interosseous nerve (PIN) and the radial tunnel in 30 Thai cadavers. J Hand Surg Am. 1993;18(1):107–12. https://doi.org/10.1016/0363-5023(93)90253-Y. PMID: 8423293.
50. Pan Y, Hung LK. The course of the terminal posterior interosseous nerve and its relationship with wrist arthroscopy portals. J Wrist Surg. 2016;5(4):315–9. https://doi.org/10.1055/s-0036-1584899.
51. Zilles K, Tillmann BN. Anatomie. Springer; 2010.
52. Glenesk NL, Kortz MW, Lopez PP. Anatomy, head and neck, posterior cervical nerve plexus. In: StatPearls [Internet]. StatPearls Publishing; 2023. Available from https://www.ncbi.nlm.nih.gov/books/NBK538514/.
53. Shen S, Macori F, Liu J, et al. Cervical plexus. Radiopaedia.org; 2024. https://doi.org/10.53347/rID-30693.
54. Overland J, Hodge JC, Breik O, Krishnan S. Surgical anatomy of the spinal accessory nerve: review of the literature and case report of a rare anatomical variant. J Laryngol Otol. 2016;130(10):969–72. https://doi.org/10.1017/S0022215116008148.
55. Roberts SO, Cardozo A. A detailed review of the spinal accessory nerve and its anatomical variations with cadaveric illustration. Anat Sci Int. 2024;99(3):239–53. https://doi.org/10.1007/s12565-024-00770-w.
56. Koliarakis I, Manatakis DK, Tsitsipanis C, Drakonaki E, Tsamandouras I, Tsiaoussis J. Spinal accessory nerve anatomy in the posterior cervical triangle: a systematic review with meta-analysis. Clin Anat. 2024;37(1):130–9. https://doi.org/10.1002/ca.24119.
57. Radhakrishnan A. The accessory nerve (CN XI). TeachMeAnatomy; 2023. https://teachmeanatomy.info/head/cranial-nerves/accessory/
58. AlShareef S, Newton BW. Accessory nerve injury. In: StatPearls [Internet]. StatPearls Publishing; 2022. https://www.ncbi.nlm.nih.gov/books/NBK532245/.
59. Chan PK, Hems TE. Clinical signs of accessory nerve palsy. J Trauma. 2006;60(5):1142–4. https://doi.org/10.1097/01.ta.0000174718.83440.75.

3 Anatomy of the Lumbosacral Plexus and Its Terminal Branches

The lumbar and sacral plexuses are complex networks of spinal nerves that provide motor and sensory innervation to the lower trunk, pelvis, and lower limbs. The lumbar plexus, formed by the ventral rami of T12–L4 within the psoas major muscle, primarily innervates the anterior and medial compartments of the thigh. Unlike the brachial plexus, it lacks further trunks or cords but includes anterior and posterior divisions from L2 to L4. Main branches include the iliohypogastric, ilioinguinal, genitofemoral, lateral femoral cutaneous, femoral, and obturator nerves innervating muscles of the lower limb and extensive cutaneous regions.

The sacral plexus (L4–S4), with contributions from the lumbosacral trunk (L4–L5), is located anterior to the piriformis muscle and gives rise to major nerves of the gluteal region and lower limb. These include the superior and inferior gluteal nerves, sciatic nerve, posterior femoral cutaneous nerve, and smaller branches such as the nerve to obturator internus and quadratus femoris. The sciatic nerve, the largest nerve in the body, bifurcates into the tibial and common peroneal nerves, supplying nearly all muscles of the lower leg and foot.

Certain anatomical routes, such as the greater and lesser sciatic foramina and the tarsal tunnel, accommodate nerve passage and branching. Variations, such as the presence of the psoas minor muscle or the accessory obturator nerve, are clinically significant. Pathologies like sciatica can arise from structural or positional factors, often causing radiating pain and functional impairment without necessarily involving permanent damage. Understanding these neuroanatomical relationships is crucial for clinical assessments, surgical planning, and managing neuropathies of the lower extremity.

3.1 Lumbar Plexus

The **lumbar plexus** is formed by the ventral rami of spinal nerves T12–L4, located within the psoas major muscle.

In contrast to the brachial plexus, the lumbar plexus does not split into trunks or cords. However, the spinal nerves L2–L4 divide into **anterior** and **posterior divisions**.

The terminal branches of the lumbar plexus can be traced to their respective spinal nerve contributions:

- Spinal nerve T12 forms the *subcostal nerve* which supplies the pyramidalis muscle—the deep abdominal wall muscle responsible for tension of the linea alba; and the transverse abdominal muscle, via two branches.
- Spinal nerve L1—together with some fibers of T12—make up the *iliohypogastric nerve.*
- L1 forms the *ilioinguinal nerve.*
- L1 and the anterior division of L2 form the *genitofemoral nerve.*

K. Hobitsch, *Peripheral Nerve Surgery - A Compendium*,
https://doi.org/10.1007/978-3-032-03409-0_3

- The posterior divisions of L2 and L3 are making up the *lateral femoral cutaneous nerve* which innervates skin of the anterolateral thigh and part of the gluteal region.
- The posterior divisions of L2–L4 thus create the *femoral nerve*.
- Anterior divisions of L2–L4 form the *obturator nerve* which innervates muscles of the medial compartment of the thigh.
- The *accessory obturator nerve* is composed by spinal nerves L3 and L4. It is present in about 20% of the population [1] and innervates the pectineus muscle. It furthermore supplies the skin of the hip joint (Fig. 3.1).

The spinal nerves of the three caudal branches of the lumbar plexus communicate with one another to form anterior and posterior divisions. The anterior division of L2–L4 give rise to the *obturator nerve*, while the posterior division of L2–L3 form the *lateral cutaneous femoral nerve* and the posterior division of L2–L4 constitutes the *femoral nerve*.

The three nerves from T12–L2 do not form such divisions.

Fibers of the L4 and L5 spinal nerves serve as a connection to the sacral plexus. They run in a caudal direction to the sacroiliac joint where they join the sacral plexus.

The L4 nerve is also called the "furcal nerve" due to its trifurcation to the anterior division to the obturator nerve, the posterior division to the femoral nerve, and its contribution to the lumbosacral plexus [2].

The psoas minor muscle is present in approximately 46% [6] of the population. It is located anteriorly to the psoas major muscle and receives innervation from branches of L1 and L2 spinal nerves.

Smaller branches from L1–L4 arise to innervate the quadratus lumborum—a deep abdominal muscle mainly stabilizing and moving the spine as well as the pelvis.

Mnemonic: **I**nterested **I**n **G**etting **L**unch **O**n **F**riday?

Iliohypogastric, Ilioinguinal, Genitofemoral, Lateral cutaneous femoral, Femoral, Obturator

Mnemonic

2 from 1 (2 nerves from 1 root) ➔ Iliohypogastric (L1 and some contributions of T12) & Ilioinguinal (L1)

2 from 2 (2 nerves from 2 roots) ➔ Genitofemoral (L1 + L2) & Lateral cutaneous femoral (L2 + L3)

2 from 3 (2 nerves from 3 roots) ➔ Obturator & Femoral (L2–L4)

3.1.1 Overview of the Lumbar Plexus Anatomy

T12–L4 ➔ *Lumbar plexus*

L2–L4 ➔ *Anterior and posterior divisions*

T12 ➔ *Subcostal nerves*

T12–L1 ➔ *Iliohypogastric nerve*

L1 ➔ *Ilioinguinal nerve*

L1 and anterior division of L2 ➔ *Genitofemoral nerve*

Anterior division of L2–L4 ➔ *Obturator nerve*

Anterior division of L3–L4 ➔ *Accessory obturator nerve*

Posterior division of L2–L4 ➔ *Femoral nerve*

Posterior division of L2–L3 ➔ *Lateral cutaneous femoral nerve* (Fig. 3.2)

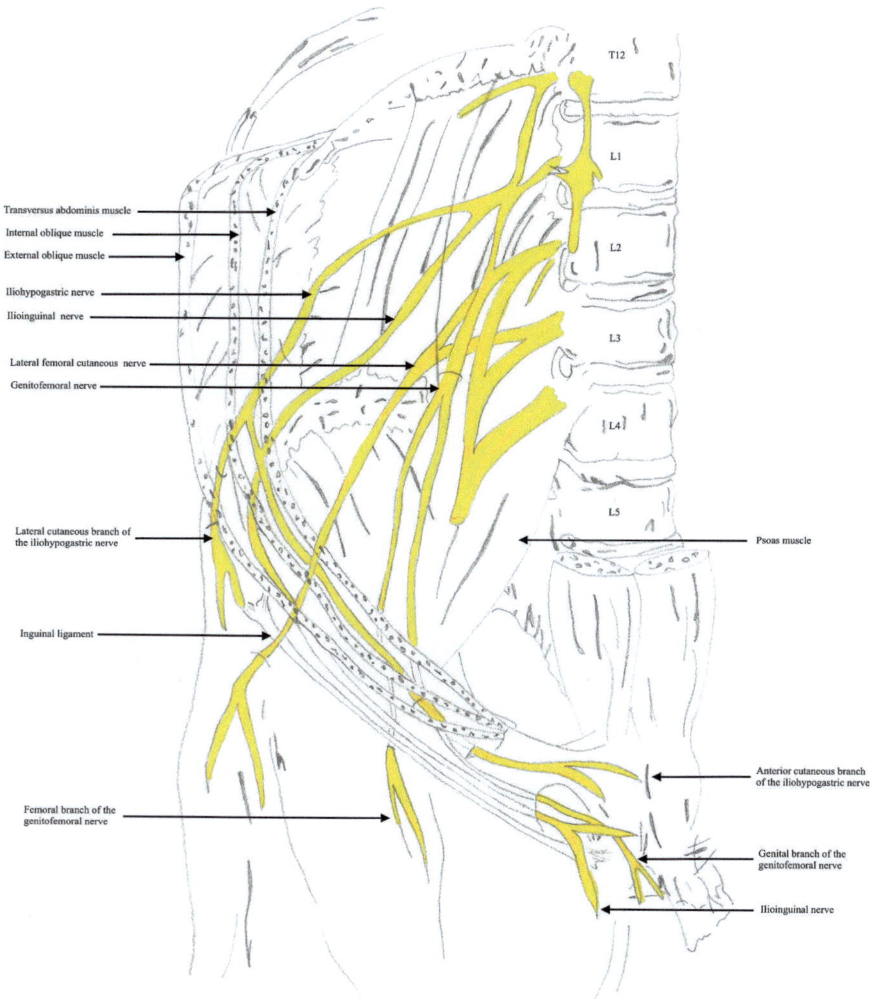

Fig. 3.1 Diagram of the anatomy of the lumbar plexus. Nerves are depicted in yellow, with labels indicating their anatomical positions

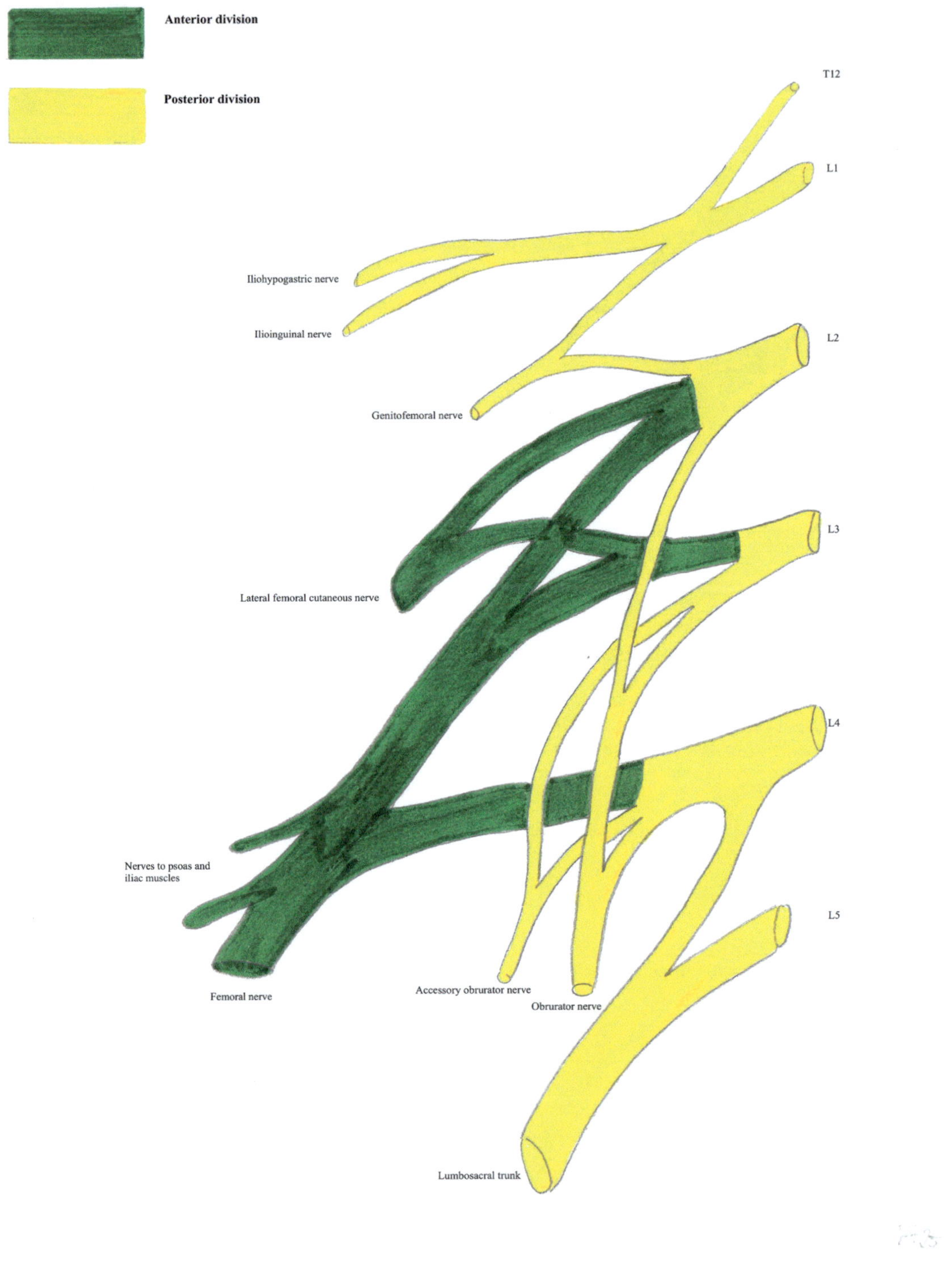

Fig. 3.2 Schematic representation of the lumbar plexus, showing anterior and posterior divisions in green and yellow, respectively

3.2 Terminal Branches

3.2.1 Iliohypogastric Nerve (T12–L1)

The **iliohypogastric nerve** emerges laterally from the psoas major muscle, courses over the iliac crest, pierces the transversus abdominal muscle, and passes around the flank. Near the anterosuperior iliac spine, a *lateral branch* emerges, perforating both the internal and external oblique muscles. Terminal branches of the iliohypogastric nerve provide innervation to the hypogastric/inguinal region and the superolateral gluteal area.

Motor Innervation

Muscular branches ➔

Internal oblique muscle: flexion of the abdomen and intraabdominal pressure

Transversus abdominis muscle: increases the intrabdominal pressure to assist forced expiration

Sensory Innervation

Lateral cutaneous branch ➔

Skin of the lateral abdomen and the posterolateral gluteal area

Anterior cutaneous branch ➔

Skin around the superficial inguinal ring at the pubic area

3.2.2 Ilioinguinal Nerve (L1)

Initially following the iliohypogastric nerve while being just below to it, the **ilioinguinal nerve** perforates the transversus abdominins and the internal oblique muscles and then passes toward the inguinal canal to join the spermatic cord. It contains mainly sensory fibers.

Motor Innervation

Muscular branches ➔

Pyramidalis muscle

> It may provide motor innervation to the internal oblique and the transversus abdominis muscles

Genital branch ➔

Cremaster muscle

Sensory Innervation

Skin of the inguinal ligament and the upper medial aspect of the thigh, as well as the mons pubis in females and the skin of the anterior part of the penis in males.

Note that the iliohypogastric nerve and the ilioinguinal nerve arise from a common trunk.

3.2.3 Genitofemoral Nerve (L1–L2)

The **genitofemoral nerve** pierces the psoas major muscle and stays anteriorly to it while it bifurcates into its two main branches—the *genital branch*, which passes through the inguinal canal, and the *femoral branch* running through the vascular triangle.

Motor Innervation

Genital branch ➔

Cremaster muscle

Sensory Innervation

Genital branch ➔

Scrotum, part of the labia majora and a small area on the medial thigh

Femoral branch ➔

Skin of the medial thigh

3.2.4 Lateral Femoral Cutaneous Nerve (L2–L3)

The **lateral femoral cutaneous nerve**—originating from the posterior divisions of the lumbar plexus—emerges lateral to the psoas major muscle and courses toward the anterior iliac spine. It then passes beneath the inguinal ligament, where it gives rise to *several branches*, before terminating in the lateral thigh. As its name suggests, this purely sensory nerve innervates the skin of the lateral aspect of the thigh.

It may also provide sensory supply to the peritoneum.

Entrapment of this nerve at the iliac crest leads to a pain syndrome called **meralgia paresthetica**.

3.2.5 Obturator Nerve (L2–L4)

The **obturator nerve** is formed by the anterior divisions of spinal nerves L2–L4, and is the only nerve of the lumbar plexus that courses medially from the psoas major muscle. It passes through the obturator canal where it divides into its two main branches —the *anterior* and the *posterior division* (Fig. 3.3).

The more superficially located anterior division, after giving off its branches—continues its course between the adductor longus and brevis muscles, ultimately terminating as the *cutaneous branch of the obturator nerve*.

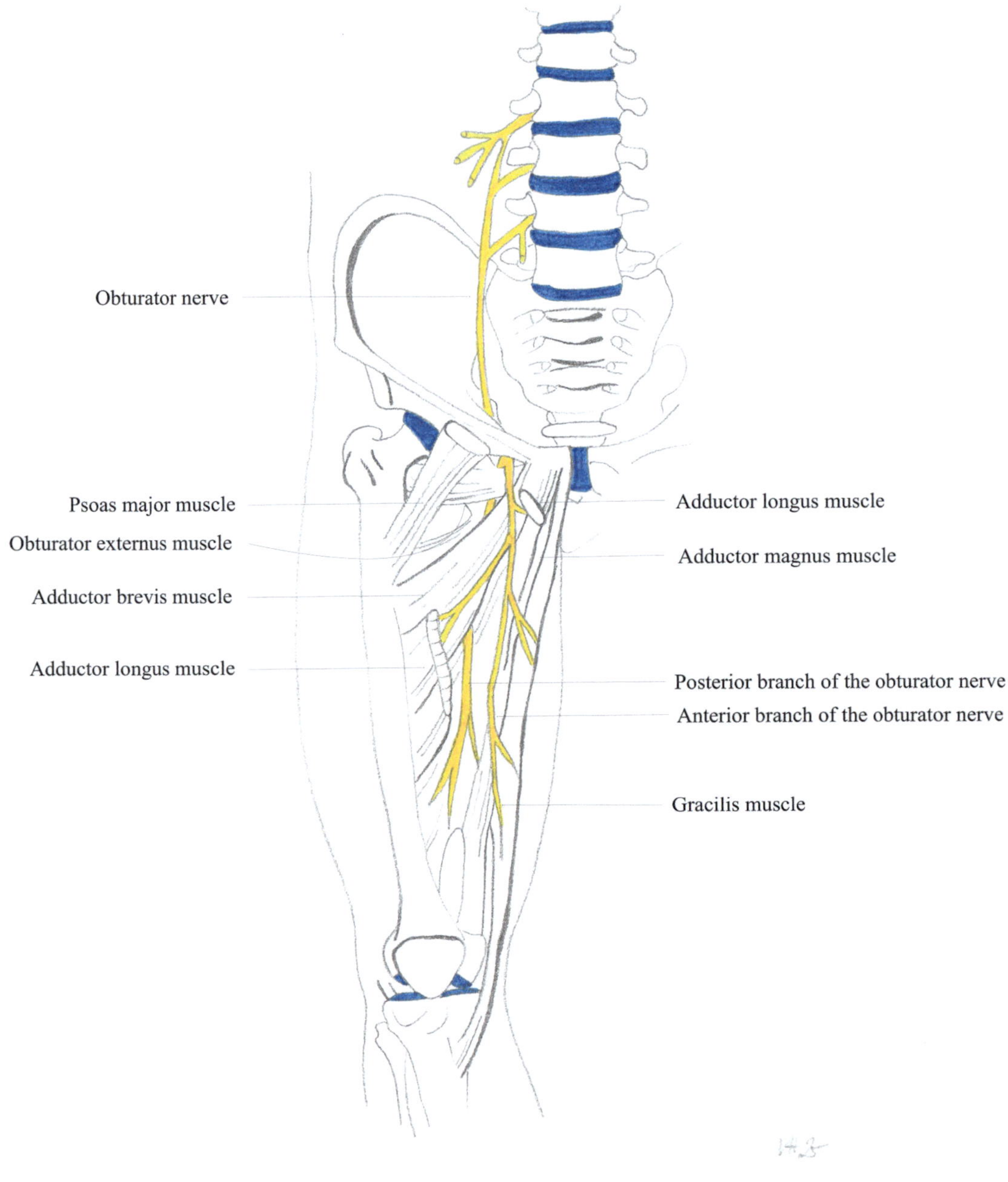

Fig. 3.3 Diagram of the human pelvic region highlighting the course of the obturator nerve

The smaller posterior division innervates a part of the adductor magnus muscle.

Motor Innervation

Anterior branch ➔

Gracilis muscle (hip adduction, knee flexion, internal rotation)

Adductor longus and brevis muscles (adduction of the thigh)

Pectineus muscle (flexion and adduction of the thigh)

Posterior branch ➔

Adductor magnus muscle (adduction and medial rotation of the thigh)

Obturator externus muscle (adduction and lateral rotation of the thigh)

Sensory Innervation

Anterior branch (proximal branch) ➔

Skin of the medial aspect of the thigh

The *accessory obturator nerve* represents an additional nerve deriving from the anterior divisions of L3 and L4 ventral rami and is present in about 10–30% of the population [14]. When existent, it typically accompanies the obturator nerve toward the obturator canal, although it does not traverse the canal itself. It rather courses superficially over the superior pubic ramus and beneath the pectineus muscle—which it innervates—before ultimately anastomosing with the obturator nerve.

3.2.6 Femoral Nerve (L2–L4)

Being the largest nerve of the lumbar plexus, the **femoral nerve** emerges laterally from the psoas major muscle—being located at a certain point between the iliac and the psoas major muscle, where it gives off a *muscular branch* to innervate the iliac muscle. It then travels beneath the inguinal ligament to reach the femoral triangle. Within the femoral triangle, the femoral nerve bifurcates into an *anterior* and a *posterior division.*

Distal to the inguinal ligament, the femoral nerve further gives off several branches, including the *medial femoral cutaneous nerve*, the *intermediate femoral cutaneous nerve,* and the *saphenous nerve.*

Other branches contain *motor fibers* that are innervating the quadriceps, the sartorius, and the pectineus muscles.

A *common branch* supplying the rectus femoris and the vastus lateralis muscle arises proximally.

In summary, the anterior division gives rise to *two motor and two sensory branches*, wheras the posterior division contributes *four motor branches*, *one sensory branch, and two articular branches.*

The sensory branch of the posterior division, known as the *saphenous nerve,* provides extensive cutaneous innervation and constitutes the terminal continuation of the femoral nerve. It accompanies the greater saphenous vein within the adductor canal (Hunter's canal, subsartorial canal) coursing inferiorly, in a groove between the adductor longus and the vastus medialis, before passing medially along the tibial bone.

As it reaches half of the tibia, it divides into two branches—a *posterior branch* which terminates at the ankle, and an *anterior branch* which continues medially to reach the hallux (Fig. 3.4).

Note, that multiple small branches exit from the saphenous nerve during its descend before it finally bifurcates into its two terminal divisions.

The saphenous nerve represents the longest nerve in the human body.

Being found in the superior part of the thigh anteromedially, the femoral triangle describes a space that contains several important structures. It is formed by the inguinal ligament superiorly, and the sartorius and the adductor longus muscle serving as a lateral and a medial border, respectively. The floor of the femoral triangle consists of the adductor longus, the pectineus, the psoas major, and the iliacus muscles. From lateral to medial it contains following structures: the femoral nerve, femoral artery, femoral vein, femoral canal (empty space), and lymphatics.

Mnemonic: NAVEL—Nerve, Artery, Vein, Empty space, Lymphatics

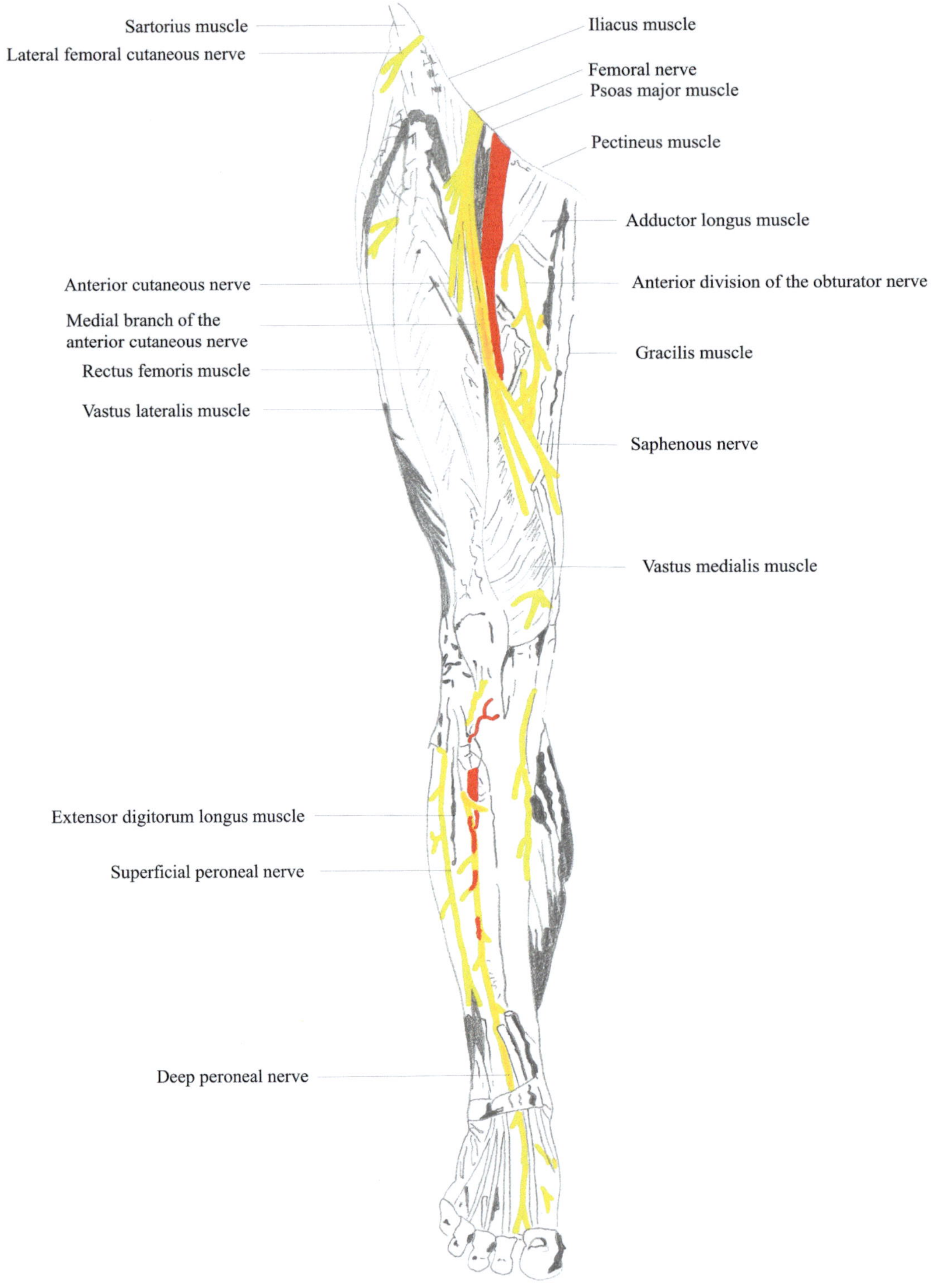

Fig. 3.4 Anatomical drawing of the femoral nerve and its associated structures

Clinically, it represents the location for catherization of the femoral artery in endovascular procedures.

Motor Innervation

Muscular branch ➔
Early branch to the psoas major and iliacus, and/or to the psoas minor (iliopsoas) muscles

Anterior division ➔
Pectineus muscle (hip flexion)
Sartorius muscle (flexion of the hip and knee, lateral rotation of the hip)

Posterior division ➔
Vastus medialis (knee extension)
Vastus lateralis (knee extension)
Intermedius muscles (knee extension)
Rectus femoris muscle (hip flexion and knee extension)

These four muscles are collectively called the quadriceps femoris.

Sensory Innervation

Anterior division:
Medial cutaneous nerve of the thigh ➔
Distal anteromedial thigh
Intermediate cutaneous nerve of the thigh ➔
Anteromedial thigh

Posterior division:
Saphenous nerve ➔
Medial side of the knee joint, lower leg, and the heel
Infrapatellar branches (from saphenous nerve) **➔**
Skin inferiorly to the patella
Two articular joint branches ➔
Nerve to the rectus femoris muscle (hip joint)
Nerve to the vastus medialis, lateralis, and intermediate (knee joint)

> Hilton's law: Nerves supplying the muscles that act upon a joint generally also provide sensory innervation to the joint itself and to the overlying cutaneous structures.

The most common lesions of the femoral nerve are herniating discs (L2–L4), pelvic fractures, and hip dislocation.

3.3 Sacral Plexus

The spinal nerves exit the spinal cord through the anterior sacral foramina to form the **sacral plexus** which is located anteriorly to the piriformis muscle within the pelvis. The plexus is primarily composed of the anterior rami of spinal nerves S1–S4, with additional contributions from L4 and L5 spinal nerves; for this reason it is often referred to as the **lumbosacral plexus** (Figs. 3.5 and 3.6).

The sacral plexus compromises five major peripheral nerves, as well as several smaller branches that innervate the pelvic floor, walls, and muscles.

There are three possible ways nerves can descend from the sacral plexus to the inferior limb:

1. Via the greater sciatic foramen to terminate into the gluteal region, above or beneath the piriformis muscle
2. Remaining within the pelvis, thereby innervating the pelvic muscles, organs as well as the perineum
3. Exiting the pelvis again via the greater sciatic foramen, then looping around the sacrospinous ligament just to reenter the pelvis through the lesser sciatic foramen

> Most of the nerves are taking the first route via the greater sciatic foramen.

The smaller branches of the sacral plexus directly innervate their target muscles, except for the *perforating cutaneous and the pelvic splanchnic nerves*.

Following branches need to be mentioned:

1. The *perforating cutaneous nerve* (S2, S3) pierces the sacrotuberous ligament—a structure, extending from the sacrum to the ischial tuberosity—to innervate the skin of the inferior gluteal region.
2. The *pelvic splanchnic nerves* (three branches) contain parasympathetic nerve fibers supplying the visceral organs such as the urinary bladder and the internal urethral sphincter; they also promote rectal motility and are responsible for the sexual function.

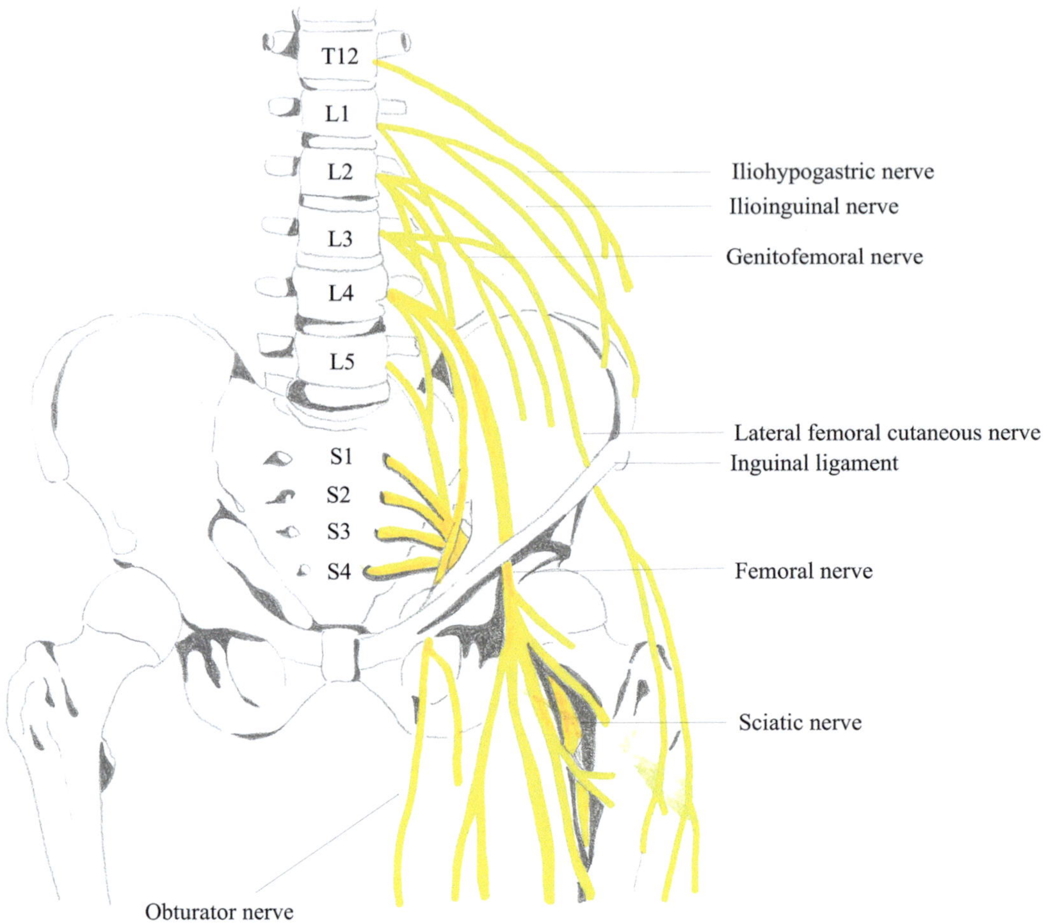

Fig. 3.5 Anatomical drawing of the sacral plexus with its associated nerves

3. The *nerve to the piriformis* derives from the posterior division of S1 and S2 spinal nerves. The piriformis muscle functions as an external hip rotator.
4. The *internal obturator nerve*, from the anterior division of L5–S2 exits through the greater sciatic foramen. It then loops around the sacrospinous ligament to re-enter via the lesser sciatic foramen to directly innervate the obturator internus and the superior gemellus muscles.
5. The *nerve to the quadratus femoris*—from the anterior division of L4–S1—exits via the greater sciatic foramen inferior to the piriformis muscle and enters the anterior surface of the quadratus femoris muscle.

The *coccygeal plexus* (S4, S5, and Co1) represents a mainly sensory plexus innervating the skin around the coccygeal region. It can give rise to up to three anococcygeal nerves.

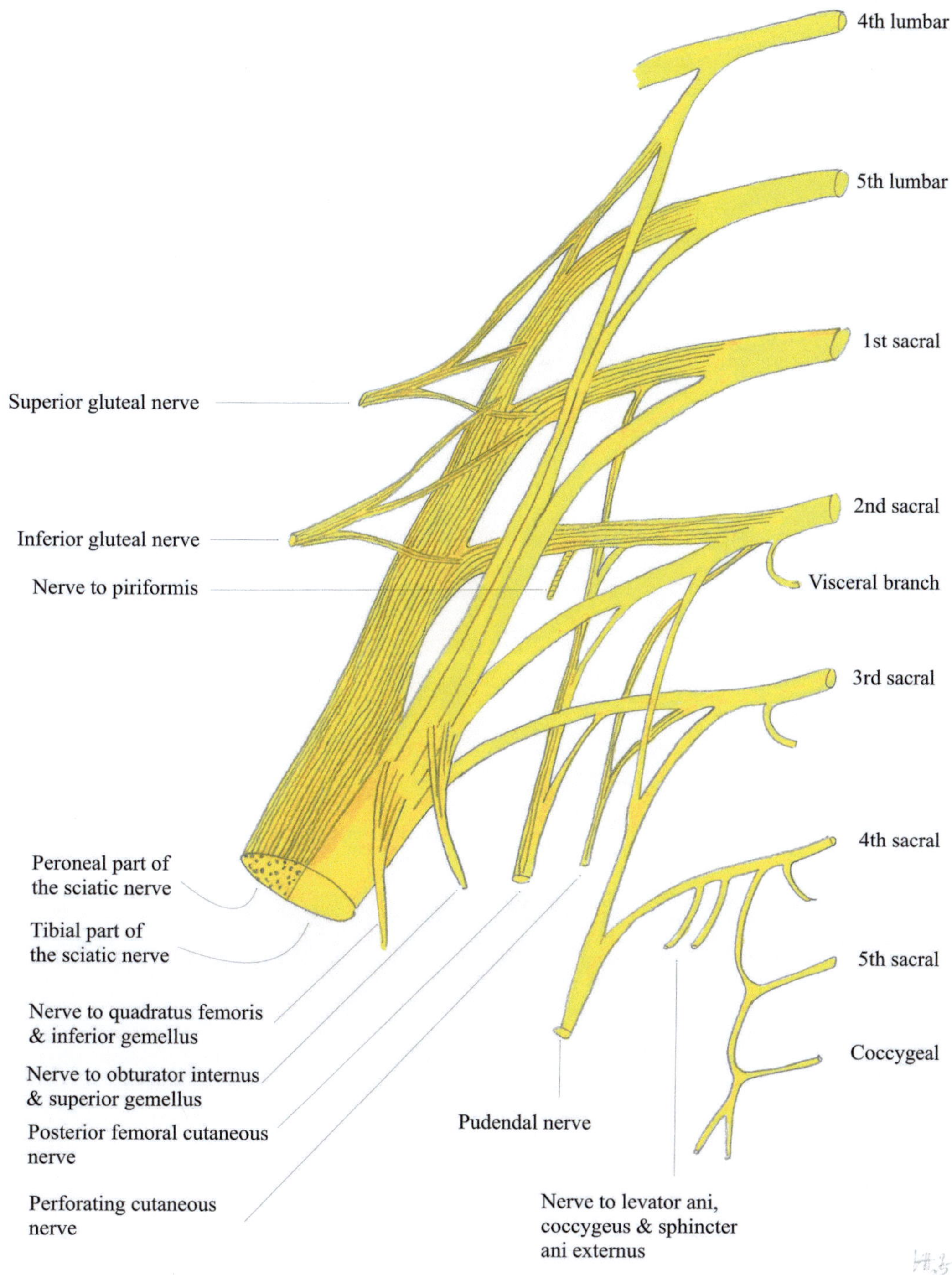

Fig. 3.6 Schematic representation of the lumbo-sacral plexus

The anterior division of the sacral plexus forms two nerves—the *nerve to the quadratus femoris and the inferior gemelli muscle* (L4–S1), and the *nerve to the obturator internus and the superior gemelli muscle* (L5–S2). Their motor innervation mainly allows external hip rotation of the mentioned muscles.

The posterior division terminates into two branches as well, the *superior gluteal nerve* (L4–S1) and the *inferior gluteal nerve* (L5–S2).

One single nerve is formed by both the anterior and the posterior division—*the femoral cutaneous nerve,* also known as the *lesser sciatic nerve* (Fig. 3.7).

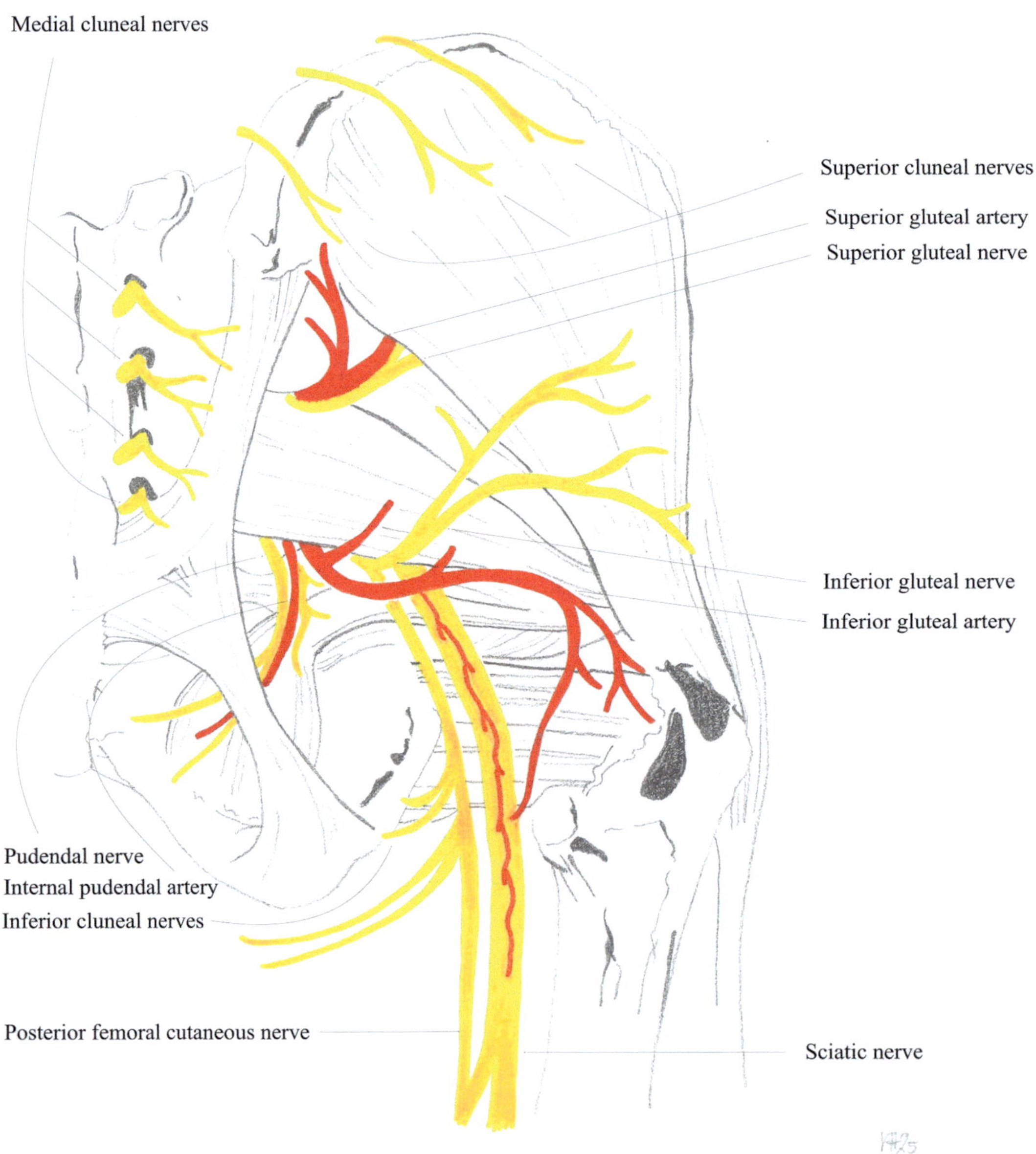

Fig. 3.7 Diagram of the anatomy of the sacral plexus and its terminal nerves

3.3.1 Overview of the Sacral Plexus Anatomy

Ventral rami of L4–S4 form the sacral plexus
Anterior branches ➔
 Nerve to quadratus femoris muscle
 Nerve to obturator internus muscle
 Pudendal nerve
 Nerves to levator ani muscle and external anal sphincter
Posterior branches ➔
 Nerve to the piriformis muscle
 Superior gluteal nerve
 Inferior gluteal nerve
 Perforating cutaneous nerve
 Pelvic splanchnic nerves
Terminal branch ➔
 Sciatic nerve (tibial and common peroneal nerves)

3.4 Terminal Branches

3.4.1 Superior Gluteal Nerve (L4–S1)

The **superior gluteal nerve** represents the first nerve of the sacral plexus and exits the pelvis— accompanying the gluteal artery and vein—via the greater sciatic foramen to enter the gluteal region superiorly to the piriformis muscle toward the tensor fasciae latae.

It acts as a purely motor nerve, innervating the gluteus medius and minimus as well as the tensor fascia latae muscles.

Besides innervating muscles that are promoting abduction, flexion, and rotation of the thigh, the superior gluteal nerve plays an important role regarding stabilization of the pelvis as it tensions the iliotibial tract, thereby reducing the burden of the femur on the standing leg.

Owing to its anatomical course, the superior gluteal nerve is suscepitble to injury from intramuscular injections which can result in weakness of hip abduction and a positive Trendelenburg sign [23].

The Trendelenburg sign is characterized by a drop of the pelvis toward the side of the lesion, resulting from insufficient stabilization by the gluteal muscles. During gait, the body compensates by tilting toward the ipsilateral side—a pattern known as Duchenne gait.

3.4.2 Inferior Gluteal Nerve (L5–S2)

The **inferior gluteal nerve** follows a course similar to that of the superior gluteal nerve, accompanying the inferior gluteal artery and vein. As it reaches the inferior border of the piriformis muscle, it divides into *multiple muscular branches*, each terminating into different regions of the gluteus maximus muscle.

Similar to the superior gluteal nerve, the inferior gluteal nerve is a motor nerve that innervates the strongest extensor of the hip joint—the gluteus maximus muscle. In addition, the gluteus maximus muscle assists in external rotation and, to a lesser extent, abduction and adduction. It is also essential for postural stability during standing as it prevents anterior tilting of the pelvis.

3.4.3 Sciatic Nerve (L4–S3)

Representing the largest nerve of the body, the **sciatic nerve** consists of two distinct components—the tibial and the common peroneal division—which maintain separated fascicles but are enclosed within a common epineurium. (Fig. 3.8).

With the exception of the sensible saphenous nerve, the sciatic nerve is the sole nerve supplying the lower leg.

It is formed by five spinal nerves at the anterior side of the piriformis muscle.

After entering the greater sciatic foramen inferior to the piriformis muscle, the sciatic nerve courses between the trochanter minor and the ischial tuberosity toward the medioposterior aspect of the thigh. At this level, it is covered by the gluteus maximus muscle and positioned superficial to the obturator internus, quadratus femoris, adductor magnus, and the two gemelli muscles.

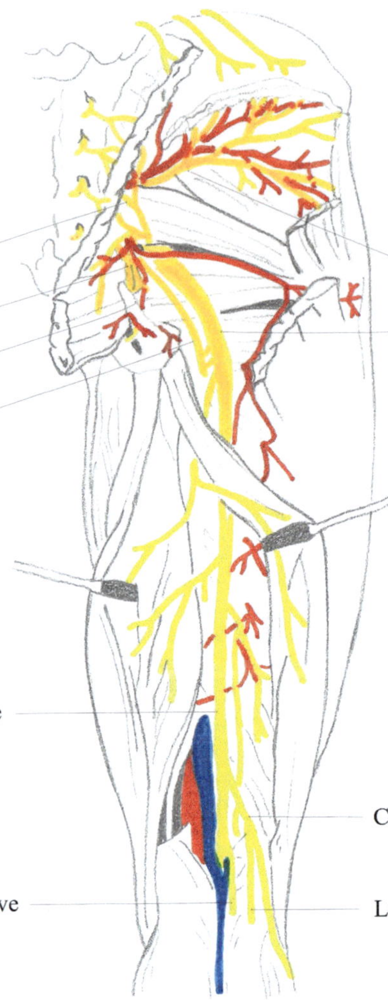

Fig. 3.8 Anatomical drawing of the human leg's posterior view, illustrating the sciatic nerve and its branches

> Always keep in mind the anatomical variations, with the sciatic nerve running superiorly to the piriformis muscle or even perforating it.

As it continues its course toward the popliteal fossa, the sciatic nerve remains in a posterior position, situated deep to the hamstring muscles. Laterally, it is related to the long and short heads of biceps femoris, while medially it is bordered by the semitendinosus and semimembranosus muscles.

At that level, it gives off *several muscular branches*, and—with consideration for anatomical variations—separates into a proper *tibial nerve* and a *common peroneal nerve* (or *common fibular nerve*), usually in the last third of the thigh—just before reaching the popliteal fossa [29].

> In approximately 11% of the population, the sciatic nerve already divides in its two proper nerves at the level of the pelvis [30].

The *tibial nerve* represents the larger branch and has a more medial location. It derives from the anterior division of spinal nerves L4–S3 innervating the posterior compartment of the lower limb. As it descends through the leg, the tibial nerve remains a medioposterior position to join the popliteal artery and vein—continuations of the femoral vessels—at the distal thigh. At this level, it gives rise to the *medial sural cutaneous nerve,* which courses between the two heads of the gastrocnemius muscle to perforate the subcutaneous fascia. It then unites with the *lateral sural cutaneous branch* of the common peroneal nerve to form the *sural nerve*. The sural nerve follows a posterolateral course along the leg, passing posterior to the lateral malleus to terminate into the dorsolateral foot.

Remaining deep to the gastrocnemius and the soleus muscles, the tibial nerve reaches the posterior side of the medial malleolus bone to finally enter the foot under the flexor retinaculum (lacinate ligament), also referred to as the tarsal tunnel. The flexor retinaculum represents a fibrous band extending from the medial malleolus to the calcaneus bones.

The tarsal tunnel contains several structures including the tibial nerve, the posterior tibial artery and veins, the tendons from the tibialis posterior, the flexor digitorum longus, and the flexor hallucis longus muscles.

Before entering the tarsal tunnel—or within the tarsal tunnel (anatomical variations)—the *medial calcaneal nerve* emerges from the tibial nerve.

Finally, it bifurcates into the *medial* and *lateral plantar nerves.*

The larger medial plantar nerve passes between the abductor hallucis and the flexor digitorum brevis and divides into *digital nerves* to innervate the first three fingers.

The lateral plantar nerve travels through the quadratus plantae and the abductor digiti minimi pedis muscle to branch into a *superficial sensory* and a *profound motor nerve*, innervating the intrinsic muscles of the foot.

The *common peroneal nerve* is formed by the posterior divisions of L4–S2 supplying the anterior compartment of the leg. After bifurcating from the sciatic nerve, the common peroneal nerve courses toward the posterior aspect of the fibular head where it gives rise to two sensory branches: the *lateral sural cutaneous nerve* and the *lateral cutaneous nerve of the calf.*

The common peroneal nerve further runs laterally from the fibular shaft deep to the peroneus longus muscle. The aponeurosis of the peroneus longus muscle—together with an aponeurosis connecting the peroneal fascia to the soleus—forms a structure called the fibular tunnel. At this level, the common peroneal nerve bifurcates into a deep and a superficial nerve.

The *deep branch of the peroneal nerve* joins the anterior tibial artery as it descends the lower leg with the extensor digitorum longus muscle positioned superficially. Its direction then shifts medially, travelling along the tibia beneath the anterior tibial muscle. Upon entering the foot via the anterior tarsal canal (formed by the superior and inferior retinaculum), it terminates by bifurcating into a *medial* (sensitive) and a *lateral* (motor) *branch*. The medial branch accompanies the dorsalis pedis artery to the first web space, while the lateral branch supplies the extensor digitorum brevis muscle.

The *superficial branch of the peroneal nerve* courses within the superficial peroneus longus and the deeper located extensor digitorum longus muscles.

As it reaches the foot— immediately proximal to the extensor retinaculum, it gives rise to two sensory branches—the *medial* and *intermediate dorsal cutaneous nerves of the foot* (Fig. 3.9).

Structural lesions of the sciatic nerve may occur, especially after hip surgeries or due to fractures, spinal disc herniation, spondylodiscitis, or pregnancy.

The most common affection presents the acute excruciating sciatic pain (sciatica). This condition reflects irritation of the sciatic nerve without structural damage, often resulting from malposition, and may be accompanied by paresthesia along the nerve's distribution. Predisposing factors are primarily occupational—particularly in individuals working in ergonomically challenging positions such as truck drivers. There is no predisposition related to gender, body habitus, or genetic factors [38].

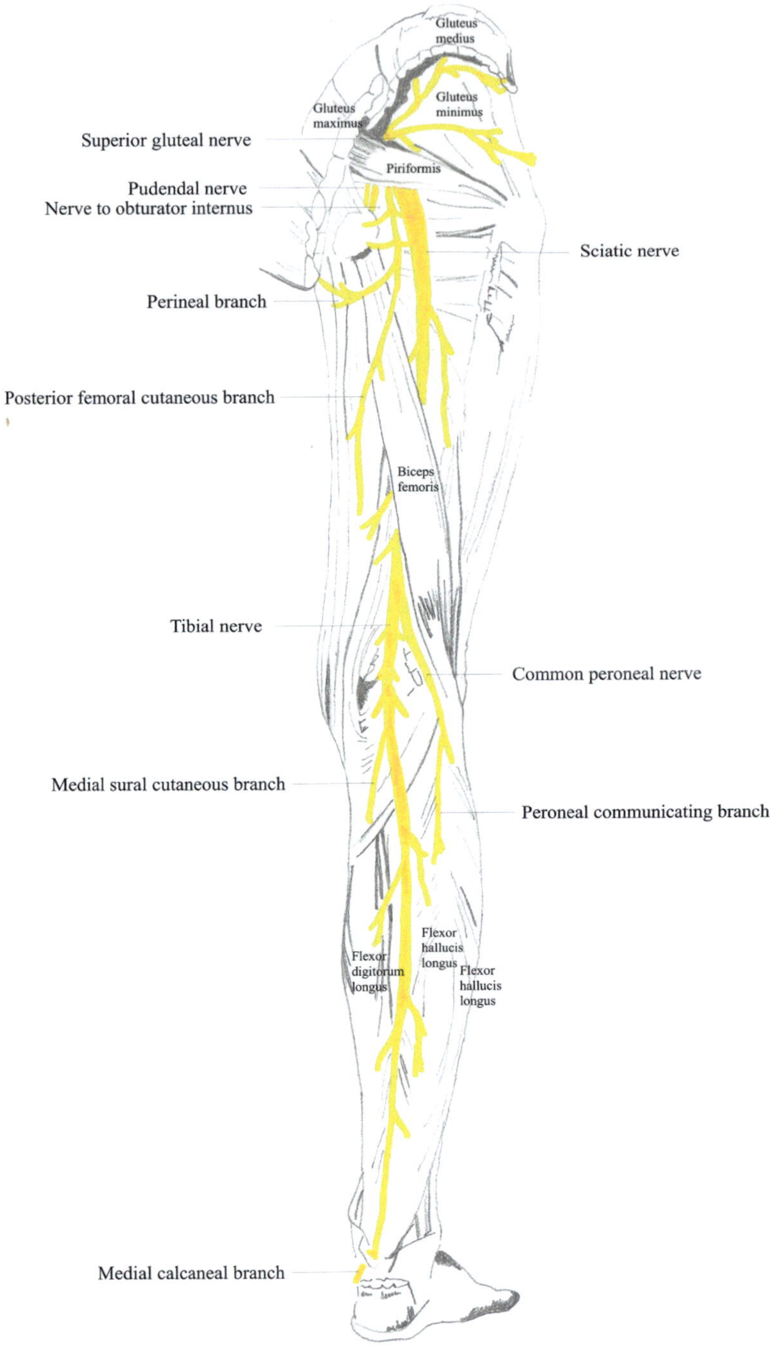

Fig. 3.9 Anatomical drawing and course of the sciatic nerve

Motor Innervation

Two large branches (one from tibial and one from common peroneal division of sciatic nerve) ➔

Hamstring muscles:

Tibial part—Semitendinous, semimembranous, long head of biceps femoris muscles

Common peroneal part—Short head of biceps femoris muscle

The two branches emerge very proximal in the pelvis and travel distal to the gluteal region.

> Lesions to these small nerves usually don't have a clinical impact as long as the two larger branches are intact.

Occasionally, the muscular branches also contribute to the innervation to the obturator internus, the gemellus superior and inferior, and the quadratus femoris muscles.

Tibial nerve ➔

Small portion of adductor magnus muscle
Popliteus muscle
Plantaris muscle
Triceps surae (gastrocnemius and soleus) muscles
Tibialis posterior muscle
Flexor digitorum longus muscle
Flexor hallucis longus muscle
Intrinsic muscles of the foot muscle

The popliteus and plantar muscles (branches are at the level of the popliteal fossa) have only little clinical significance.

Medial plantar nerve ➔

Abductor hallucis and flexor digitorum brevis muscles (S1, S2)
Flexor hallucis brevis muscle (more distally innervation)
Lumbrical muscle of the foot (L5, S1)

Lateral plantar nerve and the deep branch ➔

Intrinsic muscles (quadratus plantae, abductor digiti minimi pedis, lumbricals II–IV, dorsal interossei, both heads of the adductor hallucis).

Common peroneal nerve ➔

Short head of biceps femoris muscle.

Superficial peroneal nerve ➔

Peroneus longus and brevis muscles (L5, S1, foot eversion).

The **peroneus tertius muscle**, when present, represents a lateral extension of the extensor digitorum longus; however, it is innervated by the *superficial peroneus nerve* and contributes to extension of the lateral part of the foot.

The *accessory peroneal nerve* represents a distal branch of the superficial peroneal nerve being present in up to 35% of the population [34]. It contains motor fibers and innervates the extensor digitorum brevis muscle which is usually supplied by the deep peroneal nerve.

Deep peroneal nerve ➔

Tibialis anterior muscle (it is the main dorsiflexor of the foot)
Extensor digitorum longus muscle
Hallucis brevis muscle
Extensor hallucis longus muscle

> The deep peroneal nerve represents a relatively long motor branch, coursing along the fibular shaft, and is therefore susceptible to selective injury fractures or surgical procedures.

Lateral terminal branch of the deep peroneal nerve ➔

Extensor digitorum brevis muscle (L5–S1)

Sensory Innervation

Sural nerve ➔

Lateral aspect of lower leg, the heel and ankle, as well as the dorsolateral foot

> Due to overlapping of sensory dermatomes, injury to or resection of the sural nerve typically results sensory loss confined to the lateral aspect of the ankle.

Tibial nerve ➔

Posterolateral leg, sole of the foot

> The sole of the foot represents the most important area regarding sensation as it influences proprioception and thus walking.

Medial calcaneal nerve ➔

Medial half of the heel

Medial plantar nerves ➔

Medial sole

Lateral plantar nerves ➔

Lateral sole

Superficial and deep peroneal nerves ➔

Anterolateral leg and dorsal aspect of the foot

Lateral cutaneous nerve to the calf ➔

Lateral knee and calf

Two articular joint branches ➔

Knee joint

3.4.4 Posterior Femoral Cutaneous Nerve (S1–S3)

The purely sensitive **posterior femoral cutaneous nerve**—or **lesser sciatic nerve**—derives from the posterior division of the sacral plexus. It exits the pelvis via the greater sciatic foramen and courses between the trochanter minor and the ischial tuberosity just inferior to the gluteus maximus muscle. At this level, the *inferior cluneal nerves* (also referred to as *gluteal branches*) arise from the posterior femoral cutaneous nerve and travel medially to the inferior border of the gluteus maximus muscle, providing cutaneous innervation to the inferior gluteal region.

More inferiorly, the *perineal branches* emerge to innervate the perineum.

The remaining fascicles of the posterior femoral cutaneous nerve run toward the posterior thigh between the biceps femoris and the semitendinosus muscles, and continue their course beneath the fascia lata until they reach the popliteal fossa where its *terminal branches* end.

Lesions to this nerve are very rare.

Sensory Innervation

Inferior cluneal nerves ➔

Inferior and lateral gluteal region till the gluteal sulcus

Perineal branches ➔

Perineum and posterior parts of labia majora/scrotum

Terminal branches ➔

Dorsal aspect of thigh and the popliteal fossa

Other branches arising from the dorsal rami of spinal nerves L1–L3 are the *superior cluneal nerves,* which innervate the upper gluteal region. The *medial cluneal nerves* formed by the dorsal rami of S1–S3, provide sensory innervation to the medial aspect of the buttock.

3.4.5 Pudendal Nerve (S2–S4)

The **pudendal nerve** contains motor, sensory, and also vegetative fascicles and represents the major nerve of the pudendal plexus—a plexus, which is commonly considered as the caudal part of the lumbosacral plexus.

It may receive contributions from S1 and very rarely also from S5.

Along with the sciatic nerve, it exits the pelvis through the greater sciatic foramen, loops around the sacrospinous ligament just to re-enter the perineum via the lesser sciatic foramen, accompanied by the *nerve to the obturator internus*. It subsequently courses alongside the internal pudendal artery—one of the three pudendal arteries—within the pudendal canal (Alcock-canal) ventrally to reach the symphysis.

Within the pudendal canal, several nerves branch, the first one being the *inferior rectal nerves*, followed by the *perineal nerves* which further bifurcate into superficial (sensible) and deep (motor) branches. The superficial branches again divide into the *posterior scrotal* or the *posterior labial nerves*.

The *perineal nerve* is the largest branch of the pudendal nerve.

Representing the terminal continuation, the *dorsal penile/dorsal clitoral nerve* perforates the urogenital diaphragm and the deep transverse perineus muscle where it gives off branches to the corpus cavernosum of the penis or clitoris, where it finally ends.

The pudendal nerve plays an important role regarding the function of the pelvic floor muscles, the sphincter muscles and the function of the genitals (sexual function).

The Alcock syndrome or pudendal neuralgia represents a pain syndrome in the perineal area caused by injury to the pudendal nerve within the pudendal canal. Possible causes are injury of the perineum during birth, or by tumors in this area (e.g., rectal tumors). The pain is typically exacerbated when assuming sedentary position.

Additionally, sphincter weakness may occur leading to urinary and fecal incontinence. The sexual function can be impaired.

<u>Motor Innervation</u>

Inferior rectal nerves ➔
External anal sphincter

Deep branches of perineal nerves ➔
External urethral sphincter
Transverse perineal muscle
Bulbospongiosus muscle
Ischiocavernosus muscle

<u>Sensory Innervation</u>

Inferior rectal nerves ➔
Skin of the anal region

Posterior scrotal/labial nerves (perineal nerves) **➔**
Perineum, dorsal aspect of scrotum/labia majora

Dorsal penile/clitoridis nerves ➔
Prepuce, glans penis and corpus cavernosum penis, glans clitoridis, corpus cavernosum clitoridis

As already mentioned, multiple anatomical variations exist in the lumbosacral plexus too, especially regarding the components of the branches.

When receiving nerval contributions from T12 and only small from S3, it is considered a pre-fixed lumbosacral plexus.

Post-fixed lumbosacral plexus implies lack of T12 contribution and only small L1 but a dominant S4 spinal nerve input.

Further Reading

1. Anloague PA, Huijbregts P. Anatomical variations of the lumbar plexus: a descriptive anatomy study with proposed clinical implications. J Man Manip Ther. 2009;17(4):e107–14. https://doi.org/10.1179/106698109791352201. PMID: 20140146; PMCID: PMC2813498.
2. Harshavardhana NS, Dabke HV. The furcal nerve revisited. Orthop Rev. 2014;6(3):5428. https://doi.org/10.4081/or.2014.5428.
3. Kikuchi S, Hasue M, Nishiyama K, Ito T. Anatomic features of the furcal nerve and its clinical significance. Spine (Phila Pa 1976). 1986;11(10):1002–7. https://doi.org/10.1097/00007632-198612000-00006. PMID: 3033836.
4. Siccardi MA, Tariq MA, Valle C. Anatomy, bony pelvis and lower limb: psoas major. In: StatPearls. Treasure Island: StatPearls Publishing; 2023.
5. Anderson CN. Iliopsoas: pathology, diagnosis, and treatment. Clin Sports Med. 2016;35(3):419–33. https://doi.org/10.1016/j.csm.2016.02.009.
6. Merrighi APL, Atakiama VT, Bento de Lima FF. Occurrence of the psoas minor muscle: a literature review. Quest J. 2021;8(2):47–51. https://www.questjournals.org

7. Singh O, Al Khalili Y. Anatomy, back, lumbar plexus. In: StatPearls. Treasure Island: StatPearls Publishing; 2023.
8. Mirjalili SA. Chapter 45 - anatomy of the lumbar plexus. In: Tubbs RS, Rizk E, Shoja MM, Loukas M, Barbaro N, Spinner RJ, editors. Nerves and nerve injuries. Academic Press; 2015. p. 609–17. https://doi.org/10.1016/B978-0-12-410390-0.00047-0.
9. Tagliafico A, Bignotti B, Cadoni A, Perez MM, Martinoli C. Anatomical study of the iliohypogastric, ilioinguinal, and genitofemoral nerves using high-resolution ultrasound. Muscle Nerve. 2015;51(1):42–8. https://doi.org/10.1002/mus.24277. PMID: 24797303.
10. Klaassen Z, Marshall E, Tubbs RS, Louis RG Jr, Wartmann CT, Loukas M. Anatomy of the ilioinguinal and iliohypogastric nerves with observations of their spinal nerve contributions. Clin Anat. 2011;24(4):454–61. https://doi.org/10.1002/ca.21098. Epub 2011 Jan 3. PMID: 21509811.
11. Reinpold W, Schroeder AD, Schroeder M, Berger C, Rohr M, Wehrenberg U. Retroperitoneal anatomy of the iliohypogastric, ilioinguinal, genitofemoral, and lateral femoral cutaneous nerve: consequences for prevention and treatment of chronic inguinodynia. Hernia. 2015;19(4):539–48. https://doi.org/10.1007/s10029-015-1396-z. Epub 2015 Jun 17. PMID: 26082397.
12. Ariyasinghe C, Hacking C, Stewart M, et al. Lateral femoral cutaneous nerve. Radiopaedia.org; 2025. https://doi.org/10.53347/rID-38862.
13. Koh M, Markovich B. Anatomy, abdomen and pelvis, obturator nerve. In: StatPearls. Treasure Island: StatPearls Publishing; 2023.
14. Akkaya T, Comert A, Kendir S, Acar HI, Gumus H, Tekdemir I, Elhan A. Detailed anatomy of accessory obturator nerve blockade. Minerva Anestesiol. 2008;74(4):119–22.
15. Samani K. The femoral nerve. TeachMeAnatomy; 2025. https://teachmeanatomy.info/lower-limb/nerves/femoral-nerve/
16. Stofferin H, Pfitscher K, Hörmann R, Gmeiner R, Thaler M. The anatomical course of the femoral nerve with regard to the direct anterior approach for total hip arthroplasty. J Arthroplast. 2024;39(5):1341–7. https://doi.org/10.1016/j.arth.2023.11.028. Epub 2023 Dec 1. PMID: 38043744.
17. Refai NA, Black AC, Tadi P. Anatomy, bony pelvis and lower limb: thigh femoral nerve. In: StatPearls. Treasure Island: StatPearls Publishing; 2023.
18. Shahid S. Femoral nerve. Kenhub; 2023. https://www.kenhub.com/en/library/anatomy/femoral-nerve
19. Miniato MA, Black AC, Varacallo MA. Anatomy, back, lumbosacral trunk. 2023 Oct 12. In: StatPearls [Internet]. Treasure Island: StatPearls Publishing; 2025. PMID: 30969700.
20. Matejcík V. Anatomical variations of lumbosacral plexus. Surg Radiol Anat. 2010;32(4):409–14. https://doi.org/10.1007/s00276-009-0546-3. Epub 2009 Aug 21. PMID: 19696958.
21. Knipe H, Nithiyananthan K, MacManus D, et al. Sacral plexus. Radiopaedia.org; 2025. https://doi.org/10.53347/rID-29885.
22. Willick SE, Margherita AJ, Carter GT. Isolated superior gluteal nerve injury: two case reports. Muscle Nerve. 1998;21(7):951–3. https://doi.org/10.1002/(sici)1097-4598(199807)21:7<951::aid-mus17>3.0.co;2-t. PMID: 9626259.
23. Tempski J, Kotlarek A, Pękala J, Fibiger G, Krager E, Łazarz D, Rosa M, Glądys K, Walocha JA, Pękala P. Variability and clinical anatomy of the superior gluteal nerve-a systematic review and meta-analysis. J Anat. 2025;246(4):467–78. https://doi.org/10.1111/joa.14174.
24. Pinho AR, Leite MJ, Lixa J, Silva MR, Vieira P, Nery-Monterroso J, Bezerra MC, Alves H, Madeira MD, Pereira PA. Superior gluteal Nerve anatomy and its injuries: aiming for a more secure surgical approach of the pelvic region. Diagnostics. 2023;13(14):2314. https://doi.org/10.3390/diagnostics13142314.
25. Mahadevan V. Pelvic girdle and lower limb. In: Standring S, editor. Gray's anatomy: the anatomical basis of clinical practice. 40th ed. Elsevier; 2008. p. 1327–429.
26. Apaydin N. Chapter 47 - variations of the lumbar and sacral plexuses and their branches. In: Tubbs RS, Rizk E, Shoja MM, Loukas M, Barbaro N, Spinner RJ, editors. Nerves and nerve injuries. San Diego: Academic Press; 2015.
27. Giuffre BA, Black AC, Anatomy JR. Sciatic Nerve. 2023 Nov 16. In: StatPearls [Internet]. Treasure Island: StatPearls Publishing; 2024. PMID: 29494038.
28. Adibatti M, Sangeetha V. Study on variant anatomy of sciatic nerve. J Clin Diagn Res. 2014;8(8):AC07–9. https://doi.org/10.7860/JCDR/2014/9116.4725.
29. Tomaszewski KA, Graves MJ, Henry BM, Popieluszko P, Roy J, Pękala PA, Hsieh WC, Vikse J, Walocha JA. Surgical anatomy of the sciatic nerve: a meta-analysis. J Orthop Res. 2016;34(10):1820–7. https://doi.org/10.1002/jor.23186.
30. Kirschner JS, Foye PM, Cole JL. Piriformis syndrome, diagnosis and treatment. Muscle Nerve. 2009;40(1):10–8. https://doi.org/10.1002/mus.21318.
31. Desai SS, Cohen-Levy WB. Anatomy, bony pelvis and lower limb: tibial nerve. In: StatPearls. Treasure Island: StatPearls Publishing; 2023.
32. Knipe H, Campos A, Yu Y, et al. Tibial nerve. Radiopaedia.org; 2025. https://doi.org/10.53347/rID-24724.
33. Ryan W, Mahony N, Delaney M, O'Brien M, Murray P. Relationship of the common peroneal nerve and its branches to the head and neck of the fibula. Clin Anat. 2003;16(6):501–5. https://doi.org/10.1002/ca.10155.
34. Tzika M, Paraskevas GK, Kitsoulis P. The accessory deep peroneal nerve: a review of the literature. Foot (Edinb). 2012;22(3):232–4. https://doi.org/10.1016/j.foot.2012.05.003.
35. Hardin JM, Devendra S. Anatomy, bony pelvis and lower limb: calf common peroneal Nerve (com-

mon fibular nerve). In: StatPearls. Treasure Island: StatPearls Publishing; 2022.
36. Van den Bergh FR, Vanhoenacker FM, De Smet E, Huysse W, Verstraete KL. Peroneal nerve: Normal anatomy and pathologic findings on routine MRI of the knee. Insights Imaging. 2013;4(3):287–99. https://doi.org/10.1007/s13244-013-0255-7.
37. Davis D, Taqi M, Vasudevan A. Sciatica. In: StatPearls. Treasure Island: StatPearls Publishing; 2024.
38. Hicks BL, Lam JC, Varacallo MA. Piriformis syndrome. In: StatPearls. Treasure Island: StatPearls Publishing; 2023.
39. Jiamjunyasiri A, Tsutsumi M, Muro S, Akita K. Origin, course, and distribution of the posterior femoral cutaneous nerve and the spatial relationship among its branches. Anat Sci Int. 2023;98(4):540–7. https://doi.org/10.1007/s12565-023-00721-x.
40. Kinter KJ, Newton BW. Anatomy, abdomen and pelvis, pudendal nerve. In: StatPearls. Treasure Island: StatPearls Publishing; 2023.
41. Schraffordt SE, Tjandra JJ, Eizenberg N, Dwyer PL. Anatomy of the pudendal nerve and its terminal branches: a cadaver study. ANZ J Surg. 2004;74(1–2):23–6. https://doi.org/10.1046/j.1445-1433.2003.02885.x.
42. Juenemann KP, Lue TF, Schmidt RA, Tanagho EA. Clinical significance of sacral and pudendal nerve anatomy. J Urol. 1988;139(1):74–80. https://doi.org/10.1016/s0022-5347(17)42297-x.
43. Amarenco G, Lanoe Y, Ghnassia RT, Goudal H, Perrigot M. Syndrome du canal d'Alcock et névralgie périnéale [Alcock's canal syndrome and perineal neuralgia]. Rev Neurol. 1988;144(8–9):523–6.
44. Kaur J, Leslie SW, Singh P. Pudendal nerve entrapment syndrome. In: StatPearls. Treasure Island: StatPearls Publishing; 2023.

Clinical Examination

4

*This comprehensive clinical examination guide outlines the assessment of neuromuscular and neurological function with focus on segmental innervation and motor deficits. It includes dermatome-based sensibility testing, muscle atrophy identification, and observation of vegetative and trophic changes. Special emphasis is placed on the back and shoulder girdle, highlighting conditions such as scapula alata and dropped shoulder, including their neural correlates (*e.g.*, long thoracic, spinal accessory, and dorsal scapular nerves). Detailed motor testing procedures for upper and lower limb muscles are provided, including specific tests for the integrity of the nerves. Functional assessments in various patient positions (standing, prone, supine, sitting) are included to evaluate gait abnormalities (*e.g.*, Trendelenburg sign, foot drop) and muscle strength. This guide serves as a practical framework for localized neurological diagnostics in a clinical setting.*

4.1 Upper Extremity

4.1.1 Accessory Nerve (C2, C3, C4)

Trapezius Muscle

Origin: Superior nuchal line, occipital protruberance, and cervical processi spinosi

Insertion: Clavicula, acromium, and scapular spine

Function: Stabilizing the scapula is the main function

Descending/superior fibers ➔
Elevation and upward rotation of the shoulder, extension of the neck

Transverse/middle fibers ➔
Shoulder retraction (together with the rhomboid muscles), upward rotation of the scapular (together with the serratus anterior muscle). This allows raising the arm beyond shoulder level

Ascending/inferior fibers ➔
Lowering of the shoulder by depressing the scapula

Clinical examination: Elevating the shoulder against resistance. When crossing the hand at the back, the trapezius can be seen nicely

Injury: Dropped shoulder, lateralized scapula, inability to lift the arm above the horizontal line

Sternocleidomastoid Muscle

Origin: Manubrium of the sternum and clavicle

Insertion: Mastoid process of the temporal bone

Function: Lateral rotation of the head

Clinical examination: Rotation of the head against resistance (Fig. 4.1)

> Weakness of the trapezius muscle but a functioning sternocleidomastoid would suggest a distal lesion of the accessory nerve, e.g. in the posterior triangle of the neck

K. Hobitsch, *Peripheral Nerve Surgery - A Compendium*,
https://doi.org/10.1007/978-3-032-03409-0_4

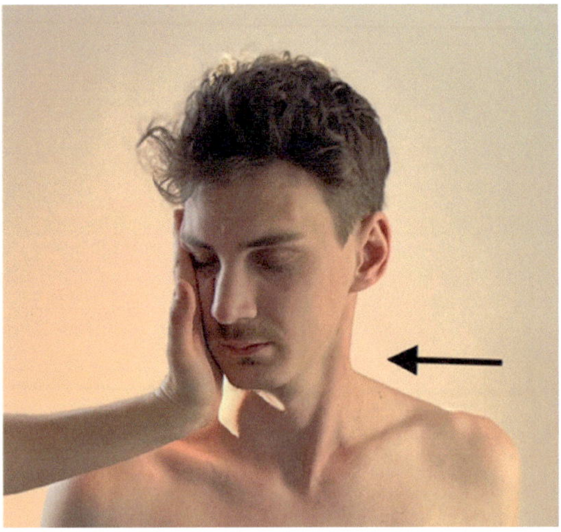

Fig. 4.1 Contraction of the sternocleidomastoid muscle can be seen while rotating the head against resistance (arrow)

4.1.2 Dorsal Scapular Nerve (C5)

Rhomboid Muscles (Rhomboid Major and Minor)

Origin: Spinal processes of vertebral body T1/2–T4/5

Insertion: Medial edge of the scapular spine

Function: Cranial and medial contraction as well as stabilization of the scapula

Clinical examination: With the palm of the hand on the lower back (thereby relaxing the trapezius), instruct the patient to push the hand against the examiner's hand while palpating the rhomboids between the scapula (Fig. 4.2)

Injury: Weakness of this muscle may suspect a proximal lesion (root avulsion) as this muscle is located close to the spine

Levator Scapulae Muscle

Origin: Transversal processes of C1–C4

Insertion: Scapular spine

Innervation: Lateral branch of the cervical plexus

Function: Cranio-medial elevation and/or retraction of the scapula

Clinical examination: Same as for the rhomboids

Injury: Lesion of the dorsal scapular nerve clinically presents with a scapula alata

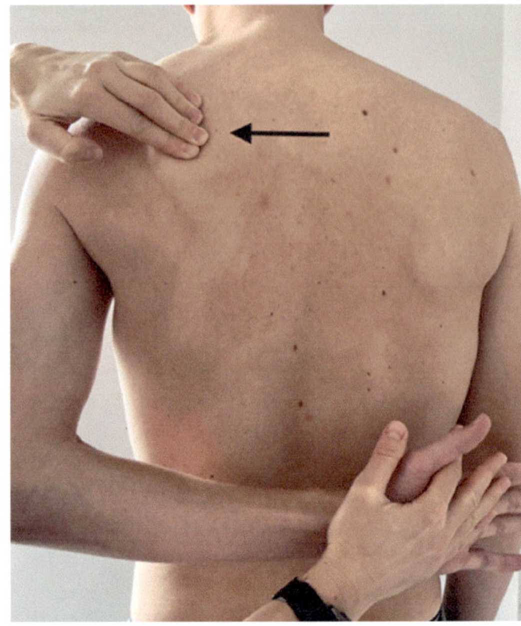

Fig. 4.2 Clinical examination of the rhomboids: Ask the patient to push away the hand away from the back against resistance. The rhomboids can be palpated at the medial border of the scapula (arrow)

4.1.3 Suprascapular Nerve (C5, C6)

Supraspinatus Muscle

Origin: Supraspinous fossa

Insertion: Greater tubercle of the humerus and the shoulder capsule

Function: Abduction (initial 20–30°) and external rotation of the upper arm (together with the deltoid muscle); it is part of the rotator cuff

Clinical examination: Abduction of the arm against resistance while palpating the supraspinatus fossa

Jobe test: Ask the patient to lift the arm to 90° with a 30° abduction and the thumb facing down (pronation). Internal rotation of the arm will minimize the effect of the deltoid muscle. If pain occurs while pressing the arm down, the test is considered being positive (Fig. 4.3)

Injury: The most common lesion of the supraspinatus muscle is the impingement syndrome which is typically caused by degenerative changes of the tendon

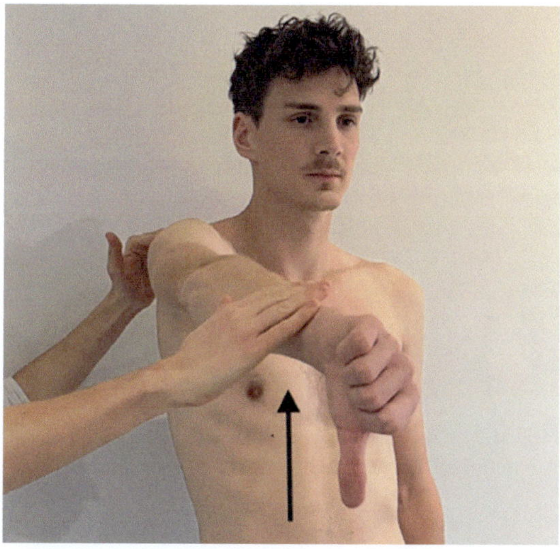

Fig. 4.3 Clinical examination of the supraspinatus muscle: Palpating the supraspinatus fossa while the patient resists downward pressure of the arm

Infraspinatus Muscle

This muscle receives accessory innervation by the axillary nerve (C4–C6)

Origin: Infraspinous fossa

Insertion: Greater tubercle of the humerus and the shoulder capsule

Function: Mainly external rotation (together with supraspinatus and deltoideus), weak abduction

Clinical examination: External rotation of the arm against resistance with the elbow flexed at 90° (Fig. 4.4)

Lesions of the suprascapular nerve are most commonly caused by trauma, such as scapular fracture or sudden shoulder disruption and typically trigger acute clinical signs. Gradual onset of symptoms may indicate nerve compression or the presence of cystic lesions. If severe pain is present, acute brachial neuritis should be considered.

> Preserved shoulder abduction in the absence of retroposition or anteflexion suggests an **injury of the deltoid muscle**, as abduction may still be possible through the action of the supraspinatus muscle.

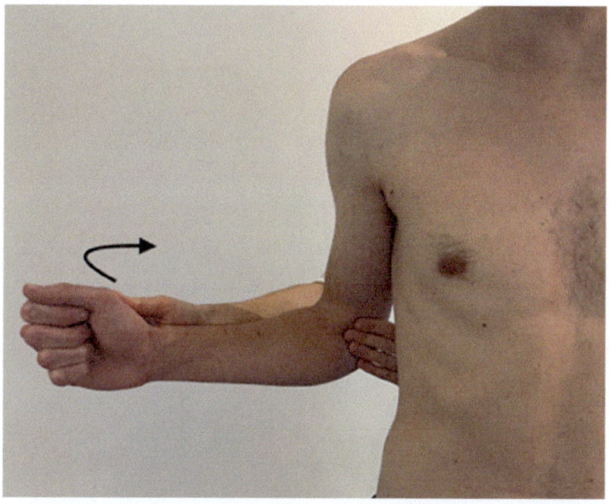

Fig. 4.4 External rotation of the 90° flexed arm (arrow) against resistance to examine the infraspinatus muscle

> External rotation with elbow flexion at 90°:
> Infraspinatus muscle (suprascapularis nerve)
> Teres minor muscle (axillary nerve)

4.1.4 Subscapular Nerve (C5, C6)

Subscapular Muscle

Origin: Subscapular fossa

Insertion: Lesser tubercle of the humerus

Function: Internal rotation of the arm and, when the arm is elevated, it also mediates adduction movement.

It is part of the rotator cuff

Clinical examination:

Lift-off test—The patients's dorsal side of the hand should be placed at the lower back, then ask the patient to push the hands away against resistance (Fig. 4.5)

Belly-press test—Put your hand in front of the patient's abdomen and ask to press against your hand with the elbow being flexed (Fig. 4.6)

Teres Major Muscle

The teres major muscle may also receive additional innervation from the thoracodorsal nerve (rare) and the axillary nerve

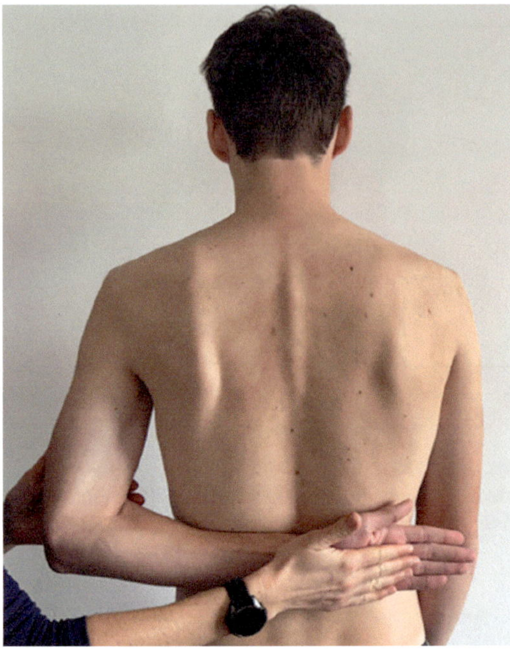

Fig. 4.5 Lift-off test: Contraction of the subscapular muscle while pushing the hand away against resistance

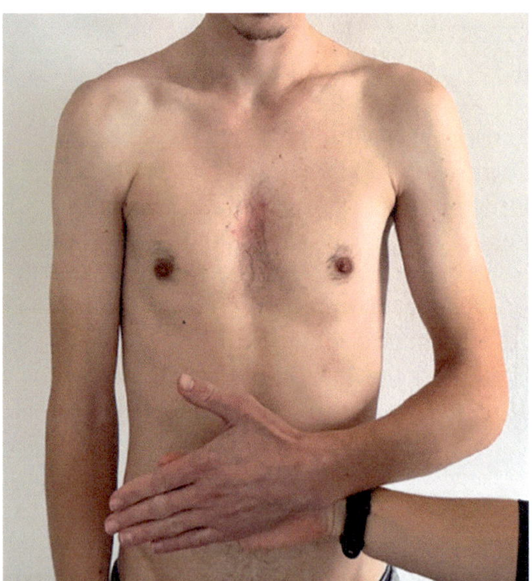

Fig. 4.6 Belly-press test: The ability to press the arm towards the abdomen without flexion of the wrist suggests a negative test as internal rotation is possible

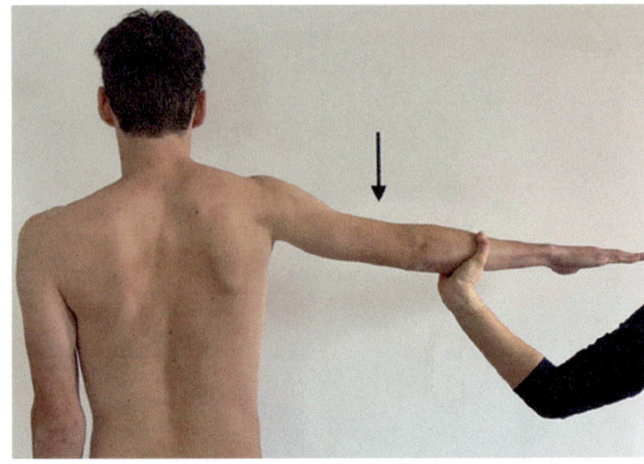

Fig. 4.7 Clinical examination of the teres major: Adduction of the elevated arm against resistance (arrow)

Origin: Inferior angle of the scapula
Insertion: Tubercular crest of the humerus
Function: Internal rotation, extension of the arm from a flexed position, adduction
Clinical examination: Let the patient adduct the elevated upper arm against resistance. The muscle belly of the teres major can be palpated (Fig. 4.7)

> **Shoulder adduction (C5, T1)**: Pectoralis major muscle (pectoral nerve)
> Latissimus dorsi muscle (thoracodorsalis nerve)
> Teres major muscle (thoracodorsalis nerve)

4.1.5 Long Thoracic Nerve (C5–C7)

Serratus Anterior Muscle

Origin: Ribs I–VIII
Insertion: Medial side of the scapula
Function: Shoulder elevation (superior part), ventral traction of the shoulder (intermediate part), and elevation of the arm (inferior part). It also acts as an accessory respiratory muscle

It forms the medial border of the axillary triangle

Clinical examination: Palpating the ribs while the arm is pushed forward (like boxing). Make sure, the shoulder girdle is placed in a forward position (Fig. 4.8)

Injury: Elevation of the arm is not possible. The Patient presents with scapula alata

MNEMONIC for innervation:

SALT (Serratus Anterior ➔ Long Thoracic nerve)

Associated nerve roots: "C5, 6, 7—raise your hands to heaven"

Scapular winging may result from weakness of the serratus anterior, rhomboid or trapezius muscles!

4.1.6 Thoracodorsal Nerve (C6–C8)

Latissimus Dorsi Muscle

Origin: T7–L5, ribs IX–XII, sacrum, and ilium

Insertion: Medial side of the humeral head

Function: Adduction and internal rotation of the arm; involved in coughing and represents an accessory respiratory muscle.

It acts as an antagonist of the deltoid muscle

Clinical examination: With the arm 90° flexed, ask the patient to adduct the arm against resistance while palpating the lower part of the scapula (Fig. 4.9)

Injury: Isolated lesions of the thoracodorsal nerve are rare, and resulting weakness can often be compensated by the other muscles. More commonly, paralysis of this nerve occurs in the context of a brachial plexus injury

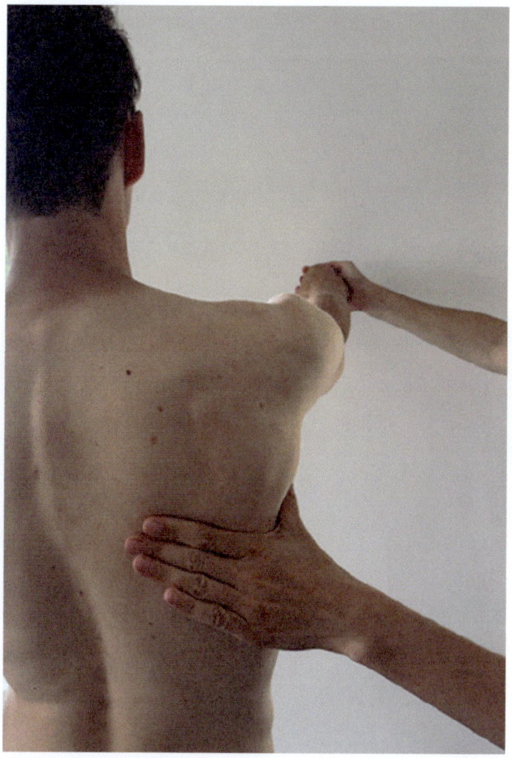

Fig. 4.8 Palpating the serratus anterior at the ribs while the patient pushes his/her arm in a forward direction

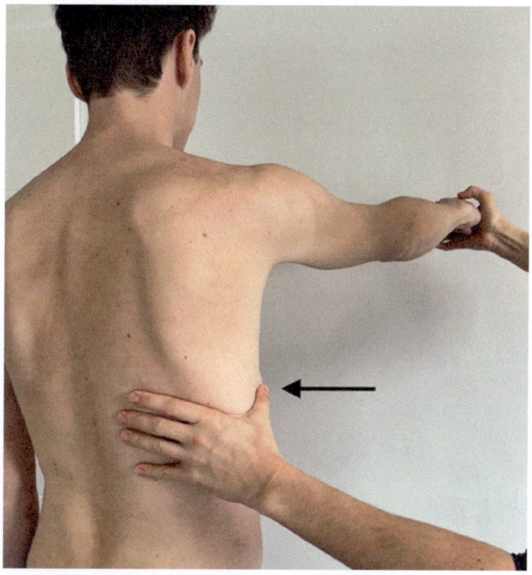

Fig. 4.9 Palpating the latissimus dorsi muscle at the lower border of the scapula (arrow) while putting resistance to the forearm into abduction and flexion movement

4.1.7 Medial (C8–Th1) and Lateral (C5–C7) Pectoral Nerves

Pectoralis Major Muscle

Origin: Clavicula (clavicular part), sternum (sternocostal part), and aponeurosis (abdominal part)

Insertion: Crest of the greater tubercle of the humerus

Function: Adduction and internal rotation of the arm at the shoulder joint. Additonally, it functions as a strong accessory inspiratory muscle, together with the pectoralis minor

Clinical examination: With the patient in supine position, ask to abduct the arm to 90° (at shoulder level), then apply a downward force to the arm (Fig. 4.10)

Pectoralis Minor Muscle

Origin: Ribs III–V

Insertion: Coracoid process of the scapula

It is located directly beneath the pectoral major muscle

Function: Antero-lateral movement but also medial rotation of the scapula

Clinical examination: With the patient in a relaxed supine position, place the heels of your hands on the coracoid process of the shoulders (Fig. 4.11). Pain elicited during the application of downward force may indicate tightness or shortening of the pectoralis minor muscle

4.1.8 Axillary Nerve (C5–C6)

Deltoid Muscle

Origin: Lateral third of the clavicle (clavicular part), acromium of the scapula (acromial part), lateral third of the scapular spine (spinal part)

Insertion: Deltoid tuberosity of the humerus

Function: Mainly abduction, but also anteversion, retroversion, internal and external rotation of the arm

Clinical examination: (Fig. 4.12)

Lateral part ➔ Shoulder abduction (from 15°)

Medial part ➔ Abduction and simultaneous retroposition of the shoulder

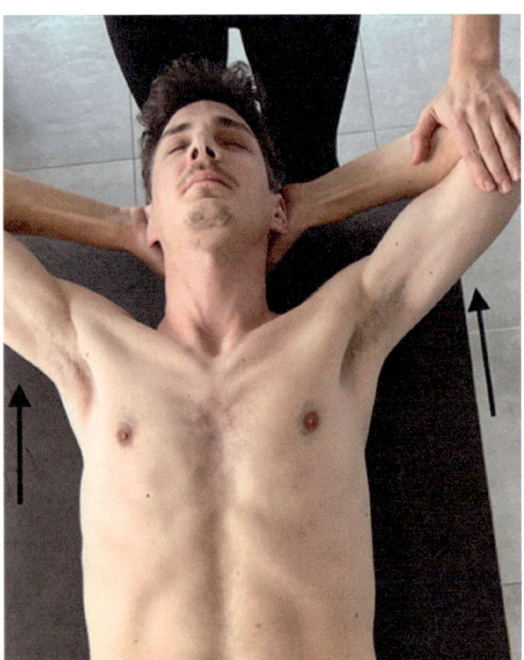

Fig. 4.10 Abduction of the arm against resistance (arrow) shows contraction of the pectoral major muscle

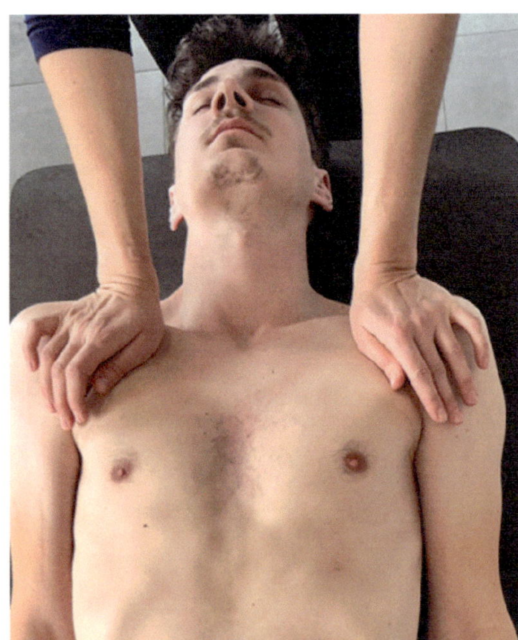

Fig. 4.11 Pain elicited when depressing the shoulders at the level coracoid process may indicate injury to the pectoralis minor muscle

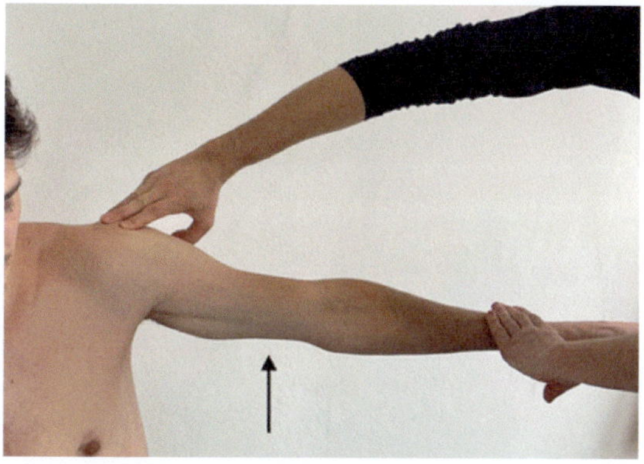

Fig. 4.12 Palpate the deltoid muscle while asking the patient to abduct the arm against resistance (arrow)

Anterior part ➔ Abduction with forward flexion of the shoulder

Injury:

Inability to abduct the arm through the initial 15° from the resting position suggests injury to the suprascapular nerve, indicating dysfunction of the supraspinatus muscle

Fractures of the humeral head or surgical procedures in this region are common causes of axillary nerve lesions

Teres Minor Muscle

Origin: Lateral edge of the scapula

Insertion: Greater tubercle of the humerus

Function: External rotation and adduction of the arm; it is part of the rotator cuff

Clinical examination: With the arm abducted in the scapular plane and the elbow flexed to 90°, instruct the patient to perform external rotation against resistance. Inability to achieve external rotation in this position constitutes a positive test (Hornblower's sign) (Fig. 4.13)

4.1.9 Musculocutaneus Nerve (C5–C7)

Biceps Brachii Muscle

Origin: Supraglenoid tubercle and coracoid process of the scapula

Insertion: Radial tuberosity

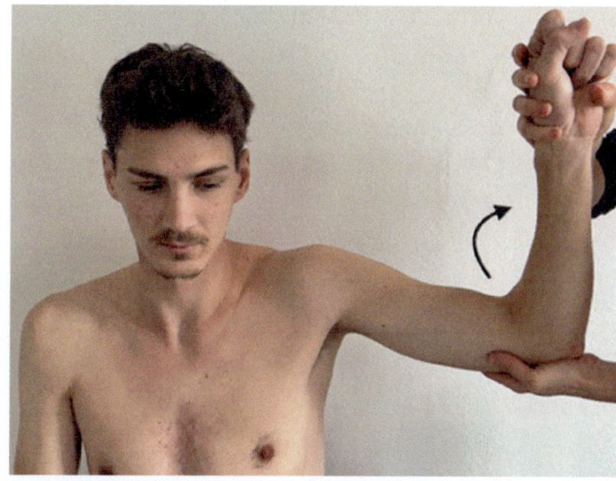

Fig. 4.13 Hornblower's sign: If external rotation of the abducted and flexed arm against resistance (arrow) is not possible, the test is considered to be positive suggesting injury of the teres minor

It is covered by the deltoid muscle

Approximately 10% of the population possesses a third head of the biceps muscle

Function: It serves as the most powerful supinator of the forearm when elbow is flexed, whereas the supinator muscle predominates during forearm extension. Additionally, it contributes to flexion of the forearm

Clinical examination: Instruct the patient to perform forearm flexion fully supinated, in order to minimize contribution of the brachioradialis (Fig. 4.14)

Brachial Muscle

Origin: Distal humerus

Insertion: Tuberosity of the ulna bone

Innervation: It may receive minor innervation from the radial nerve, likely limited to proprioception

Function: Strongest flexor of the forearm during pronation and supination

Clinical examination: Flexion of the elbow joint with the forearm being partially pronated (Fig. 4.15)

Coracobrachialis Muscle

Origin: Coracoid process

Insertion: Humeral shaft

Function: Stabilization of the humeral head, flexion, and adduction of the arm at the shoulder joint

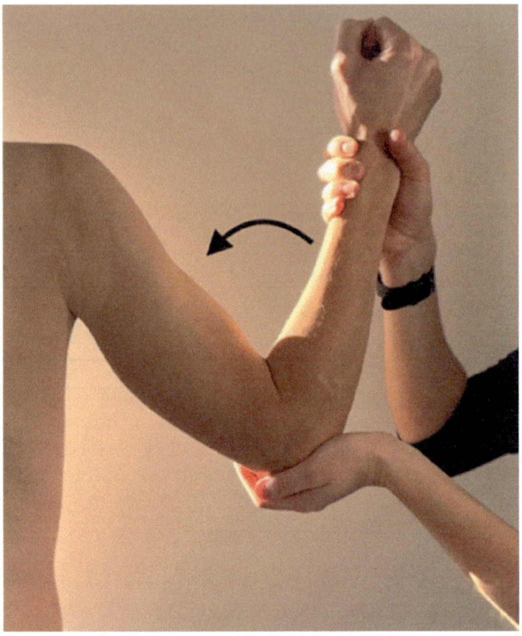

Fig. 4.14 Elbow flexion of the supinated arm against resistance (arrow) to examine biceps muscle function

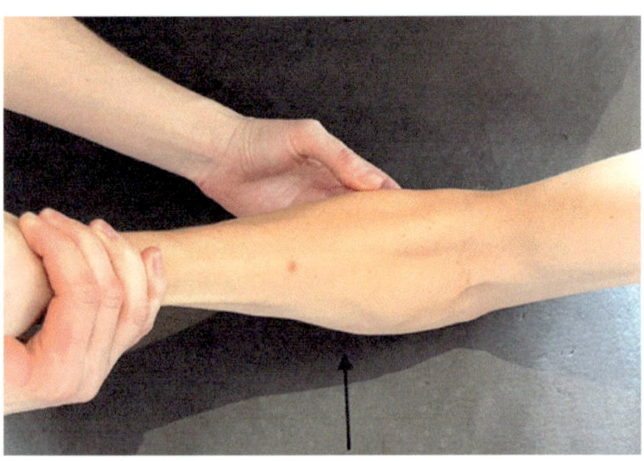

Fig. 4.15 Elbow flexion (arrow) of the partially pronated arm will reveal contraction of the brachial muscle at the lateral aspect of the proximal forearm

<u>Clinical examination</u>: By bringing the medial side of the elbow toward the eye and palpating the medial aspect of the distal upper arm—the coracobrachialis muscle can be identified deep to the biceps muscle (Fig. 4.16)

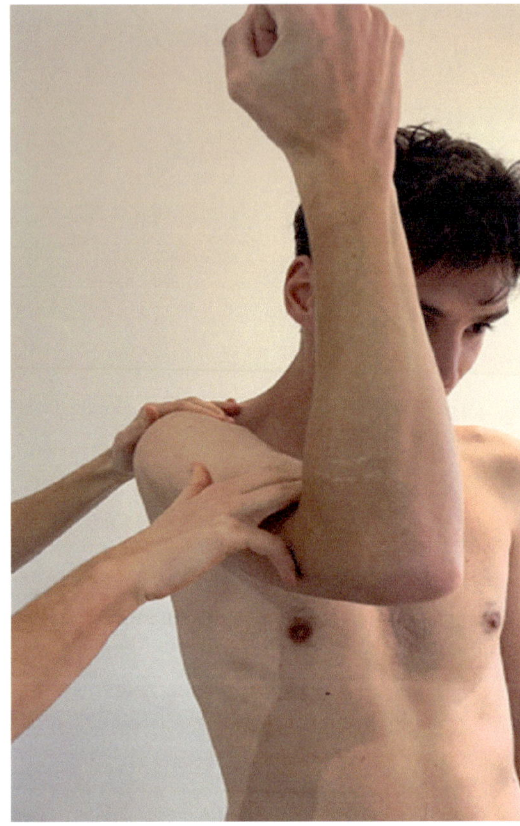

Fig. 4.16 With the elbows flexed, instruct the patient to adduct the arms at the shoulder. Pronation of the forearm during this maneuver minimizes the contribution of the biceps brachii muscle

Elbow flexion (C5–C7):
Biceps muscle (musculocutaneus nerve)
Brachial muscle (musculocutaneus and radial nerve)

Brachioradialis muscle (radial nerve): Elbow flexion with the arm pronated

Elbow extension (C5–T1):
Triceps muscle (radial nerve)

4.1.10 Median Nerve (C6–C7)

Pronator Teres Muscle

Origin: Medial epicondyle of the humerus and coracoid process of the ulnar bone

Insertion: Medial third of the radial bone

Function: Pronation and flexion of the forearm

Clinical examination: Pronation of the elbow with the forearm being extended (Fig. 4.17)

Flexor Carpi Radialis Muscle

Origin: Medial epicondyle of the humerus

Insertion: Metacarpal bones II & III

Function: Palmar flexion and abduction of the wrist, serving as the strongest wrist flexor. With the forearm extended, it also assists in pronation

Clinical examination: Flexion of the wrist toward the anterior forearm against resistance (Fig. 4.18)

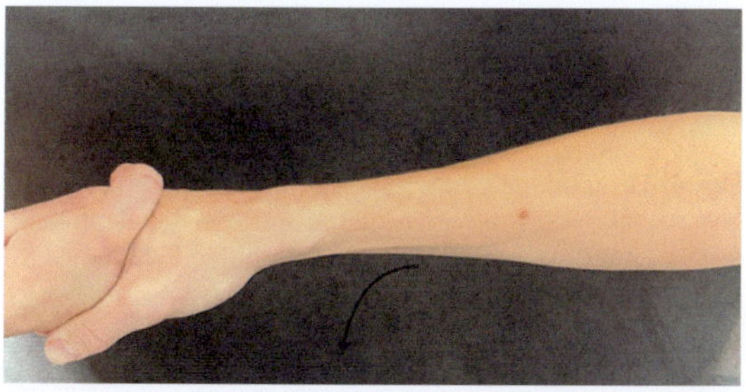

Fig. 4.17 Clinical examination of the pronator teres: Pronation of the arm against resistance (arrow)

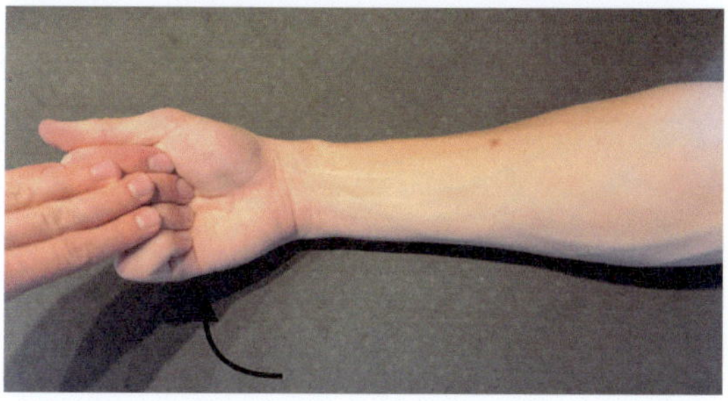

Fig. 4.18 The flexor carpi radialis can be assessed by asking the patient to perform palmar flexion of the hand against resistance (arrow)

Flexor Digitorum Superficialis Muscle

Origin:

Humeroulnar head: Medial epicondyle of the humerus and coracoid process of the ulna

Radial head: Proximal anterior border of the radius

Insertion: Medial phalanges II–V

The tendon of the flexor digitorum superficialis muscle runs beneath the transverse carpal ligament

Function: Flexion of the wrist and digits II–I. It promotes flexion of the proximal interphalangeal joint (IP)

Clinical examination: Test flexion of each finger at the metacarpophalangeal joint (MCP) with the other hand placed on the remaining fingers which are extended (Fig. 4.19)

Palmaris Longus Muscle

Cannot be tested

It is absent in approximately 15% of the population

Flexor Digitorum Profundus Muscle

Origin: Ulnar bone and interosseus membrane of the forearm

Insertion: Distal phalanges II–V

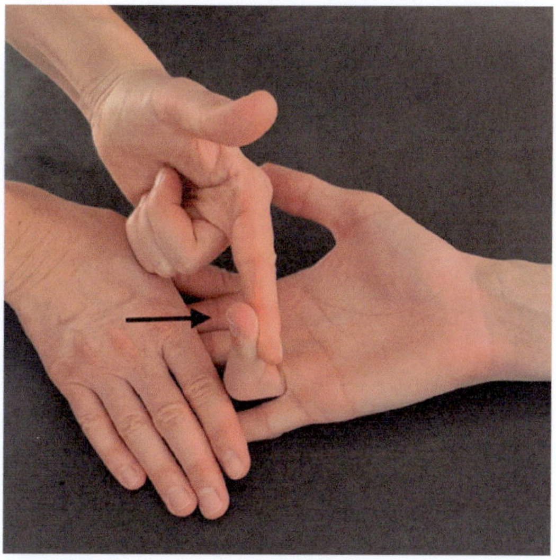

Fig. 4.19 Assess flexion of each the finger at the MCP (arrow) while stabilizing the remaining extended fingers against resistance to test the flexor digitorum superficialis muscle

The tendon of the flexor digitorum profundus muscle passes deep to the transverse carpal ligament

Function: Flexion of digits II–V at the distal interphalangeal joints

Digits II + III are innervated by the anterior interosseus branch of the median nerve

Digits III–V are innervated by the ulnar nerve

Clinical examination: To assess the flexor digitorum profundus, stabilize the metacarpophalangeal and proximal phalangeal joints of the index finger with one hand, and instruct the patient to flex the distal interphalangeal joint (DIP) against resistance (Fig. 4.20)

Flexor Pollicis Longus Muscle

Origin: Radius

Insertion: Distal phalanx I (muscle fibers course deep to the flexor retinaculum)

In approximately 40% of the population, an additional humeral head is present, inserting at the medial epicondyle. This variant is innervated by the anterior interosseus branch of the median nerve

Function: The flexor pollicis longus has a function similar to that of the flexor digitorum profundus muscle, but specific to the thumb. It facilitates flexion of the distal phalanx and contributes to thumb opposition

Clinical examination: Immobilization of the proximal joint and flexion of the distal phalanx of the thumb (Figs. 4.21 and 4.22)

A rapid method to assess function of the flexor digitorum profundus and the flexor pollicis longus muscles is to have the patient form the "**OK-sign**" by bringing the tips of the thumb and the index finger together.

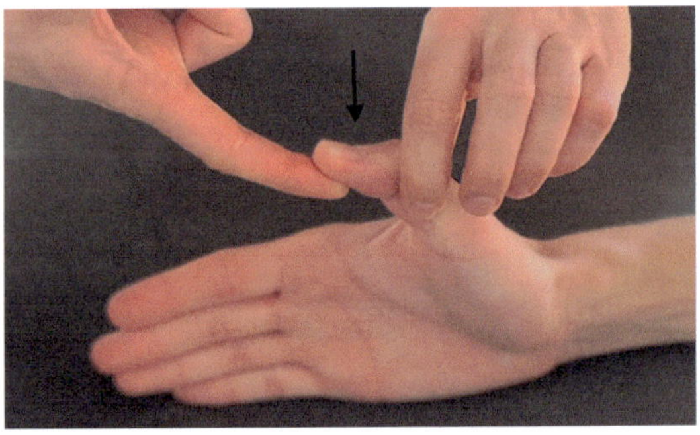

Fig. 4.21 Clinical examination of the flexor pollicis longus muscle: Flexion of the thumb at the distal phalanx (arrow) with the proximal joint immobilized

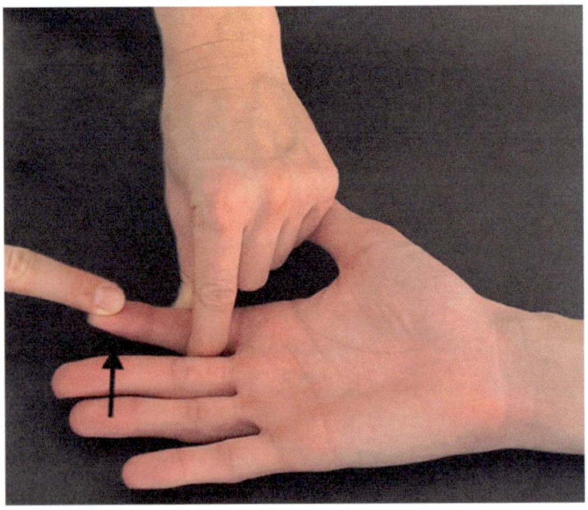

Fig. 4.20 Clinical examination of the flexor digitorum profundus muscle: Flexion of the finger at the DIP (arrow) with the MCP being immobilized

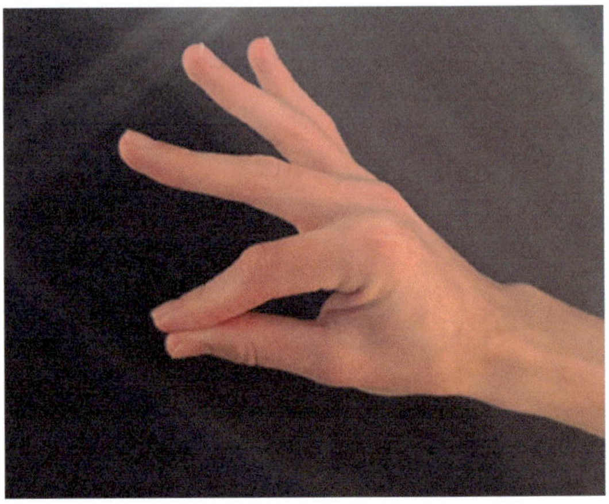

Fig. 4.22 OK-sign: Instruct the patient to put together the thumb and index finger, to assess function of the flexor digitorum profundus and the pollicis longus muscles

Abductor Pollicis Brevis Muscle

Origin: Trapezium bone and scaphoid bone as well as from the flexor retinaculum

Insertion: Proximal phalanx of the thumb

Function: Abduction of the thumb at the carpometacarpal joint away from the plane of the palm

Clinical examination: Abduction of the thumb perpendicular to the hand against resistance (Fig. 4.23)

Flexor Pollicis Brevis Muscle

Origin: Flexor retinaculum and trapezium bone

Insertion: Proximal phalanx of the thumb

The deep head of the flexor pollicis brevis muscle is innervated by the ulnar nerve, not by the median nerve.

Function: Flexion and opposition of the thumb in the metacarpophalangeal joint and flexion at the saddle joint

Clinical examination: Stabilize the distal phalanx of the thumb while instructing the patient to flex at the metacarpophalangeal joint (MCP) (Fig. 4.24)

Opponens Pollicis Muscle

Origin: Flexor retinaculum and trapezium bone

Insertion: Metacarpal bone of the thumb

This muscle is located deep to the abductor pollicis brevis muscle.

Function: Opposition of the thumb; it provides additional support to thumb adduction

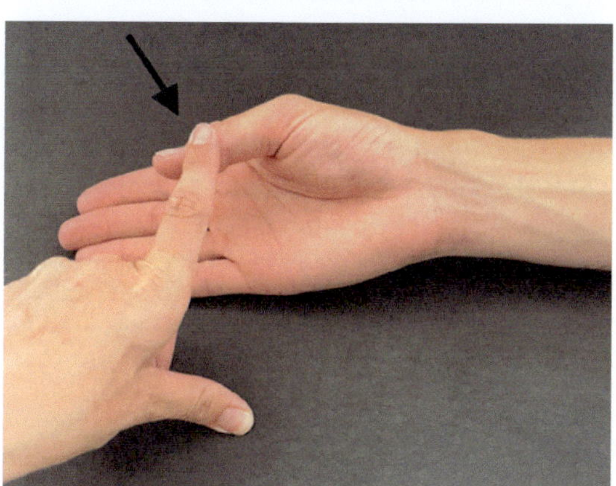

Fig. 4.23 Abduction of the thumb (arrow) perpendicular to the hand against resistance to assess function of the abductor pollicis brevis muscle

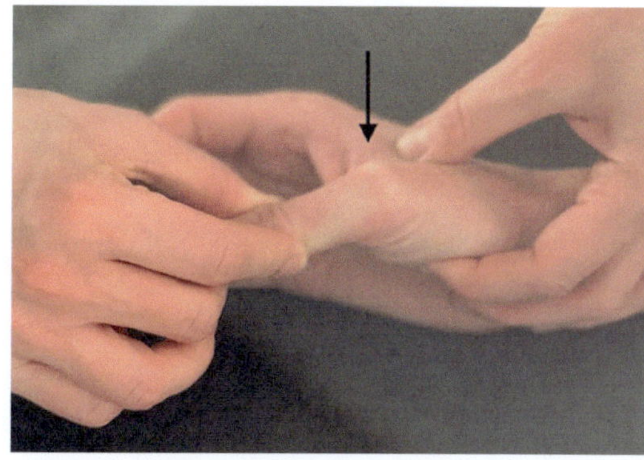

Fig. 4.24 Flexion of the thumb at the MCP (arrow) while the distal joint is immobilized to examine the flexor pollicis brevis muscle

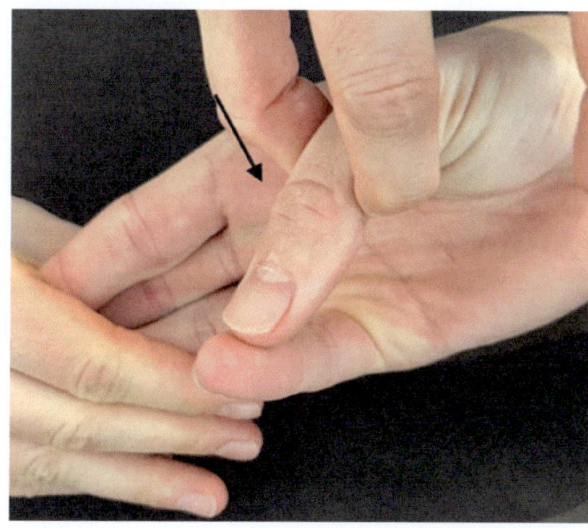

Fig. 4.25 Clinical examination of the opponens pollicis muscle: Trying to separate the thumb from the little finger (arrow) while the patient is putting maintains opposition of the two digits

Clinical examination: Instruct the patient to bring the thumb into contact with the fifth digit. Then attempt to separate the thumb from the little finger by applying opposing force (Fig. 4.25)

Opposition of the thumb is primarily mediated by the median nerve. However, in cases of median nerve injury, the ulnar nerve may mimic this movement through the action of the adductor pollicis (thumb adduction) and the flexor pollicis brevis (thumb flexion).

Lumbrical Muscles

Origin: Fibers of the flexor digitorum profundus muscle

Insertion: Metacarpophalangeal joints of digits II–V

Function: Flexion at the metacarpophalangeal joints and extension at the interphalangeal joints (gripping movements)

Innervation:

Lumbrical muscles II + III ➔ Median nerve

Lumbrical muscles IV + V ➔ Ulnar nerve

Clinical examination: Flexion of the fingers at the metacarpophalangeal joints while maintaining extension of the interphalangeal joints (Fig. 4.26)

4.1.11 Ulnar Nerve (C8–Th1)

Flexor Carpi Ulnaris Muscle

Origin: Medial epicondyle of the humerus, olecranon, and the posterior border of the ulnar bone

Insertion: Pisiforme and hamate bone, metacarpal bone V

Function: Ulnar flexion. The muscle stabilizes the pisiform bone, thereby enabling effective function of the abductor digiti minimi muscle

Clinical examination: Ulnar flexion of the wrist against resistance (Fig. 4.27)

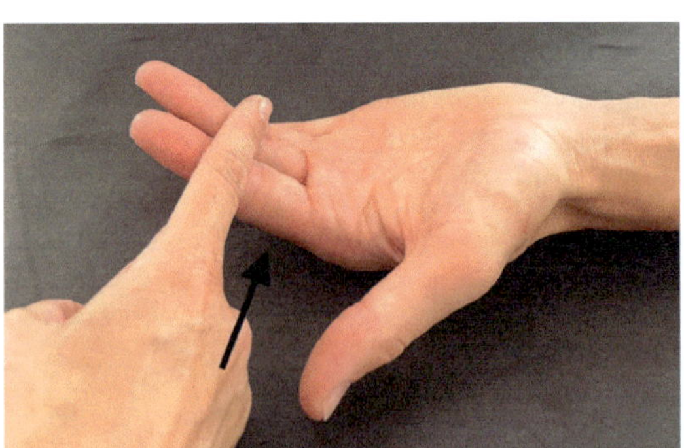

Fig. 4.26 Clinical examination of the median nerve innervated lumbricals (Dig. II + III): Flexion of the MCP joints (arrow) with the interphalangeal joints being extended

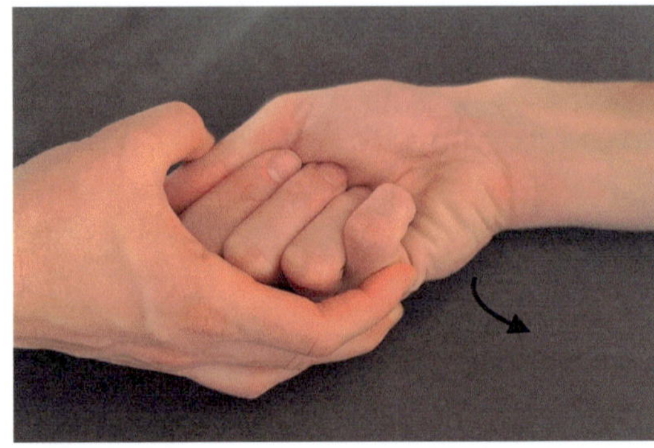

Fig. 4.27 Function of the flexor carpi ulnaris is assessed by testing ulnar flexion of the wrist against resistance (arrow)

Flexor Digitorum Profundus Muscle

Origin: Proximal anterior surface of the ulnar bone

Insertion: Distal phalanges of digits II–V

Innervation:

Digits II + III ➔ Anterior interosseus nerve of the median nerve

Digits IV + V ➔ Ulnar nerve

Function: Flexion of digits IV + V – it represents the most important flexor of the fingers

Clinical examination: Stabilize the proximal interphalangeal joint and instruct the patient to flex the distal phalangeal joint, thereby eliminating the contribution of the flexor digitorum superficialis muscle (Fig. 4.28)

Palmaris Brevis Muscle

Origin: Flexor retinaculum of the hand

Insertion: Cutaneous innervation of the hypothenar region

It spans the skin of hypothenar

Innervation: Superficial branch of the ulnar nerve

Clinical examination: Abduction of the fifth digit, accompanied by contraction of the hypothenar eminence, produces visible skin creases in the hypothenar region (Fig. 4.29)

Abductor Digiti Minimi Muscle

Origin: Piriformis bone and flexor retinaculum of the hand

Insertion: Ulnar side of the proximal phalanx of digit V

Innervation: Deep branch of the ulnar nerve

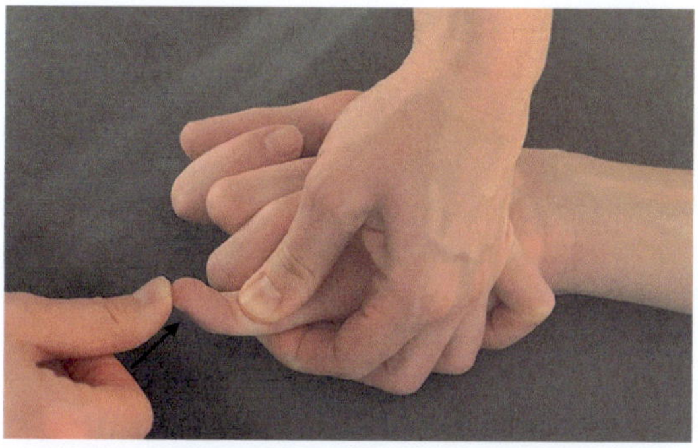

Fig. 4.28 Clinical examination of the flexor digitorum profundus muscle by flexing the DIP joint (arrow) with the PIP joint being immobilized

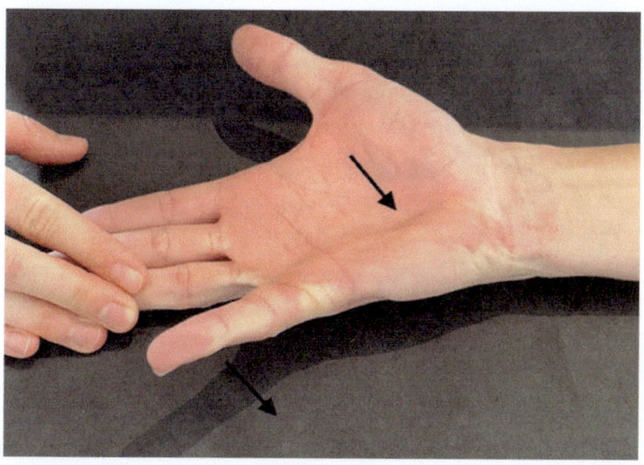

Fig. 4.29 Abduction of the fifth finger (arrow) accentuates contraction of the palmaris brevis muscle (arrow) within the hypothenar region

Function: Abduction and flexion of the fifth finger

Clinical examination: Abduction of the fifth finger against resistance (Fig. 4.30)

Opponens Digiti Minimi Muscle

Origin: Hamate bone and flexor retinaculum of the hand

Insertion: Ulnar side of the metacarpophalangeal joint of digit V

Function: The fifth finger is responsible for flexion, as well as rotation and opposition, at the metacarpophalangeal joint of digit V

Clinical examination: Ask the patient to put together the tip of digit V to the thumb and try to force it apart (Fig. 4.31)

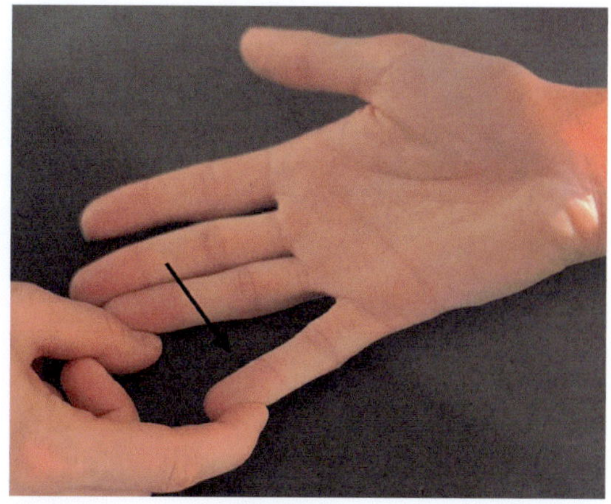

Fig. 4.30 To examine the abductor digiti minimi, ask the patient to abduct the fifth finger against resistance (arrow)

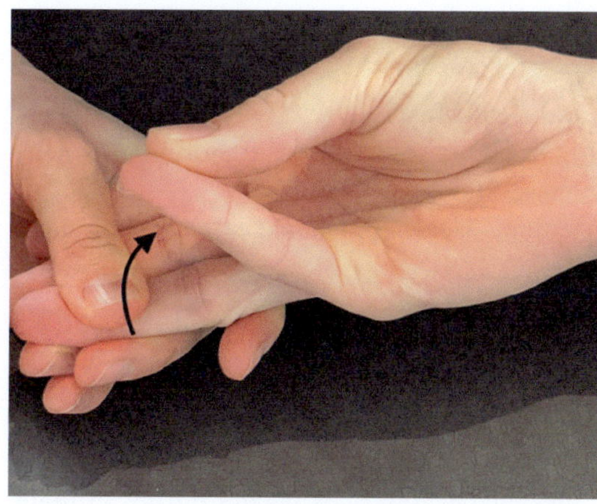

Fig. 4.31 Clinical examination of the opponens digiti minimi muscle ask the patient to approximate the tip of the fifth finger to the thumb (arrow), and then attempt to separate them by applying opposing forces

Flexor Digiti Minimi Brevis Muscle

Origin: Hamate bone and flexor retinaculum of the hand

Insertion: Ulnar side of the proximal phalanx of digit V

Function: Flexion of the fifth finger at the proximal joint

Clinical examination: Immobilize the proximal and distal interphalangeal joint and ask the patient to flex the metacarpophalangeal joint (Fig. 4.32)

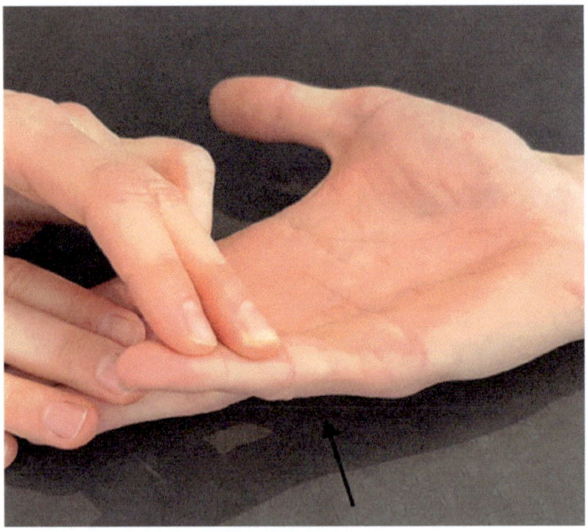

Fig. 4.32 Stabilize the proximal and distal interphalangeal joints and instruct the patient to flex the metacarpophalangeal joint (arrow) to assess function of the flexor digiti minimi brevis muscle

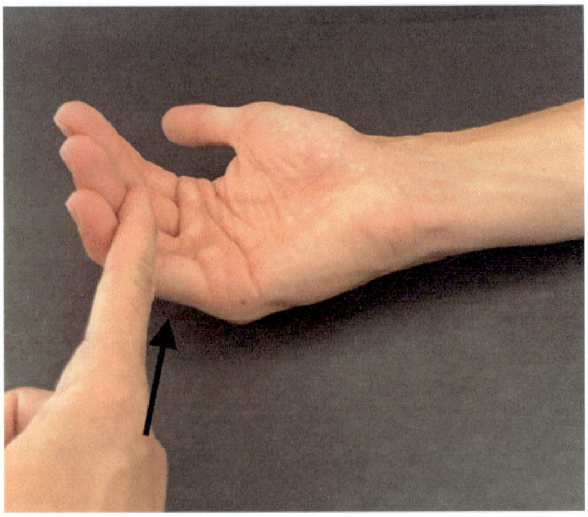

Fig. 4.33 For clinical examination of the lumbrical muscles, ask the patient to flex the fingers of the fourth and fifth digit at the metacarpophalangeal joint while maintaining extension of the interphalangeal joints (arrow)

Lumbrical Muscles

Origin: Fibers of the flexor digitorum profundus muscle

Insertion: Metacarpophalangeal joints of digits II–V

Innervation:

Lumbrical muscles II + III ➔ Median nerve

Lumbrical muscles IV + V ➔ Ulnar nerve

Function: Flexion at the metacarpophalangeal joints combined with extension at the interphalangeal joints, as occurs during gripping movements

Clinical examination: Flexing of the fingers at the metacarpophalangeal joint while keeping the interphalangeal joint extended of digit IV (Fig. 4.33)

Palmar Interossei Muscles (I–III)

Origin: Metacarpal bones I–III

Insertion: Proximal phalanges

Function: Adduction and flexion of the fingers at the metacarpal joints as well as extension of the proximal and distal phalanges

Clinical examination: Adduction of the index finger against resistance (Fig. 4.34)

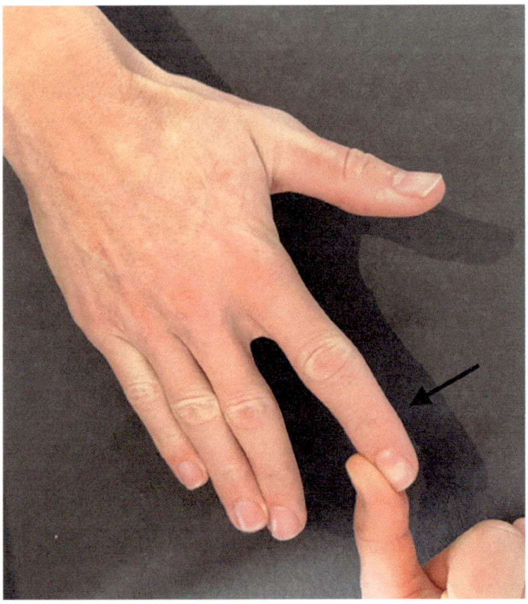

Fig. 4.34 Ask the patient to adduct the index finger against resistance (arrow) to clinically test the palmar interossei muscles I-III

Dorsal Interossei Muscles (I–IV)

Origin: Metacarpals of digits I–IV

Insertion: Proximal phalanges

Function: Abduction and flexion of the fingers at the metacarpophalangeal joints as well as extension of the proximal and distal interphalangeal joints

Clinical examination: Abduction of the index finger against resistance (Fig. 4.35)

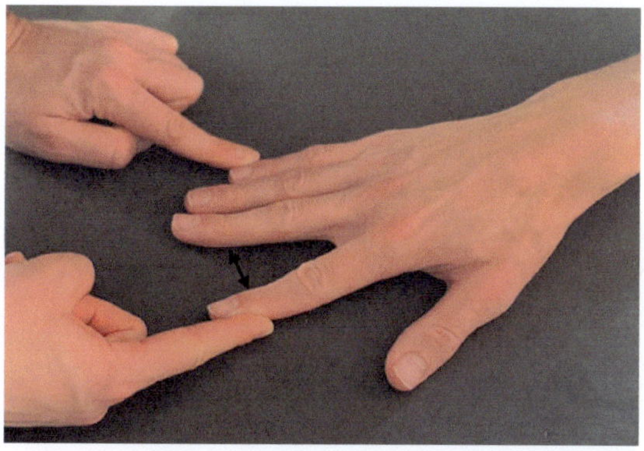

Fig. 4.35 Abduction of the index finger against resistance (arrow) to assess function of the dorsal interossei muscle

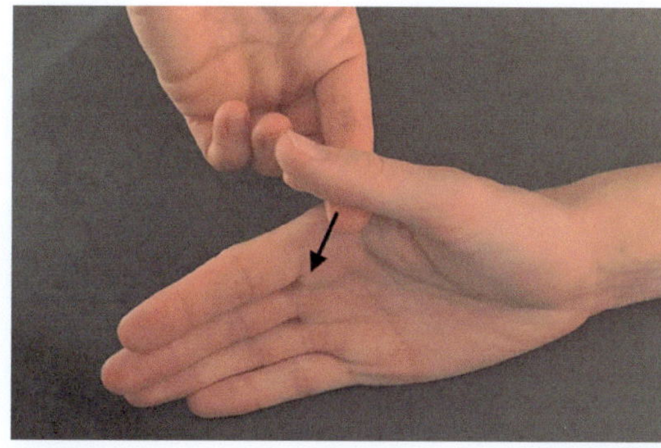

Fig. 4.36 Clinical examination of the adductor pollicis brevis muscle: Adduction of the thumb perpendicular to the palm (arrow)

In ulnar nerve lesions, atrophy of the dorsal interossei muscles may be observed, particularly pronounced in the first dorsal interosseus muscle

> Mnemonic: *PAD DAB ("Use your hand to dab with a pad") ➔ Palmar interossei ADuct, Dorsal interossei ABduct*

Adductor Pollicis Brevis Muscle

Origin: Capitate and metacarpal bone II + III
Insertion: Proximal phalanx of digit I
Function: Adduction and opposition of the thumb
Clinical examination: Instruct the patient to adduct the thumb perpendicular to the palm (Fig. 4.36)
Ulnar lesion: Positive Froment sign

Flexor Pollicis Brevis Muscle

Origin: Flexor retinaculum of the hand, the trapezium (superficial head) as well as the trapezoid and capitate bones (superficial head)
Insertion: Lateral side of the proximal phalanx
Innervation:
Deep head ➔ Deep branch of the ulnar nerve
Superficial head ➔ Recurrent branch of the median nerve
Function: Flexion of the thumb at the carpometacarpal and metacarpophalangeal joint
Clinical examination: The examination of this muscle is not useful due to its dual innervation

4.1.12 Radial Nerve (C6–C8)

Triceps Muscle

Origin: Infraglenoid tubercle of the scapula (long head) and posterior surface of the humerus (medial and lateral head)
Insertion: Olecranon of the ulnar bone
Innervation:
Long head ➔ Branch of the axillary nerve
Medial head ➔ Possible partial innervation by the ulnar nerve
Function: Extension of the forearm assisted by the anconeus muscle
Clinical examination: Instruct the patient to extend the elbow against resistance, with the shoulders abducted to 90° minimize the effects of gravity (Fig. 4.37)

Anconeus Muscle

Origin: Lateral epicondyle of the humerus
Insertion: Lateral olecranon and proximal quarter of the posterior shaft of the ulna
Function: The anconeus muscle functions as a weak extensor to support triceps muscle function, and performs a pronation movement
Clinical examination: This muscle is usually not tested

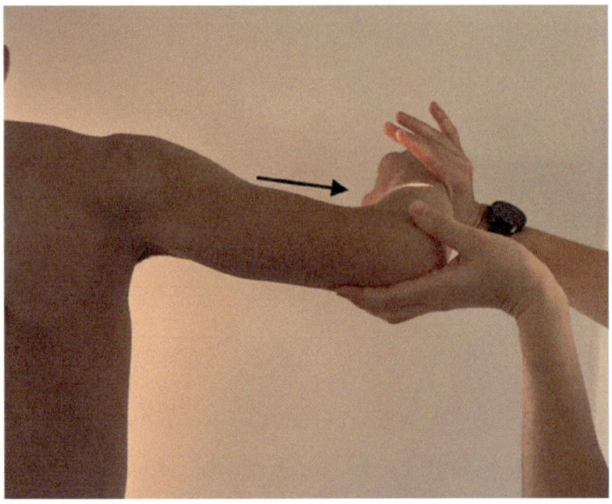

Fig. 4.37 Extension of the forearm against resistance (arrow) with the arm positioned parallel to the ground to test the triceps muscle function

Brachioradialis Muscle

Origin: Lateral edge of the humerus

Insertion: Styloid process of the radius

Function: Flexion of the forearm

Clinical examination: Flexion of the elbow against resistance with the arm in semi-pronation to eliminate the function of the biceps muscle. The brachioradialis can be palpated on the anterior surface of the proximal forearm (Fig. 4.38)

> *Mnemonic:* The **B**rachio**R**adialis follows the BR rule:
> *Function*: **B**eer mug **R**aising muscle (muscle is best tested in this position—with the arm in semi-pronation)
> *Innervation*: **B**reaks **R**ule because it is a flexor muscle although innervated by the **R**adial nerve which usually innervates extensor muscles
> *Relation*: **B**ehind the **B**rachio**R**adialis lies the **R**adial nerve in the cubital fossa

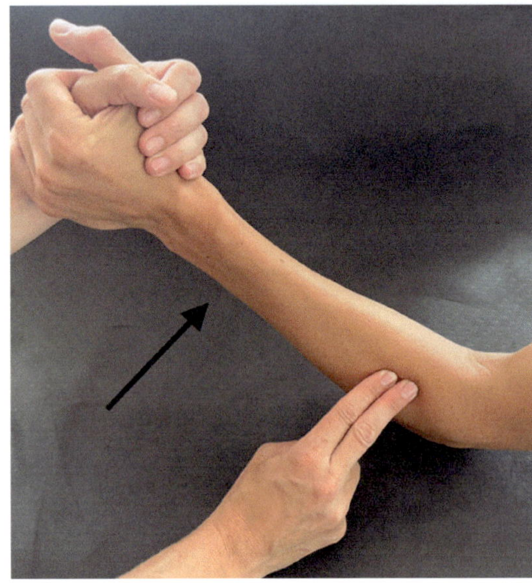

Fig. 4.38 Palpate the brachioradialis with the arm in flexed and semi-pronated against resistance (arrow)

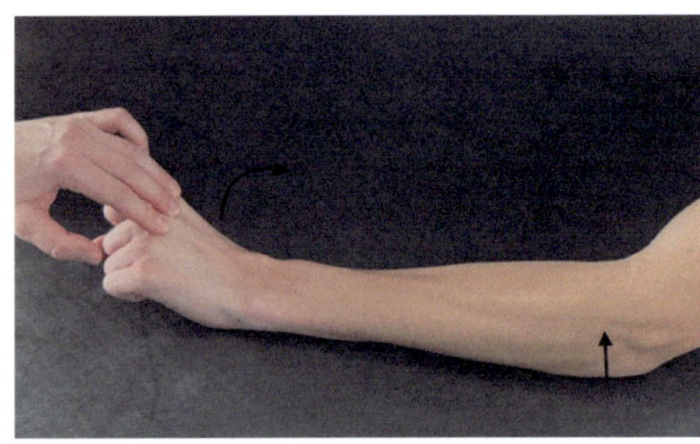

Fig. 4.39 To assess the extensor carpi radialis muscle, instruct the patient to perform wrist extension combined with radial abduction (arrow)

Extensor Carpi Radialis Longus and Brevis Muscles

Origin: Distal third of the humerus

Insertion: Dorsal aspect of the third metacarpal

Function: The muscle contributes to wrist extension and radial abduction, elbow flexion, and assists in fist closure

Clinical examination: Extension and radial abduction of the wrist against resistance in pronation leads to contraction of the muscles that can be palpated lateral and distal to the brachioradialis muscle (Fig. 4.39)

Injury: Pain, particularly during wrist extension and finger flexion, is commonly referred to as "tennis elbow"

Supinator Muscle
Origin: Lateral epicondyle of the humerus
Insertion: Upper third of the radius

In the proximal third of the radius, the radial nerve is situated between the fascial layers of the supinator muscle
The deep branch of the radial nerve pierces the supinator muscle

Function: Supination of the forearm
Clinical examination: Supination against resistance with the forearm in extension (to eliminate the biceps brachii action) (Fig. 4.40)

Extensor Carpi Ulnaris Muscle
Origin: Lateral epicondyle of the humerus
Insertion: Metacarpal bone V
Innervation: Posterior interosseus nerve
Function: Ulnar adduction and extension of the wrist
Clinical examination: Wrist extension and ulnar abduction against resistance (Fig. 4.41)

Extensor Digitorum Communis Muscle
Origin: Lateral epicondyle of the humerus
Insertion: Proximal and distal phalanges
Innervation: Posterior interosseus nerve
Function: Extension of digits II–V at the metacarpophalangeal joint
Clinical examination: Extension of the fingers at the metacarpophalangeal joint while stabilizing the distal phalangeal joint (Fig. 4.42)

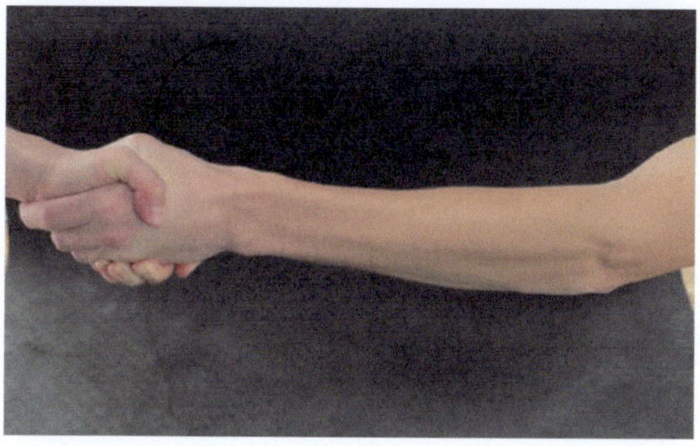

Fig. 4.40 Clinical examination of the supinator muscle: Supination against resistance with the arm extended (arrow)

Extensor Digiti Minimi Muscle
Origin: Lateral epicondyle of the humerus
Insertion: Proximal and distal phalanx of digit V
Function: Extension of the fifth finger
Clinical examination: Extension of the fifth finger at the metacarpophalangeal joint with the distal phalangeal joints being flexed (Fig. 4.43)

Abductor Pollicis Longus Muscle
Origin: Posterior side of the ulna and radius
Insertion: Base of the metacarpal bone I
Function: Abduction and extension of the thumb; it also supports abduction of the hand (radial deviation)
Innervation: Posterior interosseus branch of the radial nerve
Clinical examination: Ask the patient to abduct the thumb parallel to the palm (Fig. 4.44)

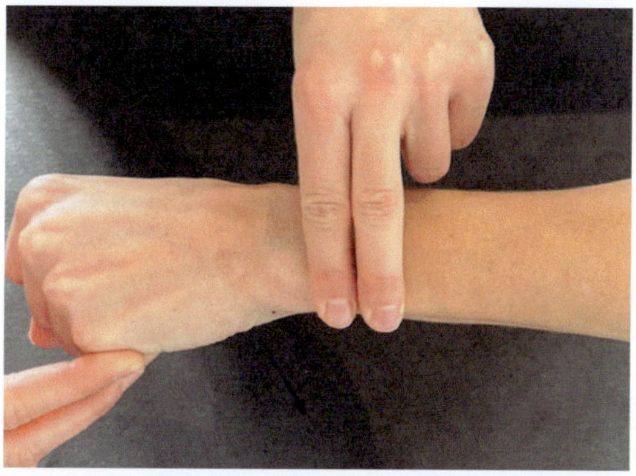

Fig. 4.41 Clinical examination of the extensor carpi ulnaris: Extension and ulnar abduction of the hand (arrow) against resistance

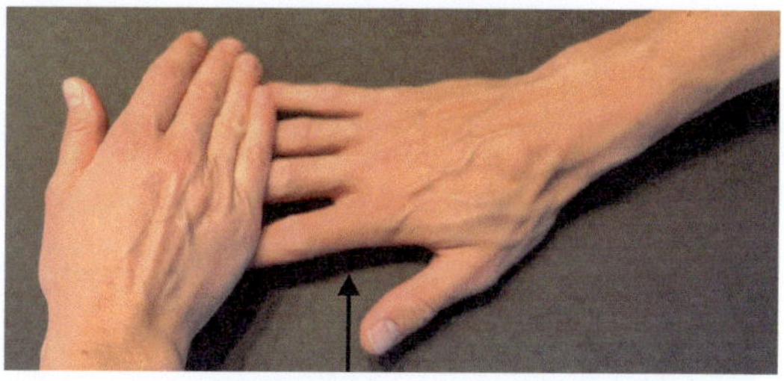

Fig. 4.42 Clinical examination of the extensor digitorum communis muscle: Extension of the fingers at the MCP joint against resistance (arrow)

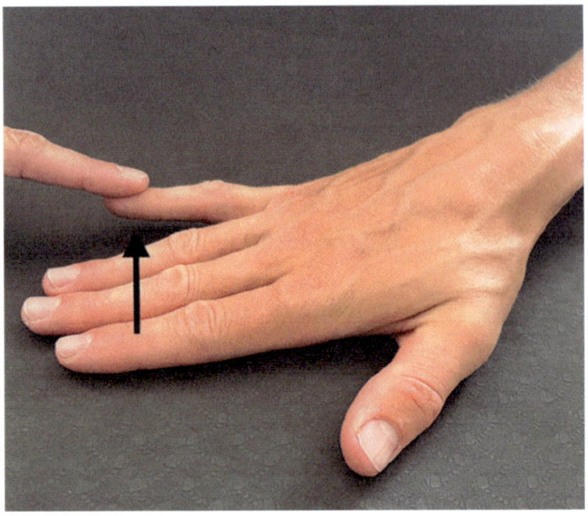

Fig. 4.43 Clinical examination of the extensor digiti minimi muscle: Extension of the fifth finger at the MCP joint against resistance (arrow)

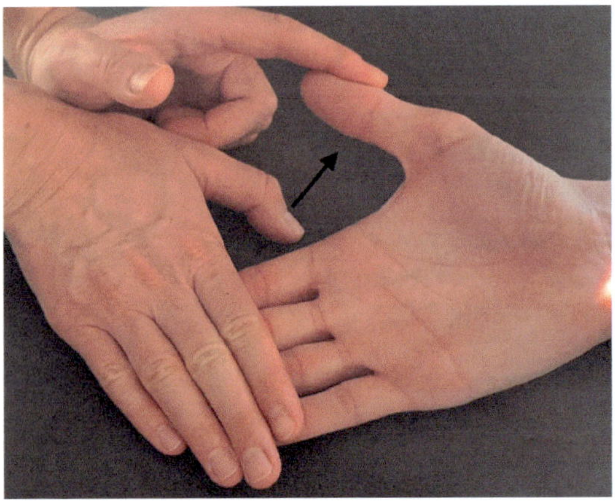

Fig. 4.44 Abduction of the thumb in plane to the hand against resistance (arrow) to assess function of the abductor pollicis longus muscle

> **Abductor pollicis brevis** (median nerve) ➔ Abduction of the thumb perpendicular to the palm
>
> **Abductor pollicis longus** (radial nerve) ➔ Abduction of the thumb in plane to the palm (in a radial direction)

Extensor Pollicis Longus Muscle

Origin: Posterior side of the ulna and radius

Insertion: Dorsal side of the distal phalanx of the thumb

Function: Thumb extension at the interphalangea joint of the thumb

Clinical examination: Extension of the thumb at the metacarpophalangeal joint against resistance (Fig. 4.45)

Extensor Pollicis Brevis Muscle

Origin: Posterior side of the radius

Insertion: Proximal phalanx of the thumb

Function: Extension of the thumb at the carpometacarpal and metacarpophalangeal joints

Clinical examination: Extension of the thumb at the distal phalangeal joint against resistance (Fig. 4.46)

> The fibers of the abductor pollicis longus, extensor pollicis longus and extensor pollicis brevis muscles form the **anatomical snuff box**, a triangular depression on the radial and dorsal aspect of the hand.

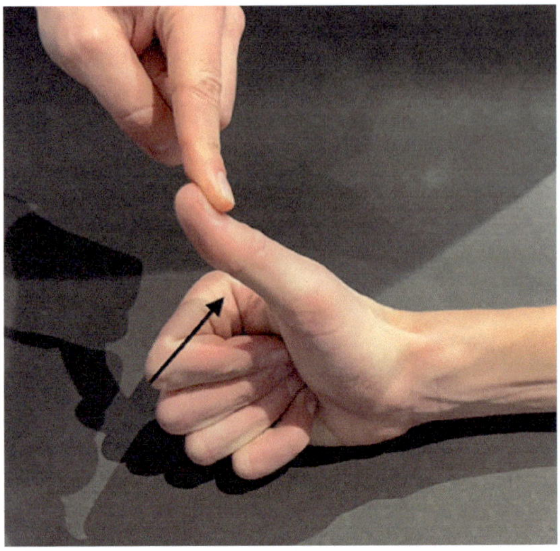

Fig. 4.45 Clinical examination of the extensor pollicis longus muscle: Extension of the thumb at the MCP joint against resistance (arrow)

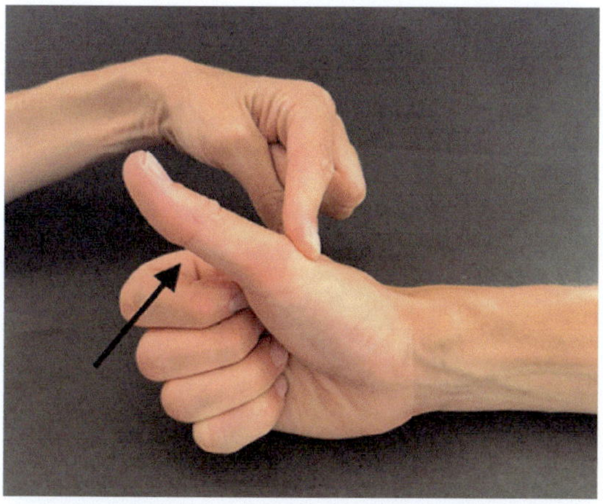

Fig. 4.46 Clinical examination of the extensor pollicis brevis: Extension of the thumb at the DIP joint against resistance (arrow)

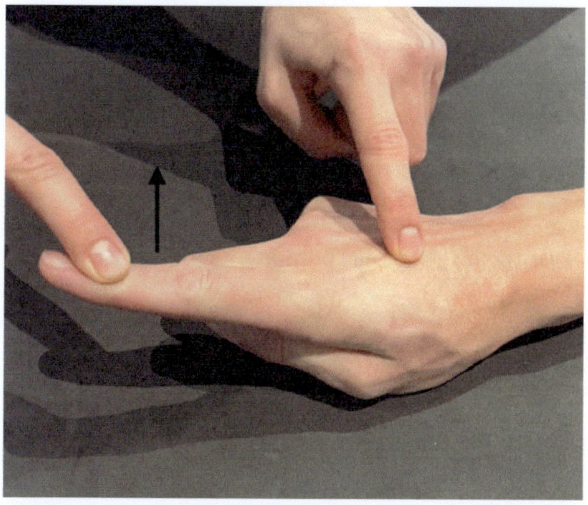

Fig. 4.47 Clinical examination of the extensor indices muscle: Extension of the index finger at the MCP joint against resistance (arrow)

Extensor Indicis Muscle

Origin: Posterior side of the ulna

Insertion: Dorsal aspect of the proximal phalanx of the index finger

Function: Extension of the index finger at the metacarpophalangeal joint

Clinical examination: Extension of the index finger against resistance (Fig. 4.47)

4.2 Lower Extremity

Observation of the patient's gait and inspection of overall posture can already provide valuable diagnostic clues regarding the affected nerve, or at least help to localize the lesion to a specific neuroanatomical level.

4.2.1 Superior Gluteal Nerve (L4–S2)

Gluteus Medius Muscle

Origin: Gluteal surface of the ileum, between the iliac crest and the posterior gluteal line

Insertion: Lateral surface of the greater trochanter of the femur

Function: Abduction and internal rotation of the thigh; it further assists in stabilizating the pelvis

Clinical examination: Abduction against resistance with the patient lying on the unexamined side (Fig. 4.48)

Gluteus Minimus Muscle

Origin: Gluteal surface of the ileum, between the anterior and inferior gluteal lines

Insertion: Anterior surface of the greater trochanter of the femur

Function: Abduction and internal rotation of the thigh; it further assists in stabilizing the pelvis

The gluteus minimus muscle is located deep to the gluteus medius muscle and functions as a synergist as it shares the same function

Clinical examination: Same as for gluteus medius muscle

The **Trendelenburg gait** is indicative of weakness of the gluteus medius and minimus muscles manifesting clinically in a pelvic drop at the affected side.

Tensor Fasciae Lata Muscle

Origin: Anterior iliac crest

Insertion: Lateral condyle of the tibia

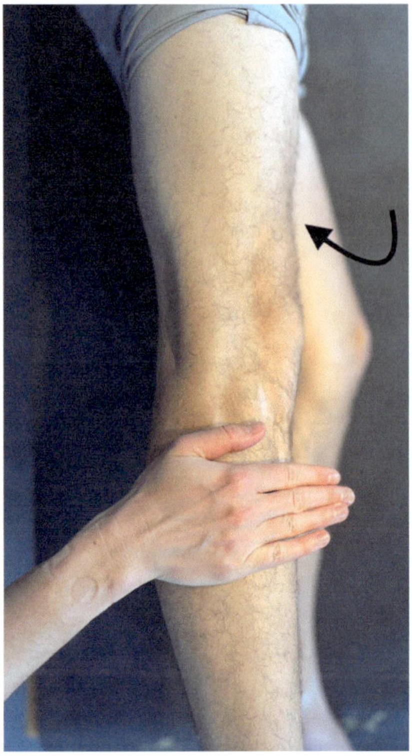

Fig. 4.48 Clinical examination of the gluteus medius muscle: Abduction of the leg against resistance (arrow)

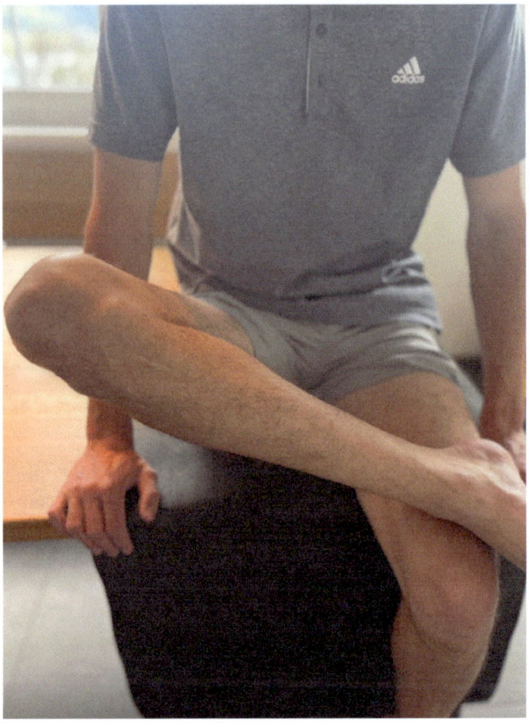

Fig. 4.49 Piriformis provocation test: The patient is instructed to place the ankle of the affected leg over the contralateral knee and bend forward. Reproduction of pain in the gluteal and priformis region indicates a positive test

It represents the most superficial muscle of the antero-lateral compartment of the thigh

Function: Internal rotation and weak abduction of the thigh, external rotation of the leg at the knee joint, and stabilization of the hip and the knee joint

Clinical examination: With the patient positioned on the non-examined side, the pelvis is stabilized. The tested thigh is placed in slight flexion, and the patient is instructed to perform abduction of the thigh against resistance

Piriformis Muscle

Origin: Anterior aspect of the sacrum

Insertion: Greater trochanter of the femur

Function: External rotation, abduction and extension of the thigh; it further assists in stabilizing the hip joint

Clinical examination: With the patient in a seated position, the ankle of the examined leg is placed over the contralateral knee. The patient is then instructed to bend forward. Elicitation of pain in the gluteal or piriformis region, suggests irritation of the piriformis muscle (Fig. 4.49)

4.2.2 Inferior Gluteal Nerve (L5–S2)

Gluteus Maximus Muscle

Origin: Gluteal surface of the ileum

Insertion: Gluteal tuberosity of the femur

Function: Extension and external rotation of the thigh

Superior part—additional abduction of the thigh

Inferior part—additional adduction of the thigh

Being a strong extensor of the leg, it is involved in the stepping or climbing movement

Clinical examination: With the patient in prone position and the knee flexed to reduce hamstring muscle involvement, the patient is asked to extend the hip by lifting the leg off the examination table. During this maneuver, the examiner palpates the gluteus maximus muscle to assess for contraction and strength (Fig. 4.50)

4.2.3 Femoral Nerve (L2–L4)

Iliac Muscle, L1–L3

Origin: Superior two-thirds of the iliac fossa

Insertion: Lesser trochanter of the femur

Function: Flexion of the thigh

Clinical examination: In supine position, ask the patient to bring the knee toward the ipsilateral rib, keeping the leg slightly externally rotated and the knee flexed. Palpate the iliac fossa to assess contraction of the iliac muscle (Fig. 4.51)

Psoas Major Muscle

Origin: Vertebrae of T12–L4

Insertion: Lesser trochanter of the femur

Innervation: Anterior rami of L1–L4 and some contributions from the femoral nerve

Function: Flexion and lateral rotation of the thigh

Clinical examination: With the patient in supine position and the leg slightly flexed, externally rotated, and abducted, apply gentle downward pressure on the leg to assess muscle strength of the psoas major (Fig. 4.52)

The iliac and psoas muscles constitute the iliopsoas, the most powerful flexor of the hip joint, playing a critical role in activities such as running.

The psoas syndrome refers to injury of this muscle, typically resulting from overuse, and, less commonly, from trauma. Patients commonly

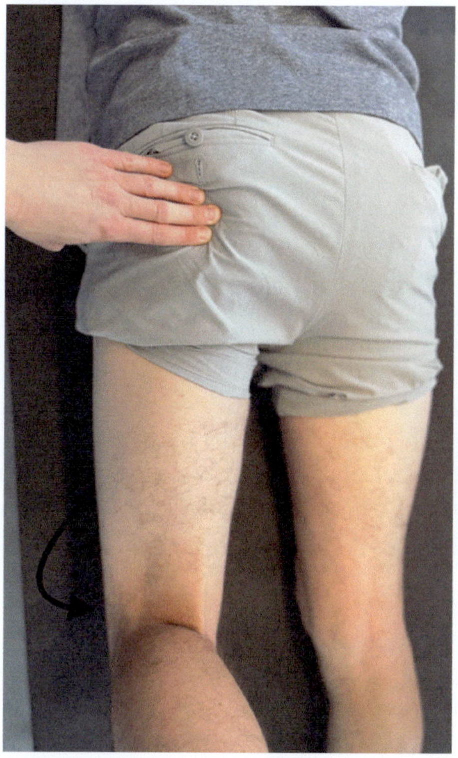

Fig. 4.50 Clinical examination of the gluteus maximus muscle: In prone position, ask the patient to lift the flexed leg (arrow) and palpate the gluteal region to assess contraction of the examined muscle

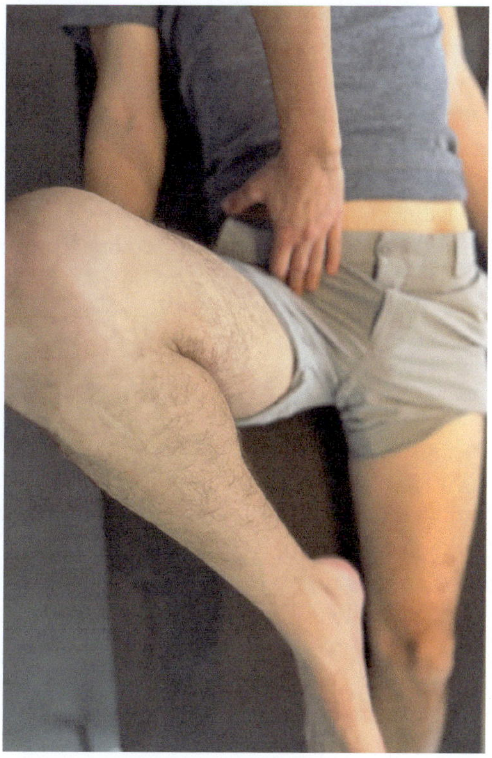

Fig. 4.51 Palpate the iliac muscle within the iliac fossa while the patient's leg is externally rotated and flexed at both the hip and knee

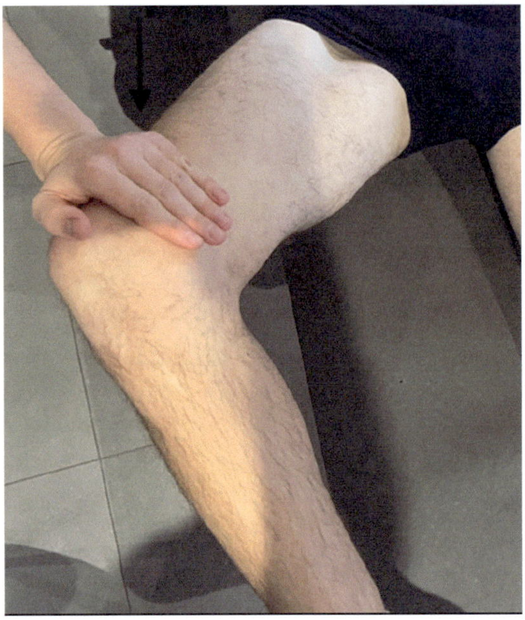

Fig. 4.52 Clinical examination of the psoas major muscle: In supine position, push the patient's slightly flexed, externally rotated and abducted leg in a downward direction

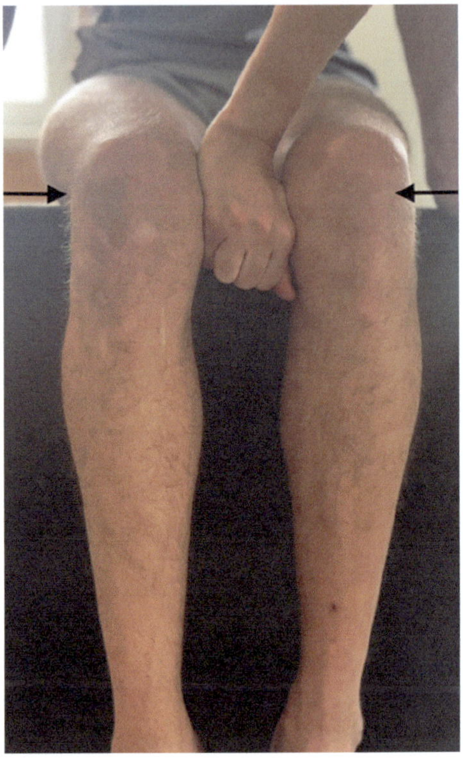

Fig. 4.53 Clinical examination of the pectineus muscle: Place a fist between the patient's knees and instruct the patient to adduct the thighs (arrow) by pressing the knees together against the resistance provided by the fist

report pain in the hip and/or inguinal region, occasionally accompanied by lower back pain. It is most frequently observed in athletes including runners, dancers, and jumpers and is generally not associated with overt paresis. Management is typically conservative, though it should be considered in the differential diagnosis of hip and lower back pain.

Psoas Minor Muscle

Origin: Vertebrae of T12–L1

Insertion: Iliopubic eminence

Innervation: Spinal nerve L1

Function: Flexion of the trunk at the vertebral column; it also assists in hip flexion, along with the poses major muscle

Injury: The psoas minor is a relatively weak muscle and injury of lesion of this muscle does not result in appreciable functional impairment

Pectineus Muscle, L1–T12

Origin: Superior pubic ramus

Insertion: Pectineal line of the femur

Innervation: Femoral (L2, L3) and the obturator nerve (L2, L3)

Function: Adduction, flexion and internal rotation of the thigh

Clinical examination: With patient in supine or sitting position and the knees slightly flexed, instruct the patient to adduct the knees together while maintaining a fist between them. In the case of muscle irritation, the patient may report pain in the region of the femoral triangle (Fig. 4.53)

Sartorius Muscle, L2–L3

Origin: Anterior superior iliac spine

Insertion: Inferior part of the medial condyle of the tibia

Function: Flexion, abduction, and external rotation of the thigh, as well as flexion and internal rotation of the leg at the knee joint

Clinical examination: With the patient in a sitting position, ask to slide the heel of the examined leg along the medial aspect of the contralateral leg (Fig. 4.54)

Quadriceps Femoris Muscles, L2–L4

Origin:

Rectus femoris ➔ Anterior superior iliac spine
Vastus intermedius ➔ Anterolateral aspect of the femur
Vastus lateralis ➔ Medial aspect of the femur
Vastus medialis ➔ Greater trochanter of the femur

Insertion:

Rectus femoris ➔ Tibial tuberosity, patella
Vastus intermedius ➔ Tibial tuberosity, patella
Vastus lateralis ➔ Tibial tuberosity, patella
Vastus medialis ➔ Tibial tuberosity, patella

Function: Flexion of the thigh, primarily mediated by the rectus femoris, combined with extension of the leg at the knee joint

Clinical examination: With the patient seated and the thigh flexed, instruct the patient to extend knee extension against applied resistance to assess quadriceps femurs strength (Fig. 4.55)

4.2.4 Obturator Nerve (L2–L4)

Note that the **obturator internus muscle** is not innervated by the obturator nerve. In contrast to the obturator externus, the obturator internus muscle abducts the flexed thigh. Nervous innervation is provided by the **nerve to the obturator (L5–S2)** – a branch of the sacral plexus.

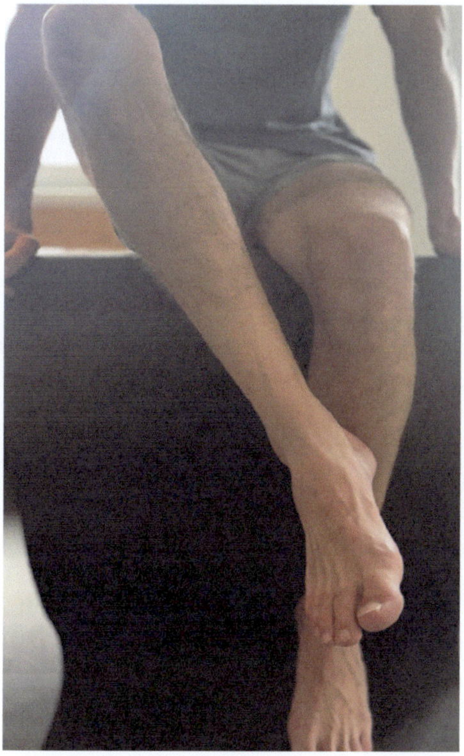

Fig. 4.54 Clinical examination of the sartorius muscle: Ask the patient to slide the heel along the non-examined leg

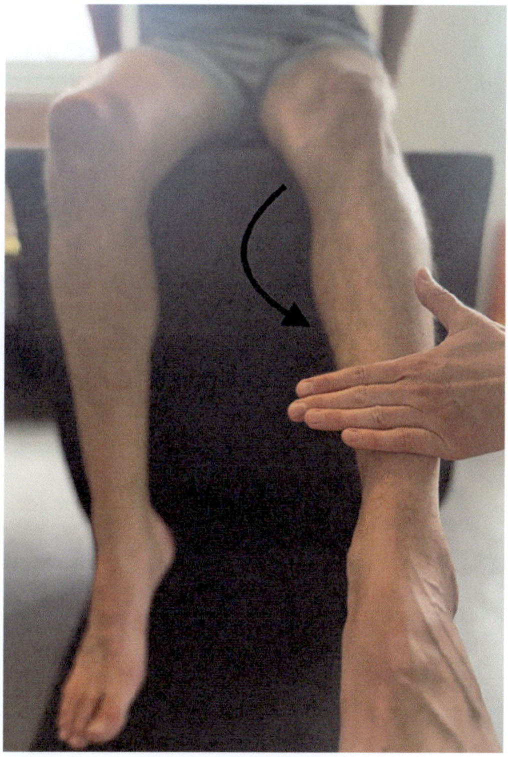

Fig. 4.55 Clinical examination of the quadriceps femoris muscle: Extension of the knee against resistance (arrow) with the thigh being flexed

External Obturator Muscle
Origin: Obturator foramen and membrane
Insertion: Trochanteric fossa of the femur
Function: External rotation and stabilization of the hip joint; it also supports adduction of the flexed thigh
Clinical examination: Ask the patient to externally rotate the flexed leg against resistance

Medial compartment of the thigh = hip adductors:

Pectineus Muscle

Adductor Magnus Muscle
Origin: Inferior part of the pubic ramus and the ischial tuberosity
Insertion: Linea aspera and adductor tuberosity of the femur
Innervation:

Hamstring part ➔ Tibial division of sciatic nerve

Adductor part ➔ Obturator nerve

Function:

Adductor part— Flexion, adduction, and external rotation of the thigh, stabilization of the pelvis

Hamstring part— Extension and internal rotation of the thigh

Clinical examination: With the patient in supine or sitting position and the knees slightly flexed, instruct the patient to adduct the knees while maintaining a fist in between. If palpation elicits pain at the origin of the adductor magnus muscle, irritation of the muscle should be suspected (Fig. 4.56)

➔ All the hip adductors (supplied by the obturator nerve) are examined the same way.

As the pectineus muscle assists in hip flexion and adduction, the clinical examination is the same as for the adductor muscle group.

Adductor Minimus Muscle
Origin: Inferior ramus of the pubis
Insertion: Linea aspera of the femur
Function: Adduction of the thigh

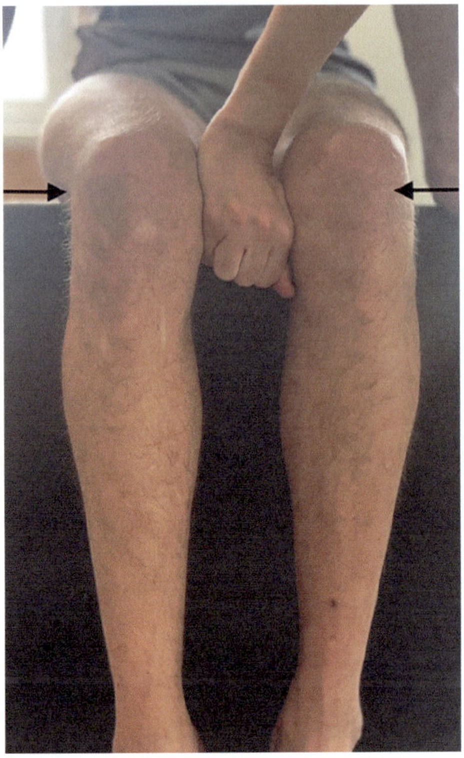

Fig. 4.56 Clinical examination of the adductor magnus muscle: Place a fist between the patient's knees and instruct the patient to adduct the thighs (arrow) by pressing the knees together against the resistance provided by the fist

The adductor minimus muscle cannot be tested alone clinically. Lesion to it may not show any clinical deficits.
It is sometimes considered as being a part of the adductor magnus muscle.

Adductor Longus Muscle
Origin: Anterior surface of the pubic body
Insertion: Linea aspera of the femur
Innervation: Anterior division of the obturator nerve L2–L4
Function: Adduction of thigh at the hip joint; it further assists in external rotation and flexion of the thigh

Adductor Brevis Muscle
Origin: Lateral aspect of the inferior ramus of the pubis
Insertion: Linea aspera of the femur

Function: Adduction of the thigh at the hip joint; it further assists in external rotation and flexion of the thigh

The adductor brevis is located posterior to the adductor longus muscle. It can be palpated between the adductor longus and gracilis muscle.

Gracilis Muscle

It represents the most superficial muscle in the medial compartment of the thigh

Origin: Ischiopubic ramus

Insertion: Medial aspect of the tibial bone just below the knee joint

It represents the only muscle of the hip adductors that crosses two joints, functioning as a biarticular muscle

Function: Flexion and internal rotation of the leg at the knee joint; however, it constitutes the weakest muscle among the thigh adductors.

Clinical examination: With the patient in prone position and the legs extended, passively abduct the legs. Next, instruct the patient to flex the knees to 90° and attempt further abduction of the thighs. Knee flexion shortens the gracilis muscle, permitting additional abduction. Restricted motion or pain during this maneuver may indicate irritation of the gracilis muscle. This test is called Phelps test (Fig. 4.57).

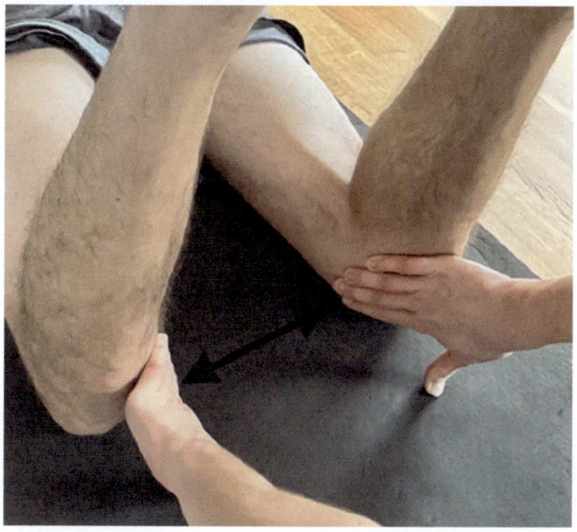

Fig. 4.57 Clinical examination of the gracilis muscle: In prone position, passively abduct the patients legs. Then instruct the patient to flex the knees and attempt further passive abduction (arrow). Pain or restricted motion may indicate muscle irritation.

4.2.5 Sciatic Nerve (L4–S3)

Thigh Group

Hamstring Muscles

These muscles receive partial innervation from small, direct branches of the sciatic nerve arising within the pelvis. Lesions of these branches are considered clinically insignificant, as they provide only supplementary innervation.

The hamstring muscles are formed by the *semitendinosus, semimembranosus, and biceps femoris muscles*:

The sciatic nerve innervates the hamstring muscles immediately after exiting the pelvis. Consequently, an isolated lesion of sciatic nerve would need to be very proximal to affect hamstring function. Although smaller distal branches of the sciatic nerve also contribute motor fibers to the hamstring muscles, lesions of these branches are generally clinically not recognizable provided the major branches remain intact.

The hamstring muscles belong to the posterior compartment of the thigh.

Hamstring Muscles

Origin: Ischial bone

Insertion: Popliteal fossa

Innervation:

Semitendinous, semimembranous and the long head of the biceps femoris muscle (medial hamstrings) ➔ Tibial division of the sciatic nerve

Short head of the biceps femoris muscle ➔ Common peroneal portion of the sciatic nerve

Function: Extension of the thigh and flexion of the knee joint thereby playing an important role in activities such as walking, running, and jumping

Clinical examination:

Instruct the patient to flex the knees against resistance while sitting or in prone position.

Tendons of the hamstring muscles can be palpated in the popliteal fossa (Fig. 4.58)

Injury: The most common pathology affecting this muscle group constitutes the proximal hamstring tendinopathy

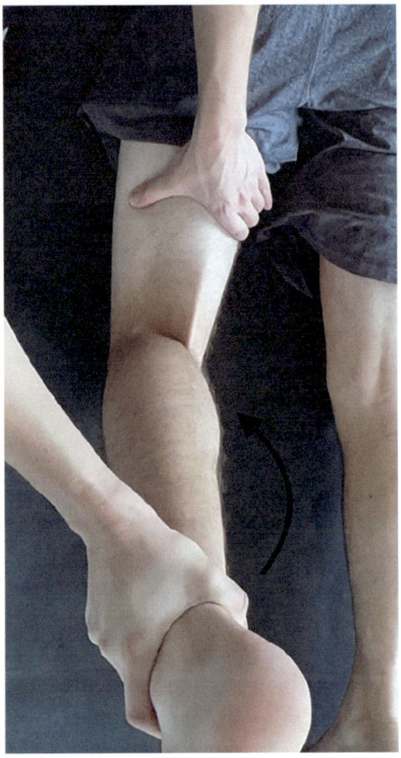

Fig. 4.58 Clinical examination of the hamstrings: With the patient being in a prone position, instruct to flex the knees (arrow) against resistance

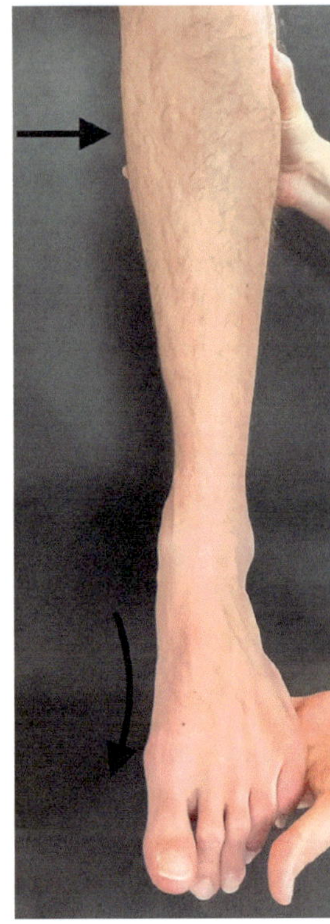

Fig. 4.59 The gastrocnemius muscle can be palpated (arrow) when asking the patient to perform plantarflexion of the foot (arrow) with the knees being extended

More distally, the sciatic nerve provides further innervation to following muscle groups:

- The posterior compartment of the leg as well as the plantar aspect of the foot are innervated by the **tibial nerve**.
- The anterior and lateral compartments of the leg receive nerve fibers from the **common peroneal nerve**.

4.2.5.1 Tibial Nerve (L4–S3)

Popliteus and Plantaris Muscles

They have only minor clinical significance

Gastrocnemius Muscle (S1, S2)

Origin: Distal part of the femur

Insertion: Calcaneus bone of the foot

Innervation: Tibial nerve (L4–S3)

Function: Foot inversion, plantar flexion and toe flexion; plantarflexion occurs primarily when the knee is extended

Clinical examination: With the patient in a sitting position, instruct the patient to perform plantar flexion of the foot with the knee extended. Contraction of the target muscle can be palpated during this maneuver (Fig. 4.59)

Injury: Gastrocnemius muscle lesions typically involve rupture and are most commonly observed in athletes. Clinically, they present with sudden pain, swelling, and weakness during plantar flexion of the foot

Soleus Muscle (S1, S2)

Origin: Proximal third of tibial and fibular bone

Insertion: Calcaneus bone

The soleus muscle lies beneath the gastrocnemius muscle

Innervation: Tibial nerve (L4–S3)

Function: Foot inversion, plantar flexion and toe flexion. Plantar flexion is possible with both the knee extended and flexed due to its distal insertion on the tibia

Clinical examination: With the patient seated, instruct to perform plantar flexion of the foot with the knee flexed (Fig. 4.60)

Collectively, these muscles are referred to as the **triceps surae**.

> Mild weakness of these muscles is more readily detected when the patient is asked to stand on their toes.

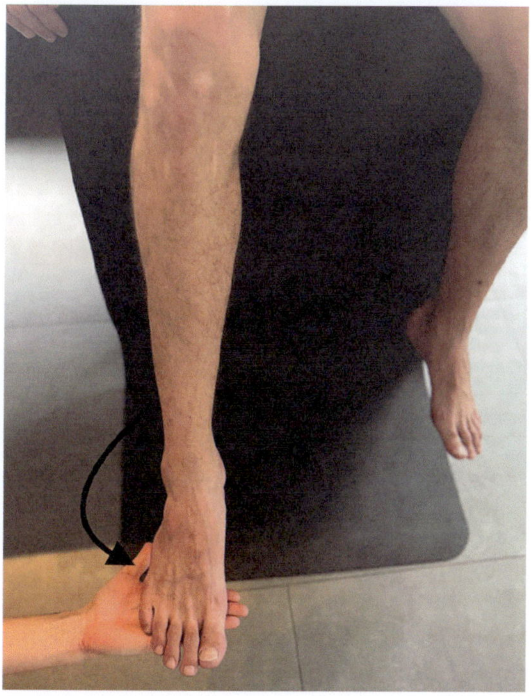

Fig. 4.60 The soleus muscle is assessed by instructing the patient to perform plantar flexion of the foot (arrow) with the knee flexed

> Due to the gastrocnemius muscle being a strong plantar flexor with the knee extended, the soleus muscle assumes primary responsibility for plantar flexor when the knee is flexed.

Tibialis Posterior Muscle (L4, L5)

Origin: Upper lateral surface of the tibia and the adjacent interosseus membrane

Insertion: Tarsal bones and the base of the metatarsal bones II–IV

Innervation: Tibial nerve (L4–S3)

Function: Facilitates foot inversion and serves as the primary muscle responsible for this movement

Clinical examination: Instruct the patient to invert the foot (Fig. 4.61)

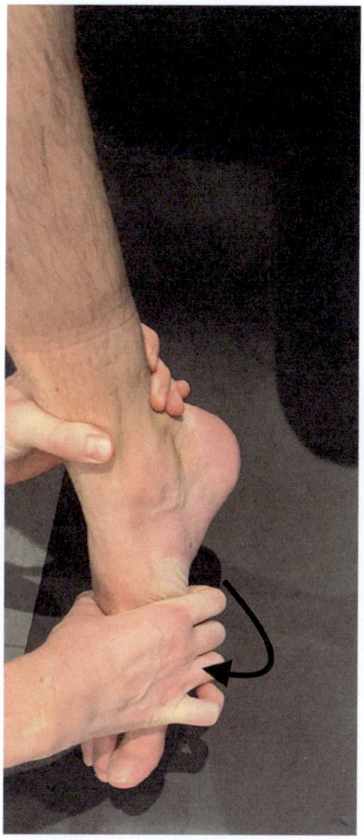

Fig. 4.61 Clinical examination of the tibialis posterior muscle: Inversion of the foot (arrow)

Injury: The tibialis posterior tendon dysfunction (PTTD), or tibialis posterior syndrome, a degenerative condition of the tendon, may develop

Flexor Digitorum Longus Muscle (L5, S1)
Origin: Posterior tibial bone
Insertion: Distal phalanges of the toes II–V
Innervation: Tibial nerve (L4–S3)
Function: Flexion of all joints of the toes except the great toe; it also supports plantarflexion and inversion of the foot
Clinical examination: Flexion of the toes (except the great toe) against resistance (Fig. 4.62)

Flexor Hallucis Longus Muscle (L5, S1)
Origin: Distal part of the posterior fibular bone
Insertion: Base of the distal phalanx of the great toe
Innervation: Tibial nerve (L4–S3)
Function: Flexion of the great toe at the metatarsophalangeal joint. In contrast to the flexor hallucis brevis muscle, it additionally flexes the toe at the interphalangeal joint and the ankle joint
Clinical examination: Flexion of the great toe against resistance (Fig. 4.63)

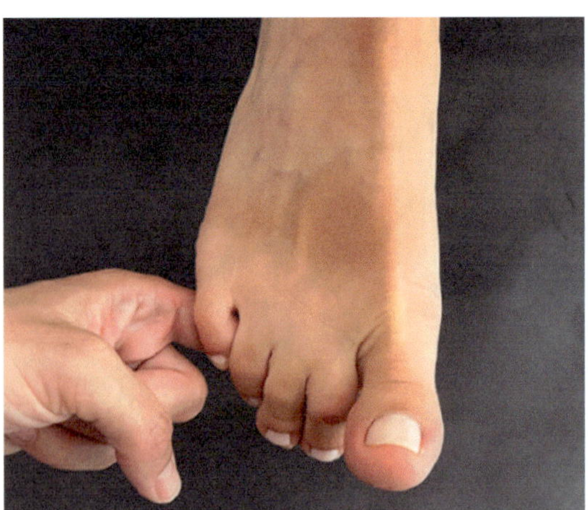

Fig. 4.62 Clinical examination of the flexor digitorum longus muscle: Flexion of the toes of digits II-V

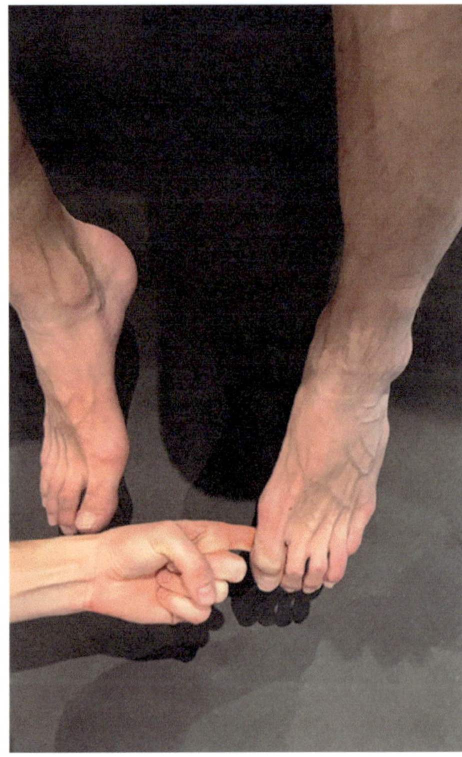

Fig. 4.63 Clinical examination of the flexor hallucis longus muscle: Flexion of the great toe

Abductor Hallucis Muscle
Origin: Medial process of the calcaneal tuberosity
Insertion: Proximal phalanx of the great toe
Innervation: Medial plantar nerve (S1–S3) of the tibial nerve
Function: Abduction and flexion of the great toe
Clinical examination: Apply lateral pressure to the great toe, directing it toward the smaller toes, and instruct the patient to actively abduct the great toe back to its neutral position to assess the strength and function of the abductor hallucis muscle (Fig. 4.64)

Flexor Hallucis Brevis Muscle
Origin: Tendon of the tibialis posterior muscle and cuneiform bone
Insertion: Proximal phalanx of the great toe
Innervation: Medial plantar nerve (S1–S3) of the tibial nerve

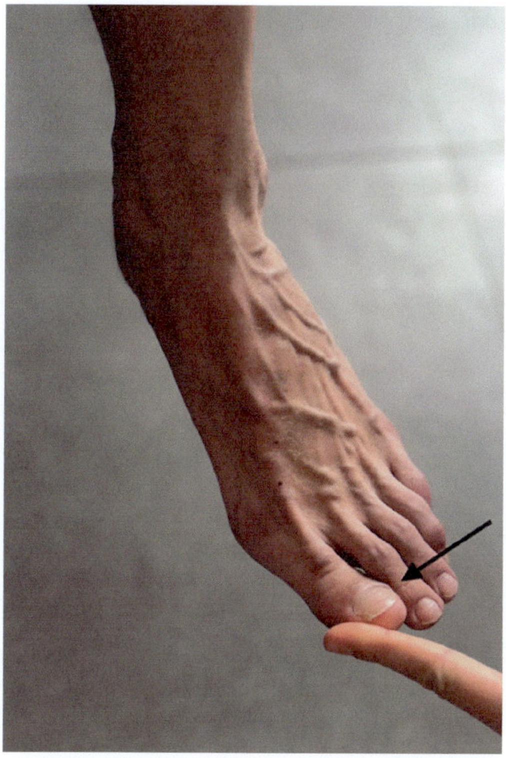

Fig. 4.64 Clinical examination of the abductor hallucis muscle: Abduction of the great toe (arrow) from an adducted position

Function: Flexion of the great toe at the metatarsophalangeal joint

Clinical examination: Instruct the patient to flex the hallux while stabilizing the remaining toes to isolate and assess function of the flexor hallucis brevis muscle.

Flexor Digitorum Brevis Muscle

Origin: Medial process of the calcaneal tuberosity

Insertion: Middle phalanx of toes II–V

Innervation: Medial plantar nerve (S1–S3) of the tibial nerve

Function: Flexion of toes II–V

Clinical examination: Instruct the patient to flex the little toe

First Lumbrical Muscle

Origin: Tendon of the flexor digitorum longus muscle

Insertion: Proximal phalanx of digit I

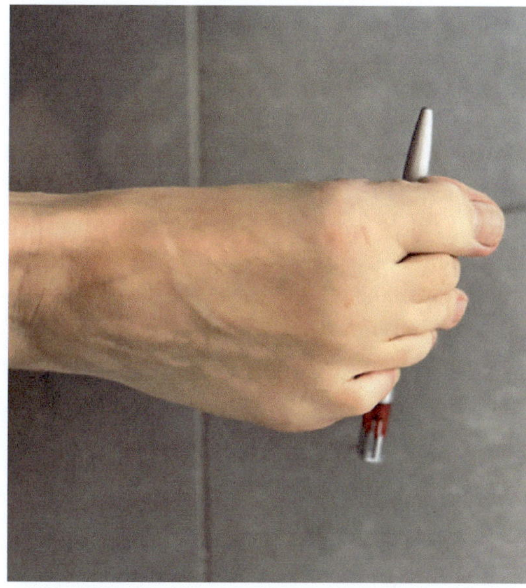

Fig. 4.65 Clinical examination of the lumbrical muscles of the foot: Ask the patient to grab something with the toes

Innervation: Medial plantar nerve (S1–S3) of the tibial nerve

Function: Flexion and adduction at the metatarsophalangeal joint, extension at the interphalangeal joint

Clinical examination: Ask the patient to grab something (pen, towel etc.) from the floor with the toes (Fig. 4.65)

Quadratus Plantae Muscle

Origin: Calcaneus bone

Insertion: Tendon of the flexor digitorum longus muscle

Innervation: Lateral plantar nerve (S1–S3) of the tibial nerve

Function: Toe flexion of the metatarsophalangeal joints II–V

Clinical examination: To assess this muscle, fully extend the toes of the patient lying in a prone position. Palpate the quadratus plantae muscle while the patient is contracting the toes

Abductor Digiti Minimi Pedis Muscle

Origin: Calcaneal tuberosity

Insertion: Proximal phalanx of digit V

Innervation: Lateral plantar nerve (S1–S3) of the tibial nerve
Function: Abduction and flexion of the toe at the metatarsophalangeal joint
Clinical examination: While stabilizing the remaining toes, ask the patient to abduct digit V

Lumbrical Muscles III–IV
Origin: From the tendons of the flexor digitorum longus muscle
Insertion: Proximal phalanx of digits II–V
Innervation: Lateral plantar nerve (S1–S3) of the tibial nerve
Function: Flexion and adduction at the metatarsophalangeal joint, extension at the interphalangeal joint
Clinical examination: Ask the patient to grab something (pen, towel etc.) from the floor with the foot

Dorsal Interossei Muscles
Origin: Proximal side of the metatarsal bones I–V
Insertion: Proximal phalanx of digits I–V
Innervation: Lateral plantar nerve (S1–S3) of the tibial nerve
Function: Flexion and abduction at the metatarsophalangeal joint II–IV, extension at the interphalangeal joint II–IV
Clinical examination: Instruct the patient to spread the toes (Fig. 4.66)

Adductor Hallucis Muscles
Origin: Metatarsal bones II–IV (oblique head) and metatarsophalangeal joints of the lateral three toes (transverse head)
Insertion: Lateral side of the proximal phalanx of the great toe
Innervation: Lateral plantar nerve (S1–S3) of the tibial nerve
Function: Adduction and flexion of the toe at the metatarsophalangeal joint
Clinical examination: Try to flex and adduct the great toe toward the smaller toes
The lateral plantar nerve provides the primarily motor innervation to the most intrinsic muscles of the foot, analogous to the ulnar nerve of the hand

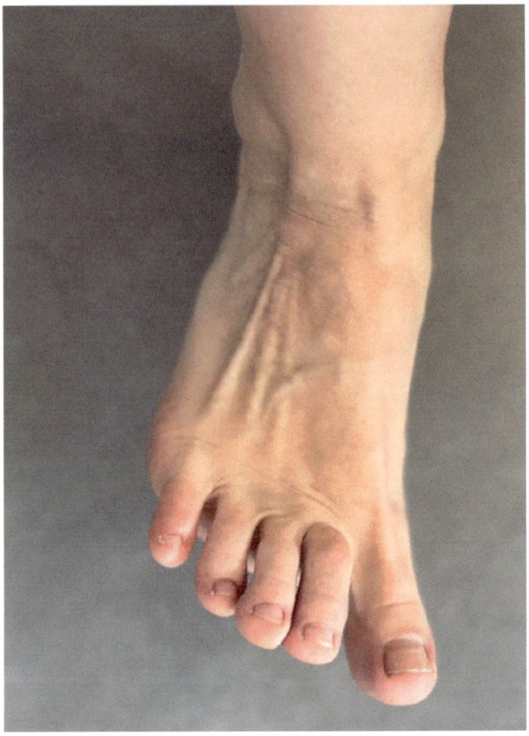

Fig. 4.66 Clinical examination of the dorsal interossei muscles of the foot: Ask the patient to spread the toes

4.2.5.2 Peroneal Nerve (L4–S2)

Short Head of the Biceps Femoris Muscle
Origin: Linea aspera and lateral supracondylar line of the femur
Insertion: Lateral aspect of the fibular head
Innervation: Common peroneal nerve (L4–S1)
Function: Knee flexion
The common peroneal nerve gives off several cutaneous and articular branches before it further divides into the superficial and deep peroneal nerve at the level of the popliteal fossa.

Peroneus Longus/Fibularis Longus Muscle
Origin: Fibula
Insertion: Metatarsal bone I and cuneiform bone
Innervation: Superficial peroneal nerve (L4–S1)
Function: Plantarflexion and foot eversion
Clinical examination for peroneus longus and brevis muscles: Eversion of the foot against resistance. The muscle can be palpated just below the lateral malleus (Fig. 4.67)

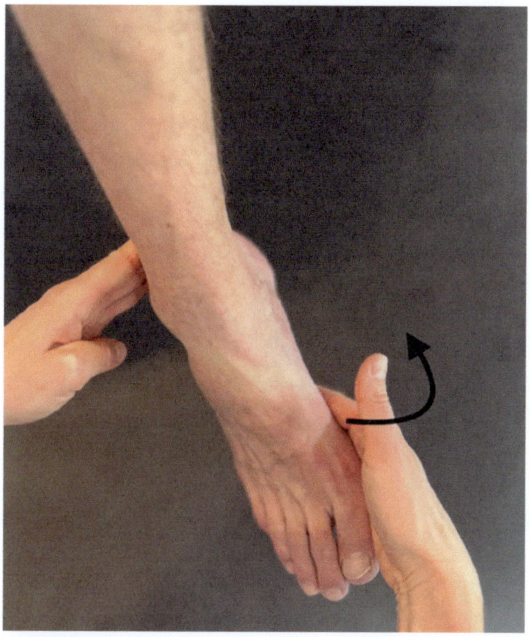

Fig. 4.67 Clinical examination of the peroneus longus muscle: Instruct the patient to evert the foot from a neutral position against resistance (arrow)

Peroneus Brevis/Fibularis Brevis Muscle

Origin: Lateral distal aspect of the fibula

Insertion: Metatarsal bone V

Innervation: Superficial peroneal nerve (L4–S1)

Function: Pronation and eversion; it further assists in plantar flexion

Tibialis Anterior Muscle

Origin: Lateral aspect of the distal third of the tibia

Insertion: Medial cuneiform bone and metatarsal bone I

The superior portion of this muscle overlies the deep peroneus nerve and the anterior tibial artery

Innervation: Deep peroneal nerve (L5–S1)

Function: Serves as the primary dorsiflexor of the foot, contributing also to inversion and weak adduction

Clinical examination: With the toes relaxed to minimize contraction of the extensor hallucis muscle, palpate the muscle belly while the patient performs dorsiflexion (Fig. 4.68)

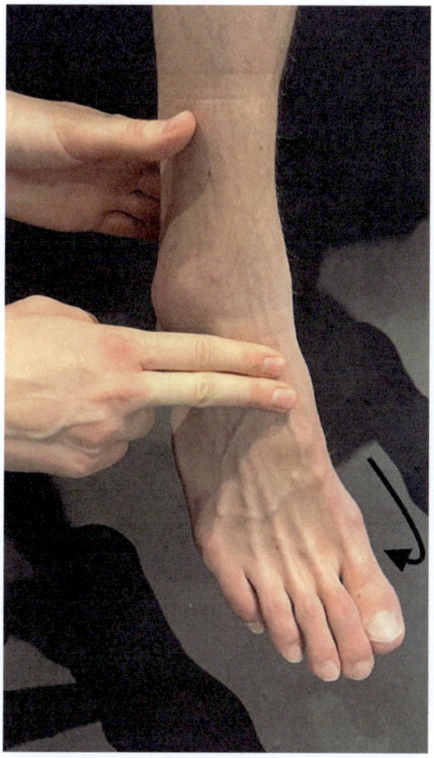

Fig. 4.68 Palpate the tibialis anterior muscle while the patient performs dorsiflexion of the foot with the toes being relaxed

Extensor Digitorum Longus Muscle

Origin: Medial surface of the proximal fibula

Insertion: Middle and distal phalanges II–V

Innervation: Deep peroneal nerve (L5–S1)

Function: Extension of toes II–V, dorsiflexion and eversion of the foot

Clinical examination: Instruct the patient to extend the lesser toes while keeping the hallux relaxed. Ask the patient to perform dorsiflexion and eversion of the foot to assess function of the extensor digitorum longus muscle (Fig. 4.69)

Occasionally, a lateral extension of the flexor digitorum longus muscle inserting onto the fifth metatarsal is present. It is considered as a distinct muscle, being named *peroneus tertius* but other than its neighboring muscle, it is innervated by the *superficial peroneal nerve*. The peroneus tertius muscle contributes to eversion and dorsiflexion of the foot.

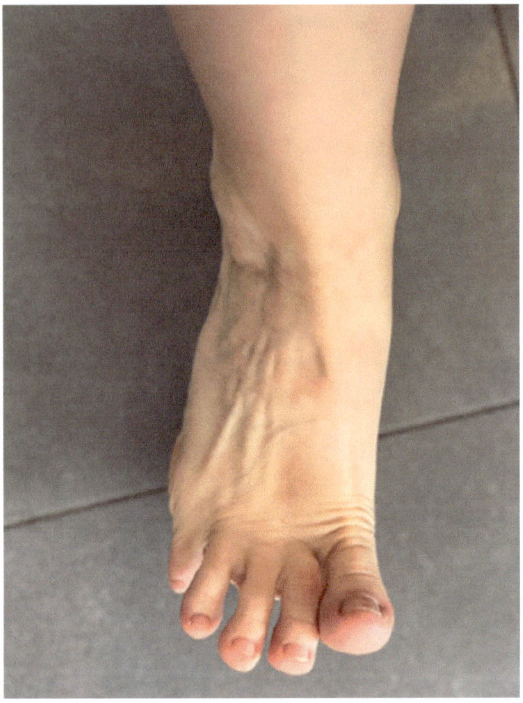

Fig. 4.69 Clinical examination of the extensor digitorum longus muscle: Instruct the patient to extend the lesser toes while performing dorsiflexion and eversion of the foot

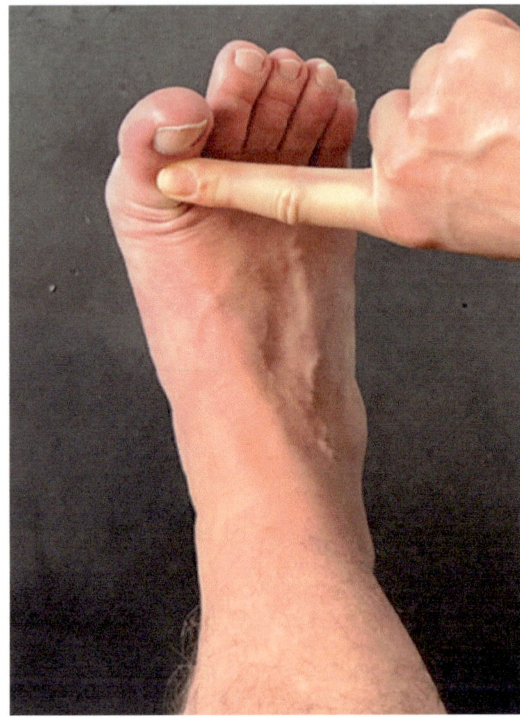

Fig. 4.70 Clinical examination of the extensor hallucis longus muscle: Ask the patient to perform extension of the great toe in combination with dorsiflexion of the foot

Extensor Hallucis Longus Muscle

Origin: Medial surface of the fibula

Insertion: Distal phalanx of the hallux

Innervation: Deep peroneal nerve (L5–S1)

Function: Extension of the toe, and dorsiflexion of the foot

Clinical examination: Extension of the hallux against resistance with concomitant dorsiflexion of the foot (Fig. 4.70)

Extensor Digitorum Brevis Muscle

Origin: Surface of the calcaneus bone

Insertion: Proximal phalanx of the first toe and tendons of the extensor digitorum longus muscle of toes II–IV

Innervation:

Lateral terminal branch of the deep peroneal nerve (L5, S1)

In approximately 20% of the population, an accessory peroneal nerve—a distal branch of the superficial peroneal nerve—may be present and may take over the innervation of the extensor digitorum brevis muscle

Function: Extension of the toes at the metatarsal phalangeal joint

Clinical examination: With the foot placed firmly on the ground, thereby minimizing compensatory activation of adjacent extensor muscles, the patient is instructed to extend the toes

4.3 Overview of the Clinical Examination

Sensibility according to the dermatome

Muscular atrophy is more evident in the smaller muscles

Vegetative symptoms, trophic changes

Back: Inspection (Fig. 4.71)

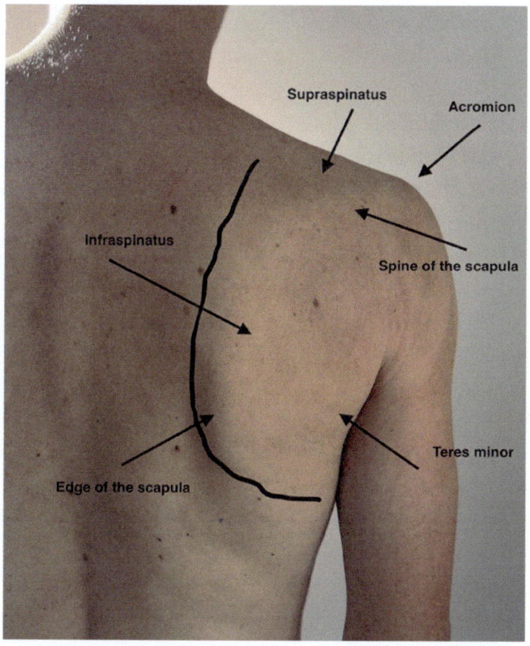

Fig. 4.71 Anatomical image representing the surface anatomy of the muscles at the dorsal aspect of the scapula. The arrows indicate the associated location of each structure on the skin surface

Winging Scapula (Scapula Alata)

- **Medial deviation of the shoulder**:
  Serratus anterior muscle paresis due to long thoracic nerve involvement. It becomes particularly evident during the wall-press test, in which the patient presses the extended and elevated (90°) arm against the wall.
- **Lateral deviation of the shoulder**:
  Rhomboidei muscles paresis due to involvement of the dorsal scapular nerve. It is characterized by lateral displacement of the medial border of the scapula away from the thoracic wall. This finding becomes more prominent when the arm is in abduction.
- **Lateral deviation of the shoulder**:
  Trapezius muscle paresis due to spinal accessory nerve lesion. The medial border of the scapula is displaced laterally from the thoracic wall. No clinical accentuation can be observed when moving the arm.

- **Other causes of scapula alata**:
  Neuralgic shoulder amyotrophy (Parsonage-Turner-Syndrome), limb girdle muscular dystrophy (LGMD), facioscapulohumeral muscular dystrophy (FSHD), oto-facio-cervical syndrome.

Dropped Shoulder

- Axillary nerve lesion (deltoideus muscle)
- Lower cervical radiculopathy
- Lesion of the spinal accessory nerve

Spinal Accessory Nerve CN XI

- Trapezius muscle ➔ To evaluate all three portions of the trapezius muscle, position the patient with the arms elevated to approximately 120° abduction. Standing behind the patient, gently apply anterior pressure to the elbows while observing contraction to the upper, middle, and lower fibers of the trapezius, which act to stabilize the scapula
- Sternocleidomastoid muscle ➔ Instruct the patient to turn the head to the lateral side against resistance

Dorsal Scapular Nerve (C5)

- Levator scapulae muscle ➔ Elevation and backward movement of the shoulder
- Rhomboidei muscles ➔ Backward adduction of the arms

Suprascapular Nerve (C5, C6)

- Subscapular muscle ➔ Lift off test and internal rotation of the humerus
- Teres major muscle ➔ Internal rotation of the humerus

Long Thoracic Nerve (C5–C7)

- Serratus anterior muscle ➔ Ask the patient to push the arm forward like boxing, thereby palpating the dorsal ribs

Shoulder Abduction

- Deltoid muscle (lateral part) ➔ Axillary nerve
- Medial part of the deltoid muscle —if an additional retroposition of shoulder is performed ➔ Axillary nerve
- Anterior part of the deltoid muscle —if the arms are additionally pushed anteriorly ➔ Axillary nerve
- Supraspinatus muscle is assessed by palpating the supraspinatus fossa during abduction ➔ Suprascapular nerve

If arm abduction is preserved but forward flexion (anteflexion) and retroposition are impaired, a lesion of the deltoid muscle should be suspected. This is explained by the fact that abduction of the arm can also be accomplished by the supraspinatus muscle.

External Rotation with Elbow Flexion to 90° and Adduction of the Arm
- Infraspinatus muscle ➔ Suprascapular nerve
- Teres minor muscle ➔ Axillary nerve

Shoulder Adduction with Elbow Flexion to 90° and Adduction of the Arm (C5–T1)
- Pectoral major muscle ➔ Pectoral nerve
- Latissimus dorsi muscle ➔ Thoracodorsal nerve
- Teres major muscle ➔ Thoracodorsal nerve

Elbow Flexion (C5–C7)
- Biceps brachii muscle ➔ Musculocutaneous nerve
- Brachialis muscle ➔ Musculocutaneous and radial nerve
- Brachioradialis muscle (examined with the arm in pronation) ➔ Radial nerve

Elbow Extension (C5–T1)
- Triceps muscle ➔ Radial nerve

Examination of the Hand
Median Nerve
- Flexor carpi radialis muscle ➔ Flexion of the hand (C6, C7)
- Flexor digitorum superficialis muscle ➔ Flexion of the fingers at the MCP joint while maintaining the remaining joints in extension (C8, T1)
- Flexor digitorum profundus muscle (anterior interosseus nerve)* ➔ Flexion of the DIP joint of digit II (C8, T1)
- Flexor pollicis longus muscle (anterior interosseus nerve)* ➔ Flexion of the DIP joint of the thumb

*Ok-sign: Quick examination of the anterior interosseus nerve

- Abductor pollicis brevis muscle ➔ Palmar abduction of the thumb against resistance
- Flexor pollicis brevis muscle ➔ Flexion of the thumb at the MCP joint while maintaining the DIP joint in extension
- Opponens pollicis muscle ➔ Moving the thumb toward digit V
- Lumbrical muscles I–III ➔ Flexion of the fingers at the PIP joint of digit II–V with the MCP joint maintaining in extension

Ulnar Nerve
- Flexor carpi ulnaris muscle ➔ Flexion and ulnar abduction of the wrist
- Palmar and dorsal interossei muscles ➔ Finger spreading (abduction) and bringing them together again (adduction)
- Palmaris brevis muscle ➔ Adduction of digit V with contraction observed at the hypothenar region
- Abductor digiti minimi muscle ➔ Abduction of digit V
- Opponens digiti minimi muscle ➔ OK-sign
- Lumbrical muscles IV–V ➔ Extension of digit IV at the PIP joint while the MCP joint is stabilized

Radial Nerve
- Extensor carpi radialis longus and brevis muscle ➔ Extension and radial abduction of the wrist
- Extensor carpi ulnaris muscle ➔ Extension and ulnar abduction of the wrist
- Extensor digitorum communis muscle ➔ Extension of the fingers at the MCP joint
- Abductor pollicis longus muscle ➔ Abduction of the thumb at the plane of the hand
- Extensor pollicis longus and brevis muscle ➔ Extension of the thumb at the MCP joint and the DIP joint

Standing Position and Gait
- Trendelenburg's sign (dropping of the pelvis when standing on one leg) ➔ Weakness of the gluteus medius and minimus muscle (superior gluteal nerve)
- Foot drop (characterized by a steppage gait) ➔ Usually weakness of anterior tibialis muscle (deep peroneal nerve)

Other causes: Sciatic nerve lesion, common peroneal nerve lesion, L5 nerve root damage (disc herniation)
Rarely: CNS (stroke, tumor), vascular injury

Prone Position

- Gluteus maximus muscle, L5–S2 (inferior gluteal nerve) ➔ Elevating the extended leg against resistance

Supine Position

- Iliopsoas muscle, L1–L3 (femoral nerve) ➔ Flexion of the thigh against resistance

Sitting Position

Adduction of the Hip Against Resistance

- Pectineus muscle, L2, L3 ➔ Femoral and obturator nerve
- Adductor magnus muscle, L2–L4 ➔ Obturator nerve
- Adductor minimus muscle, L2–L4 ➔ Obturator nerve
- Adductor longus muscle, L2–L4 ➔ Obturator nerve
- Adductor brevis muscle, L2–L4 ➔ Obturator nerve

Abduction of the Hip Against Resistance

- Gluteus medius muscle, L4–S2 ➔ Superior gluteal nerve
- Gluteus minimus muscle, L4–S2 ➔ Superior gluteal nerve
- Tensor fascia latae muscle, L4–S2 ➔ Superior gluteal nerve

Knee Flexion Against Resistance

- Hamstring muscles, L4–S3 ➔ Tibial division of the sciatic nerve

Knee Extension Against Resistance

- Quadriceps femoris muscle, L2–L4 ➔ Femoral nerve

Plantar Flexion, Toe Flexion, and Foot Inversion

- Gastrocnemius, L4–S3 ➔ Tibial nerve
- Soleus, L4–S3 ➔ Tibial nerve

Best exanimated with the patient standing on the toes

Foot Inversion Without Toe Flexion

- Tibialis posterior muscle, L4, L5 ➔ Tibial nerve

Flexion of the Toes

- Toe I, L5, S1: Flexor hallucis longus and brevis ➔ Tibial nerve
- Toes II-V: Flexor digitorum longus and brevis ➔ Tibial nerve

Dorsiflexion of the Foot

- Tibialis anterior muscle, L5, S1 ➔ Deep peroneal nerve

Foot Eversion

- Peroneus longus and brevis muscles, L4–S1 ➔ Superficial peroneal nerve

Extension of the Toes and Dorsiflexion of the Foot

- Toe I: Extensor hallucis longus muscle, L5, S1 ➔ Deep peroneal nerve
- Toes II–V: Extensor digitorum longus muscles, L5, S1: Deep peroneal nerve

Further Reading

1. Kretschmer T, editor. Nervenchirurgie: trauma, tumor, kompression. Berlin: Springer; 2014.
2. Russell SM. Examination of peripheral nerve injuries: an anatomical approach. 2nd ed. New York: Thieme; 2015.

3. Popinchalk SP, Schaffer AA. Physical examination of upper extremity compressive neuropathies. Orthop Clin North Am. 2012;43(4):417–30. https://doi.org/10.1016/j.ocl.2012.07.011.
4. Kapandji AI. The clinical evaluation of the upper limb joints' function: back to Hippocrates. Hand Clin. 2003;19(3):379–86. https://doi.org/10.1016/s0749-0712(03)00029-5.
5. Bickley LS. Bates' guide to physical examination and history taking. 12th ed. Lippincott Williams & Wilkins, a Wolters Kluwer business; 2017. https://apn.lwwhealthlibrary.com/book.aspx?bookid=1876&sectionid=0.
6. Geeky Medics. Upper limb neurological examination | OSCE guide | NEW | UKMLA | CPSA | PLAB 2 [Video]. YouTube; 2024. https://www.youtube.com/watch?v=4uAAjYzi7SY.
7. AMBOSS DACH. AMBOSS DE [YouTube channel]. YouTube; 2016. https://www.youtube.com/@ambossDACH/featured.

5 Diagnostic Tools

The principal diagnostic tools for assessing peripheral nerve injuries and neuromuscular disorders include electromyography (EMG), electroneurography (ENoG), nerve sonography, MR-neurography, and intraoperative techniques.

EMG provides qualitative insights into muscle innervation by measuring motor unit action potentials (MUAPs), aiding in differentiation between myopathies and neuropathies, lesion chronicity, and prognosis.

ENoG quantitatively assesses nerve conduction, distinguishing demyelinating from axonal lesions using parameters like conduction velocity, amplitude, and latency. Sensitive neurography offers an enhanced localization and discrimination of pre-versus postganglionic lesions.

Nerve ultrasound is a dynamic, accessible tool capable of visualizing structural nerve changes, including compressions, discontinuities, and tumor-like lesions.

MR-neurography excels at deep-tissue nerve visualization, grading nerve injury, and differentiating tumor types using contrast and signal patterns.

Intraoperative diagnostics, including direct nerve stimulation and nerve action potentials (NAPs), assist in evaluating nerve continuity and guiding surgical decisions. Collectively, these tools offer complementary data crucial for precise diagnosis, prognosis, and therapeutic planning in peripheral nerve pathologies.

5.1 Electromyography, EMG

Electromyography (**EMG**) assesses the electrical activity of a muscle in response to stimulation of its corresponding nerve using thin needle electrodes. The effective recording radius is approximately 2.5 mm, providing a localized qualitative assessment of the muscle (only a small part of the muscle is measured). It can be used to differentiate between *neuropathy* and *myopathy*.

It further represents a helpful tool for evaluating a potential reinnervation after peripheral nerve lesions (Figs. 5.7 and 5.8).

Additionally, it may tell us a lot about the prognosis, the age, or the localization of a possible lesion (nerve, nerve root, or systemic disease).

EMG can further differentiate between an axonal lesion and conduction blocks, as well as between complete and incomplete lesions— distinctions that are not always clinically apparent.

For identifying whether a lesion is acute or chronic, we use the *motor unit action potential* (MUAP) of the EMG.

MUAP: Upon entering the muscle, each motor neuron divides into multiple terminal branches, with each branch forming a motor end plate, that innervates an individual muscle fiber. Consequently, a single action potential in

K. Hobitsch, *Peripheral Nerve Surgery - A Compendium*,
https://doi.org/10.1007/978-3-032-03409-0_5

a motor neuron induces depolarization in all the muscle fibers of its motor unit (Figs. 5.1, 5.2 and 5.3).

The sum of these depolarizations can be detected on the EMG. The size of the amplitude thereby correlates with the number of innervated muscle fibers.

Myopathy
- No/barely spontaneous activity
- Potentials are low and shortened
- Small amplitude due to the decreased size of motor units

Neuropathy
- Pathological spontaneous activity due to loss of inhibition with positive waves and fibrillation on the EMG; potentials are high and prolonged
- High amplitude despite the decreased size of the motor unit as the remaining motor units are bigger due to compensatory hypertrophy which leads to a higher amplitude

Fibrillations (clinically not visible) are only present in neuropathy, whereas *fasciculations* (clinically visible) can be seen in both, neuropathy and myopathy [9].

Nerve lesion:

- Functional muscle weakness (paresis) if ≥50% of axons are damaged
- Detection of the EMG if ≥10% of axons are damaged [2, 3]
- Main finding for denervation: Fibrillations and sharp positive waves, which are a sign of pathological spontaneous activity (Figs. 5.4, 5.5, and 5.6)

> Detectable 14 days after injury and can be still seen 20 years later! They are therefore not useable as a prognostic tool!

Immediately after nerve injury, the EMG recordings distal to the lesion may appear normal. With the onset of Wallerian degeneration, which occurs between 3–9 days post-injury, electrophysiological changes become detectable, typically emerging 10–14 days after the lesion [4].

A conduction block can be differentiated from an axonal injury after 7–10 days in the EMG.

Spontaneous EMG activity, such as fibrillation potentials or fasciculations, is typically rhythmic, whereas volitional muscle activity is irregular and non-rhythmic.

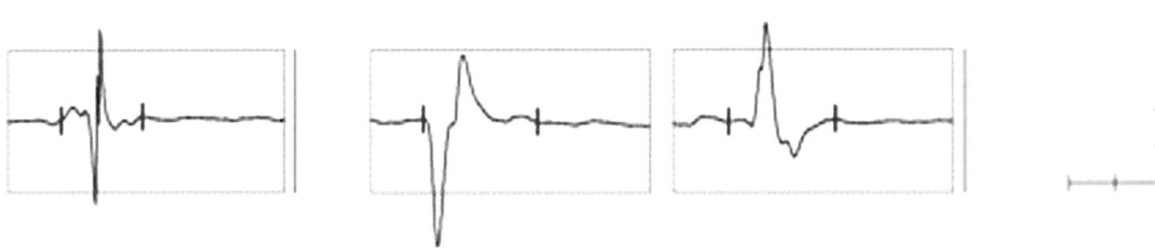

Fig. 5.1 Electromyography (EMG) signals showing normal muscle activity (MUAP) for the right peroneus longus muscle (left) and the right extensor digitorum braves muscle (right)

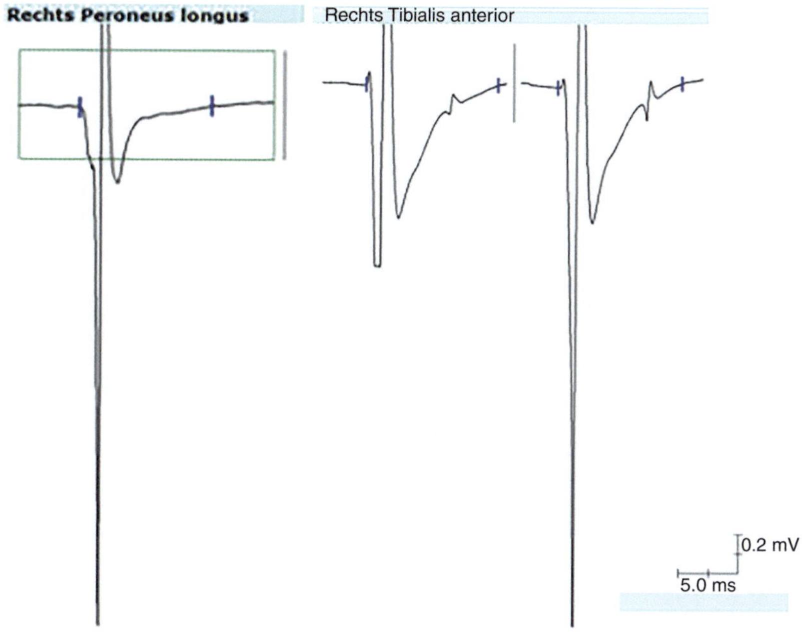

Figs. 5.2 and 5.3 Chronic neurogenic MUAPs in a 67 years old patient with an axonal lesion of the right common peroneus nerve. The potentials are >7 mV. The figures show the MUAPs of the right peroneus longus muscle (left) and the right anterior tibialis muscle (right)

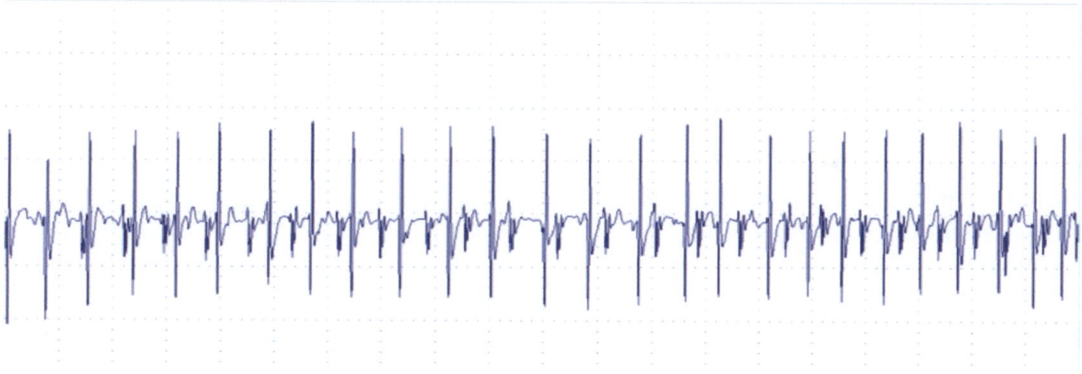

Fig. 5.4 With maximal innervation, sparse discharges with an increased discharge rate (26/s) in an incomplete axonotmesis of the tibialis anterior muscle in a 67 years old male patient

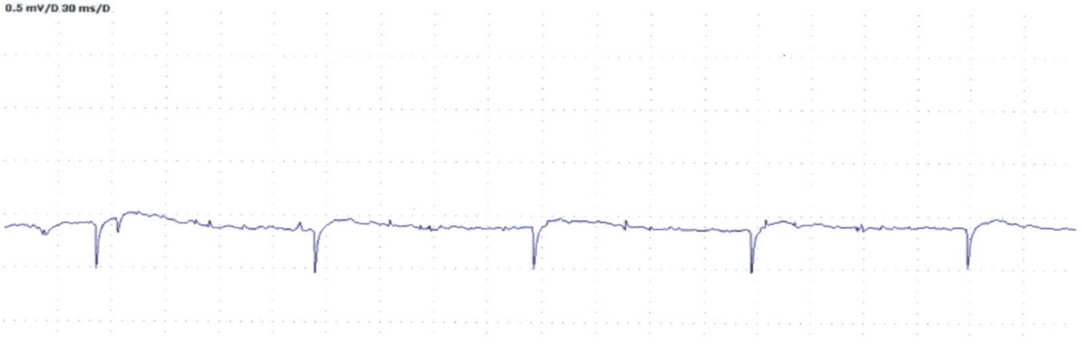

Fig. 5.5 Pathological spontaneous activity: Positive sharp waves of the right tibialis anterior muscle in axonal damage of the common peroneal nerve over the fibular head in a 67 years old male patient

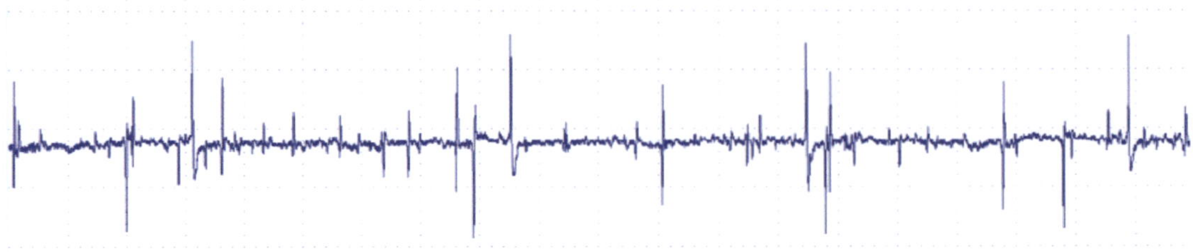

Fig. 5.6 Pathological spontaneous activity: Fibrillation potentials of the right tibialis anterior muscle in axonal damage of the common peroneal nerve over the fibular head in a 67 years old male patient

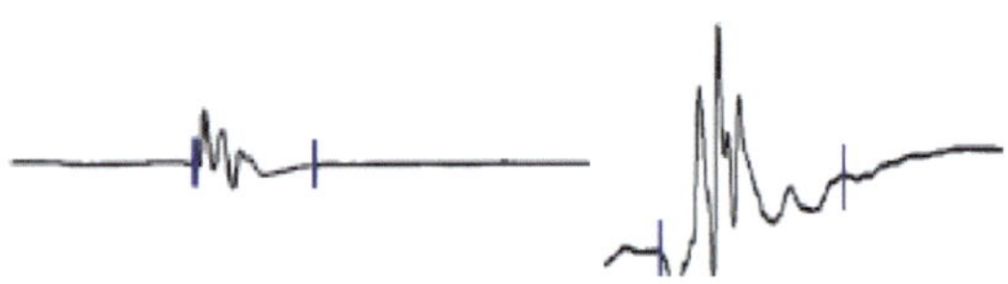

Figs. 5.7 and 5.8 Reinnervation of the left extensor digitorum brevis muscle in a traumatic distal axonal injury of the deep peroneal nerve at the ankle observed in a 57 years old male patient

5.2 Electroneurography, ENoG

As its name suggests, **electroneurography (ENoG)** evaluates the nerve itself. This technique involves stimulating the nerve at two distinct points and recording the response using surface electrodes. ENoG allows measurement of key parameters including conduction velocity, amplitude, and the latency of the action potential:

Conduction velocity (CV) ➔ Reduced in cases of demyelination, conduction block, muscular disease or atrophy, neuromuscular transmission disorder (e.g., myasthenia gravis, relaxation medication), or as a result of measuring errors

A conduction block clinically results in paresis and is classically caused by compression injury

Amplitude ➔ Reduced in cases of axonal lesion, as the amplitude level corresponds to number of conducting fibers

Motor latency ➔ Defines the time between stimulation and muscular response

Measurements should always be performed on both sides of the body. Differences of ≥50% between sides are considered significant. In general, side-to-side comparisons within the same individual provide more reliable diagnostic information than comparisons with population-based normal values.

Consider that the measured conduction velocity reflects the fastest-conducting nerve fiber within the examined section of the nerve.

Motor neurography represents a method of applying the electrode over a muscle, thereby detecting the compound muscle action potential (CMP) of a nerve at different locations. It is used for the following:

- Nerve entrapment lesions, polyneuropathy
- To differentiate between conduction block and axonal lesion, which is possible after approximately 1 week following nerve lesion
- Lesion of the myelin sheath (reduced conduction velocity) versus axonal lesion (reduced amplitude)

Conduction velocity measured proximal and distal to the lesion is typically normal in neurapraxia. Disturbances are confined to the site of injury and are generally reversible.

In axonal lesions, a reduction in amplitude is observed (axonotmesis and neurotmesis) within the first 7–10 days due to Wallerian degeneration.

Clinically and neurophysiologically, it is not possible to distinguish between axonotmesis and neurotmesis.

Stimulation proximal to a lesion results in decreased amplitude or potentials across all measured sides.

It is not possible to differentiate between a conduction block and an axonal lesion on nerve conduction studies alone. EMG is required, which will reveal pathological spontaneous activity after approximately 14 days in the case of an axonal lesion.

If nerve compression is present, remodeling processes of the myelin sheaths occur without loss of axons. Electrophysiologically, a decreased conduction velocity is detectable (Figs. 5.9, 5.10, and 5.11).

Sensitive neurography evaluates **sensitive nerve action potentials (SNAP)**, and can be performed in either an orthodromic or antidromic direction.

In orthodromic studies, the innervated skin region is stimulated, and the SNAP is recorded proximally along the corresponding nerve.

Antidromic measurement is based on the direct stimulation of a nerve, and the detection of the SNAP distal to the nerve in the dermatome-related region.

There is no difference between latency and conduction velocity in orthodromic versus antidromic neurography. The only difference is a smaller amplitude when using surface electrodes in the orthodromic measurement versus the antidromic technique [17].

The **amplitude** defines the sum of electrical activity of all stimulated sensitive nerve fibers.

The advantage of sensitive nerve conduction velocity over motor neurography is the possibility of performing stimulation not only between a proximal and a distal point of a certain nerve, but also between the nerve and its corresponding targeted organ or dermatome. This can be explained by the fact that a "sensitive end plate" does not exist, unlike in motor neurography (motor end plate).

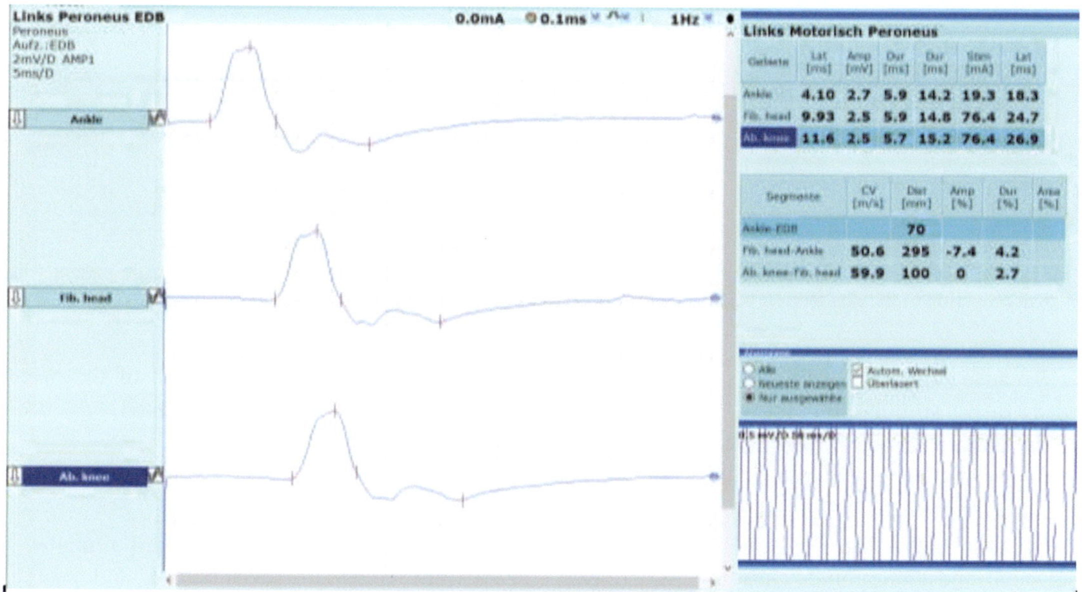

Fig. 5.9 Graphical representation demonstrating normal conduction velocity of the left common peroneal nerve in a 22 years old female patient

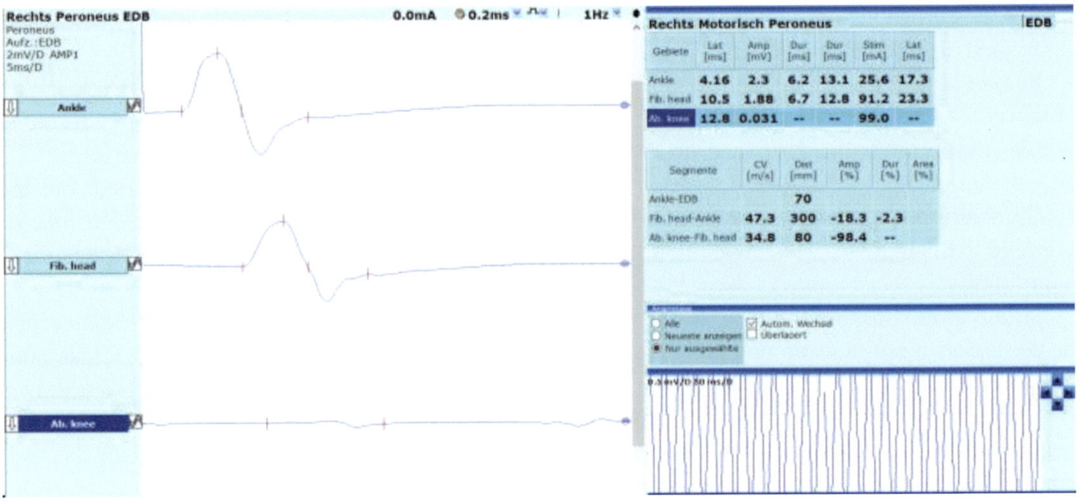

Fig. 5.10 Incomplete conduction block (neurapraxia) of the right common peroneal nerve in a 22 years old female patient

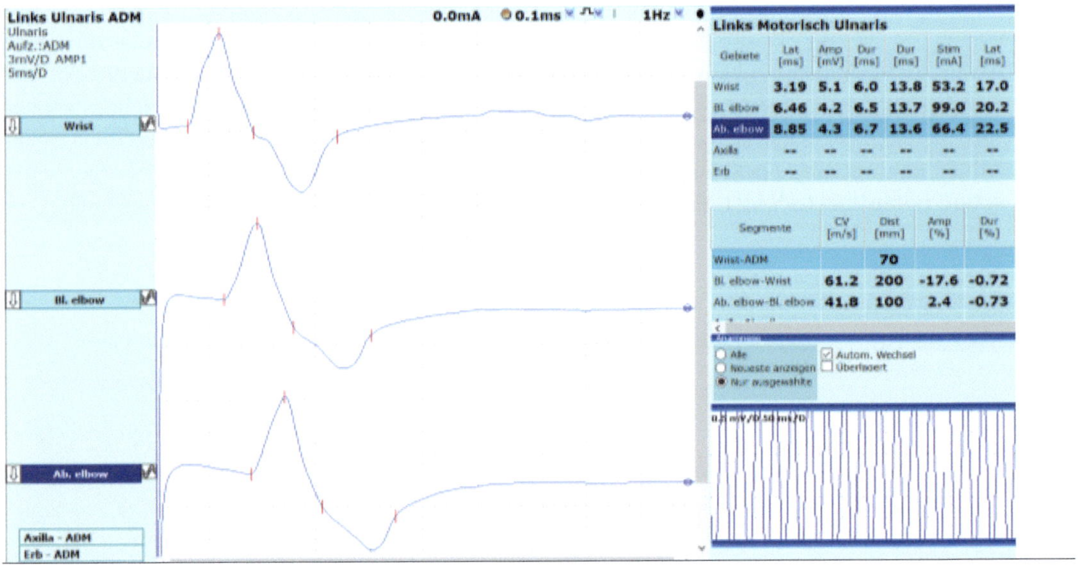

Fig. 5.11 Segmental demyelination of the left ulnar nerve at the cubital tunnel in a 52 years old female patient with evident reduction of the conduction velocity at the cubital tunnel

Because only one location along the nerve needs direct stimulation—the second point can be the targeted organ itself—sensitive neurography provides an improved accuracy in detecting distal lesions.

Another advantage is the differentiation between postganglionic lesions (decreased amplitude) and preganglionic lesions or root avulsion, where a decrease in the amplitude does not occur as only the central part of the pseudounipolar ganglionic cells is affected.

> Sensitive neurography can differentiate between brachial plexus lesion and root avulsion!

When there is a long distance between the side of stimulation and detection, the amplitude of the SNAP may decrease.

Note, that there might occur a clinical regeneration that may not be visible in neurographic measurements yet.

Somatosensory evoked potentials (SEPs, SSEPs) should also be mentioned, as they have a raison d'être in cases of axonal lesioning when SNAP cannot be measured.

The reason why SEPs work, is not clearly understood yet, but the central intensifier mechanism might be a possible explanation [18].

They are applied to observe the regeneration progress after a surgical treatment of a nerve injury as they are detected far earlier than SNAPs.

An absent regeneration is only present when both—SEPs and SNAPs—are not measurable.

To sum up, in axonal lesions, the distribution pattern in the EMG changes are pivotal for the localization of the nerve damage. The additional use of a neurography will detect diminished or even completely dropped amplitudes in all locations of stimulation, independent from the side of lesion. A motor neurography is therefore not possible, whereas the sensitive neurography can be used to differentiate between a radicular (sensitive potentials are preserved) and a peripheral lesion.

Electromyography (EMG) can detect signs of muscle reinnervation earlier than clinical examination. While electrophysiological evidence of reinnervation indicates ongoing recovery, the further course will be the progressive reinnervation and follow ups are unnecessary as the expected results of repeated electrophysiological studies will be obvious. Clinical monitoring remains essential, as functional recovery depends not only on reinnervation, but also on the restoration of sufficient muscle strength to support normal activity.

5.3 Nerve Sonography

The **ultrasound** represents an effective, accessible and cost-efficient tool, that provides both dynamic and structural information about nerves.

In patients with normal body habitus, almost all peripheral nerves—including small digital nerves—and portions of the brachial plexus can be visualized.

Ultrasound complements clinical examination and electrophysiological studies in the assessment of peripheral nerve pathology.

High-frequency probes, typically in a hockey-stick shape with frequencies around 10 MHz (range 8–18) are commonly used.

Ultrasound imaging relies on sound waves to create an image of the desired area. Tissues with higher acustic impedance, such as bones, appear hyperechoic (bright), whereas fluid-filled or softer structures appear hypoechoic (dark) (Fig. 5.19).

Nerves can be depicted in two axes, on an axial plane (cross-sectional) and on a sagittal plane (longitudinal) [21].

For nerve identification, anatomical landmarks should be used, as nerves typically run along bony or muscular borders. In axial section, the nerve has a "honeycomb appearance" while they are looking like a "bundle of straight lines" when depicting them longitudinally; due to the hyperechoic epineurium and perineurium. The hypoechoic areas are represented by the nerve fascicles [22] (Fig. 5.12).

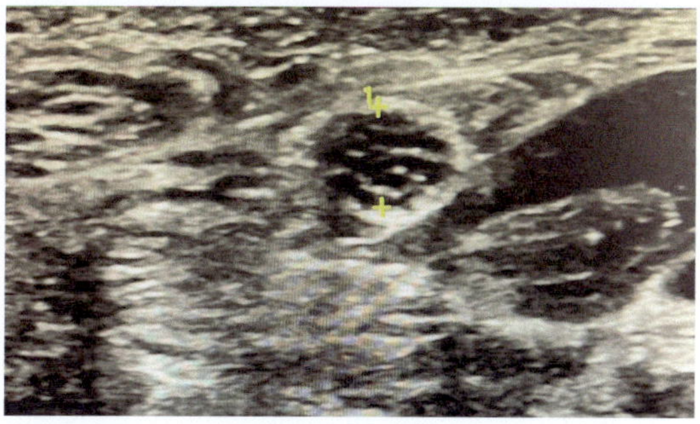

Fig. 5.12 Ultrasound image showing the cross section of a normal median nerve and its fascicles

With the use of ultrasound, a lot of pathologies can be identified—the constitution of the nerve itself (in continuity or transected, edema, or flattened), scars, and compressing structures such as tumors or foreign bodies.

Hints to Differentiate a Nerve from Other Structures:

- **Nerves** always have an interfascicular course arising from the depth and running towards the surface. They have a low anisotropy compared to tendons or muscles, which means that their echogenicity does not significantly change when tilting the transducer.
- **Tendons** are moving when moving the limb. They have a high anisotropy.
- **Vessels** can be identified when applying the Doppler imaging or by observing them collapsing when applying pressure [21].

It should be noted, that the differentiation between **arteries** and **veins** on Doppler ultrasonography is not determined by color coding (red representing flow towards the transducer and blue representing flow away from the transducer), but rather on the presence or absence of **pulsatility**. Arteries are identified by their characteristic pulsatile flow pattern, whereas veins demonstrate non-pulsatile flow.

- **Lymph nodes** are having a spherical form with a fatty hilum surrounding it.

While electrophysiological studies cannot distinguish between axonotmesis and neurotmesis in acute peripheral nerve injuries, high-resolution nerve ultrasound can provide valuable diagnostic information, potentially enabling earlier therapeutic decision-making [28].

Ultrasonographic indicators of nerve injury include hypoechogenicity, enlargement of the affected nerve, nervous structures, distension, and partial or complete discontinuity. A dehiscent gap may be visualized with or without associated hematoma or scar tissue, and nerve compression or displacement may also be observed.

Acute nerve injuries are characterized by increased intraneural vascularity, whereas chronic lesions demonstrate heightened intraneural and perineural echogenicity.

For the the quantification of nerve enlargement, reference values have been published; however these values vary considerably across literature. Furthermore, nerve values are influenced by patient-specific factors including sex, age, and body weight [27].

The cross-sectional area (CSA) ratio, which compares the nerve diameter at two anatomical sites, can serve as an indicator for focal nerve enlargement. For example, an increased median nerve CSA ratio at the wrist relative to the forearm may suggest median nerve swelling at the carpal tunnel susceptive for a carpal tunnel syndrome.

Secondary muscular changes such as edema in the acute phase or atrophy in the chronic stages may further support the diagnosis of nerve injury.

In the case of nerve compression, following changes can be observed:

- Flattening of the nervous structure at the compression site (Fig. 5.13)
- Thickened nerve proximal to the compression (intraneural swelling and venous congestion). In a sagittal plane, the nerve has an hour-glass or fusiform appearance (Fig. 5.15)
- Sudden change of the caliber ("notch sign")
- Homogenous hypoechogenic nerve structure (due to swollen fascicles) (Figs. 5.14 and 5.16)
- Intraneural hyperemia on the Doppler ultrasound

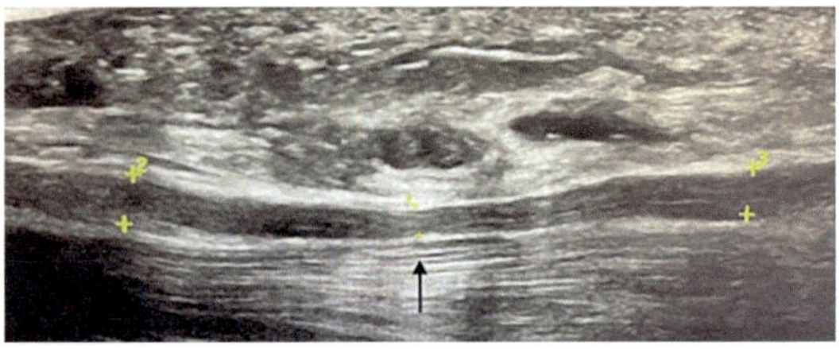

Fig. 5.13 Median nerve in carpal tunnel syndrome: The median nerve is flattened by the flexor retinaculum (arrow)

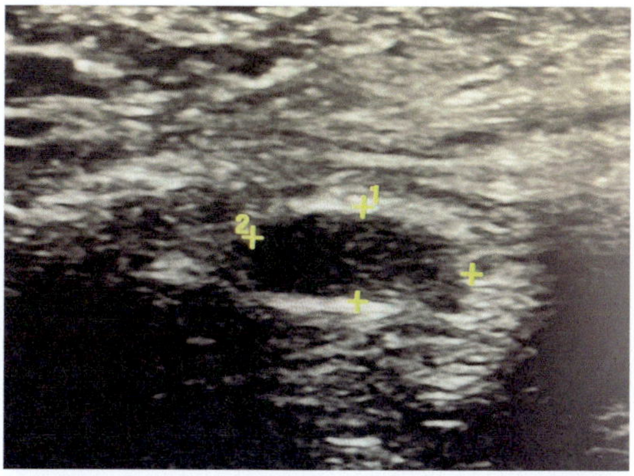

Fig. 5.14 Cross section of the median nerve in carpal tunnel syndrome. The nerve structures have a homogenous hypoechogenic appearance

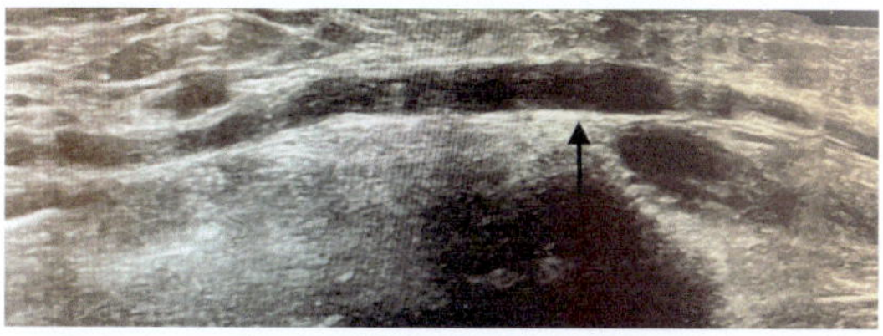

Fig. 5.15 Thickening of the ulnar nerve prior to the compression site at the cubital tunnel due to intraneural swelling and venous congestion (arrow)

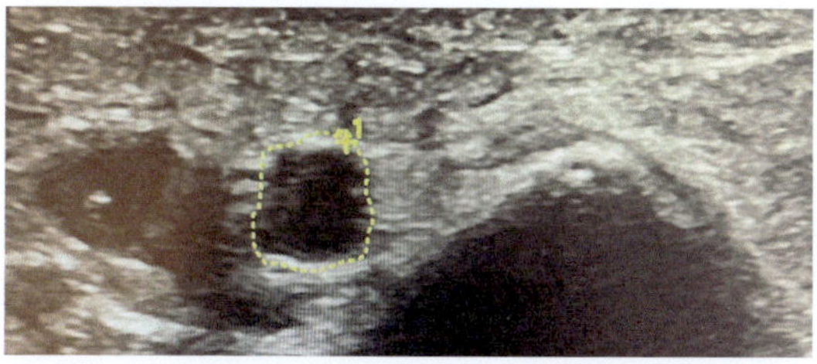

Fig. 5.16 Cross-sectional ultrasonographic image of the ulnar nerve in cubital tunnel syndrome. The nerve demonstrates a homogenous hypoechogenic appearance

Ultrasound may also be employed in the postoperative setting to identify potential complications. Normal postoperative findings following nerve repair include suture-related artifacts, edema, and small fluid collections.

Pathological changes include dehiscence, loss of continuity of the fascicles, intraneural fluid retention, and the presence of a neuroma [21] (Fig. 5.17).

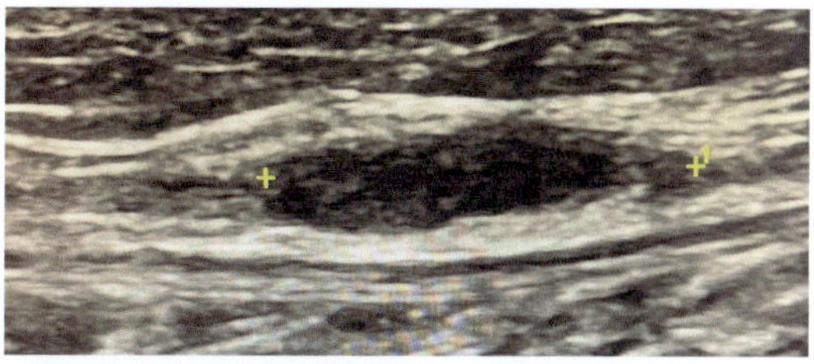

Fig. 5.17 Longitudinal ultrasonographic view of the sural nerve demonstrating a post-surgical neuroma following varicose vein stripping

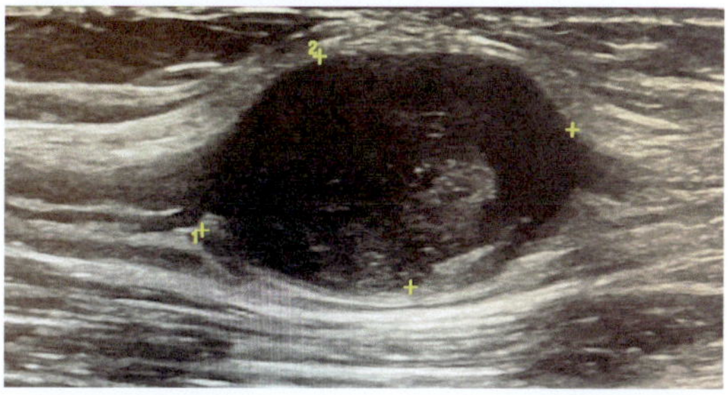

Fig. 5.18 Longitudinal ultrasonographic view of the median nerve demonstrating a schwannoma

For sonographic visualization of the brachial plexus, the common carotid artery and internal jugular vein should first be identified. The transverse process of the seventh cervical vertebra (C7)— distinguished by the absence of an anterior tubercle—serves as a key anatomical landmark. By angling the probe laterally, the anterior and medial scalene muscles can be delineated, with the brachial plexus appearing between them as a cluster resembling a "bunch of grapes".

When the ultrasound examination is performed with the patient's arm in abduction or external rotation, compressive masses may be revealed, raising suspicion for thoracic outlet syndrome (TOS). However, definitive diagnosis of TOS remains challenging due to the limited image projection caused by the overlying clavicle [29].

Schwannomas typically present as well-defined, homogenous, hypoechoic, oval-shaped lesions, positioned eccentrically along a nerve fascicle. Continuity of a fascicle entering and exiting the schwannoma may often be visualized (Fig. 5.18).

Differentiation between schwannomas and neurofibromas can be difficult. Neurofibromas, however, more commonly demonstrate a spindle-shaped morphology with loss of the normal fascicular pattern.

Malignant peripheral nerve tumors (MPNST) are typically characterized by poorly defined margins and variable morphology. The presence of sudden-onset pain combined with rapid tumor growth raises suspicion for a malignant peripheral nerve sheath tumor.

Intratumoral cystic or regressive changes may further indicate malignancy, as these features often reflect tissue destruction or necrosis resulting tumor growth outpacing neovascularization. An exception to this rule is the ancient schwannoma, a benign peripheral nerve sheath tumor that may also demonstrate regressive changes.

Morton's neuroma, by contrast, does not represent a true neoplasm. It develops as a consequence of chronic compression and repeated microtrauma of the plantar digital nerve, often associated with poor footwear. On ultrasound, Morton's neuroma typically appears as a hypoechoic mass, most commonly located within the second and third intermetatarsal space.

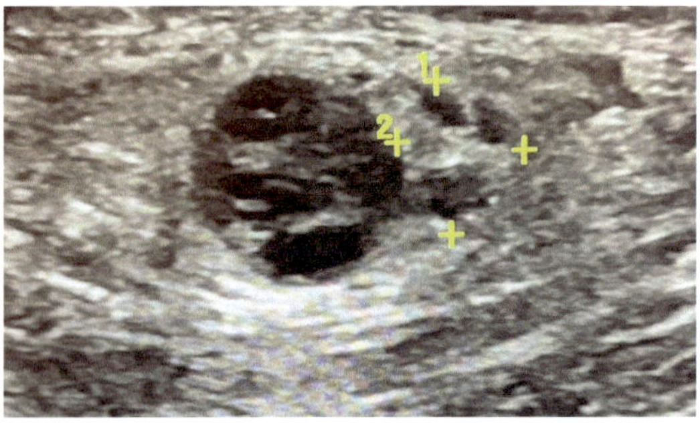

Fig. 5.19 Ultrasonographic image representing a popliteal cyst compressing the peroneal nerve (yellow)

5.4 MR-Neurography

The principle advantage of **magnetic resonance imaging** (**MRI**) over the aforementioned diagnostic modalities lies in its ability to precisely localize nerve lesions while providing a pain-free examination. In contrast to nerve sonography, the MR neurography allows for the visualization of deeper located nervous structures. Even small peripheral nerve branches, and, in some cases, individual fascicles can be identified (Fig. 5.20).

Depending on the imaging protocol and the examiner's expertise, MRI may also permit differentiation of the severity and extent of nerve injury.

Furthermore, the administration of contrast agents enhances lesion characterization and facilitates the differentiation of tumors.

> Signal enhancement of the nerve in the T2-weighted sequence represents the most important and sensitive criterion for a lesion.

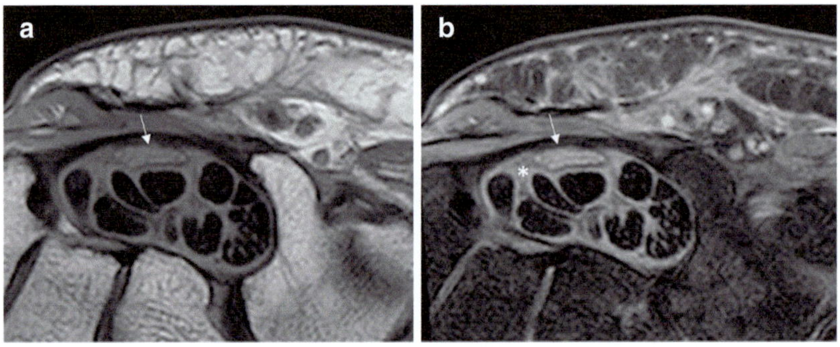

Fig. 5.20 Normal median nerve within the carpal tunnel in the setting of mild soft tissue inflammation (asterisk). The median nerve (arrows) exhibits a fascicular pattern and appears isointense to muscle on axial PD (**a**), while on PD-SPAIR (**b**), it demonstrates mildly increased fascicular signal intensity corresponding to the amount of endoneurial fluid. The endoneurium, perineurium, and epineurium structurally organize each nerve into a fascicular structure, which can be visualized on MRI and is referred to as the fascicular pattern. PD: Protron Density, PD-SPAIR: Proton Density Spectral Adiabatic Inversion Recovery

Peripheral nerve tumors classically present as spherical or oval masses, appearing homogenous and isointense relative to muscle in T1-weighted sequences and hyperintense in T2-weighted sequences.

Features suggestive for malignancy include larger size (>5 cm) with ill-defined margins, heterogenous structure, and signal intensity in the presence of necrosis. Infiltration of the adjacent structures as well as perilesional edema are additional signs.

Characteristic MRI-findings for specific peripheral nerve sheath tumors and nerve injury include:

- **Neurofibroma**: Central contrast enhancement with "target sign" (a hyperintense lesion with a central hypointense focus on T2-weighted images) or the "tail sign" (a continuity of the involved fascicle entering and exiting the tumor).
- **Schwannoma**: A hyperintense margin on T2-weighted images, marked enhancement after the administration of gadolinium, and increased signal intensity on STIR sequences. Additional features include the "fascicle sign" (multiple small ring-like structures within the lesion), and the "split-fat sign" (a thin rim of surrounding fat encasing the tumor) (Figs. 5.21 and 5.22).

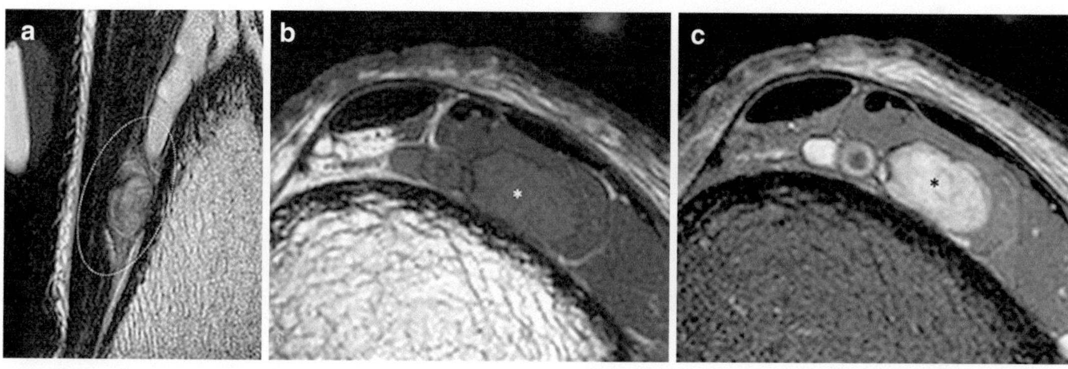

Fig. 5.21 Schwannoma of the deep peroneal nerve at the ankle demonstrates a fusiform focal enlargement in sagittal T2 (**a**) and axial T1 (**b**) plane. The lesion shows a homogeneous high signal on axial PD-SPIR (**c**)

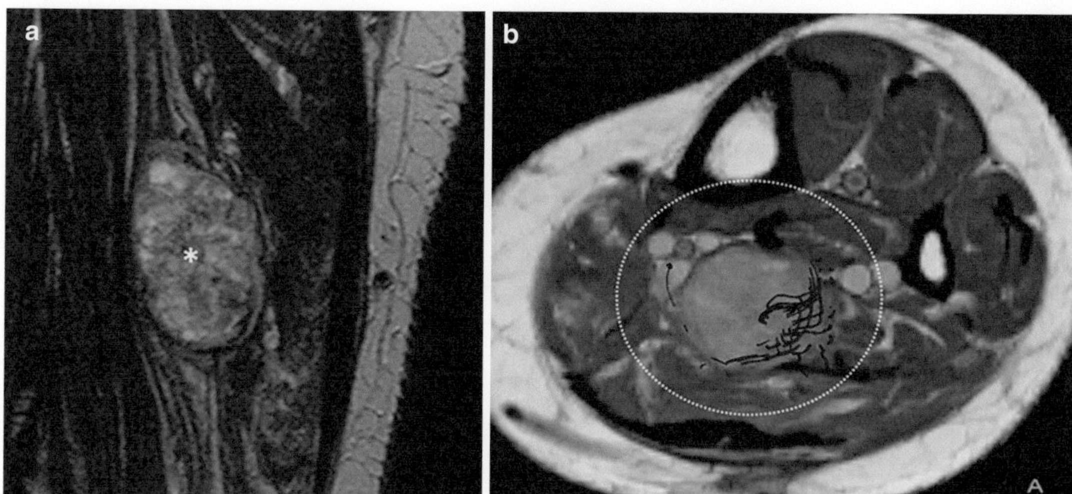

Fig. 5.22 Schwannoma of the tibial nerve (asterix) appears to be in continuity and eccentrically located in sagittal T2 (**a**). In the axial DTT (**b**) plane, the fascicles are displaced (dotted circle)

- **MPNST versus infection**: Differentiation may be challenging, however, MPNSTs typically demonstrate marked contrast enhancement, vascularization and intralesional necrosis.
- **Infection versus perineurioma**: Infectious processes are usually characterized by a strong T2-weighted signal.
- **Nerve compression**: Classically presents as a focal signal reduction at the compression site with proximal and distal nerve flattening. The affected nerve is often edematous and exhibits strong T2-weighted hyperintensity.
- **Nerve injury**:

  Neurapraxia generally does not exhibit characteristic imaging findings (Fig. 5.23).

  Axonotmesis—depending on severity—may present with swelling, intact but edematous fascicles and occasionally a neuroma-in-continuity (Fig. 5.24).

  Neurotmesis typically demonstrates a transected nerve, occasionally with formation of an end-bulb neuroma (Figs. 5.25, and 5.26).

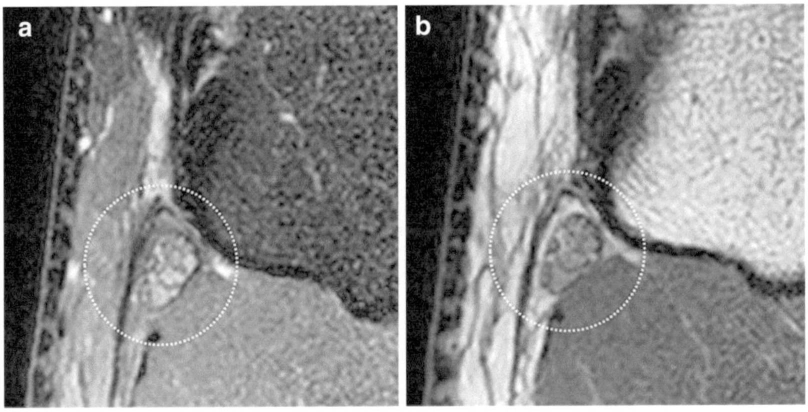

Fig. 5.23 Neurapraxia: Peroneal nerve at the fibular-head level (dotted circles in **a** and **b**), exhibiting a normal fascicular pattern with mildly increased signal intensity in some fascicles. The perineural gliding tissue and the fascia show normal anatomy as well as signal intensity. The muscles (not shown) did not present signs of denervation

Fig. 5.24 Axonotmesis: Neuroma in continuity of the radial nerve prior to its entry into the spiral groove (**a**—coronal T2). Focal nerve thickening is observed (arrows and dotted circle) with partial loss of the fascicular pattern (**b**). On the axial PD-SPAIR image (**c**), fascicles maintaining continuity are still visible (arrowhead)

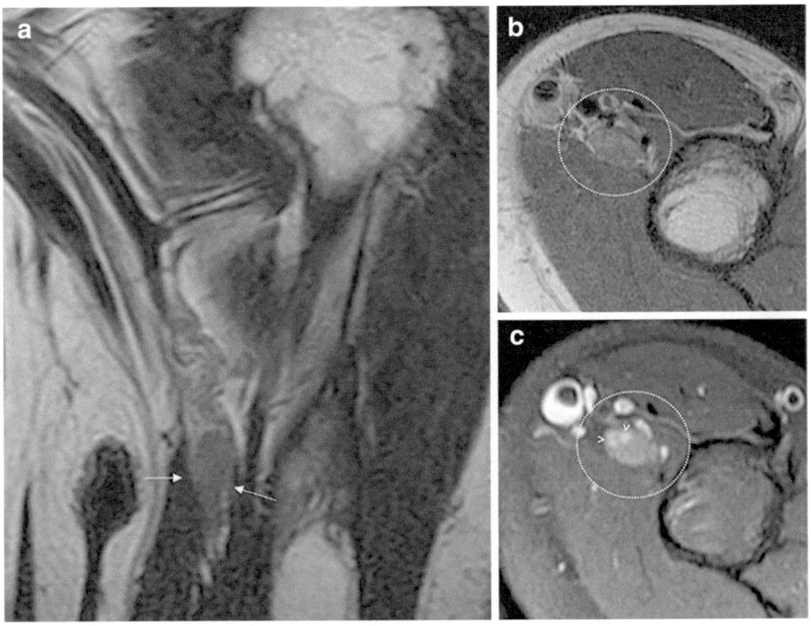

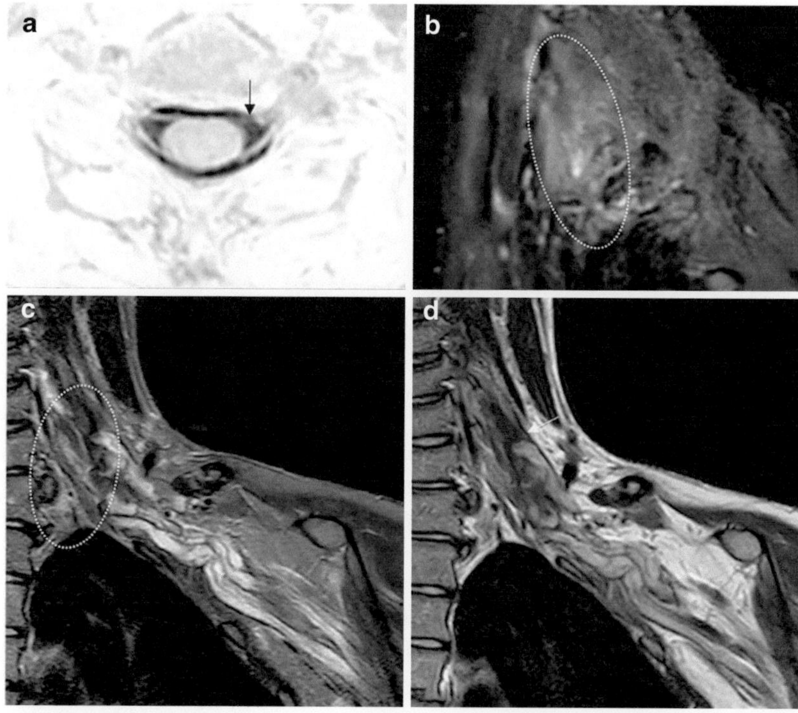

Fig. 5.25 Neurotmesis: Traumatic brachial plexus injury. Axial 3D-DRIVE (**a**) shows partial anterior avulsion of a nerve root (arrow). Sagittal STIR (**b**), coronal STIR (**c**), and coronal T2 (**d**) demonstrate rupture of the trunks of the brachial plexus. (**c**) also shows the distal stump of the superior trunk covered by fibrous tissue (arrow)

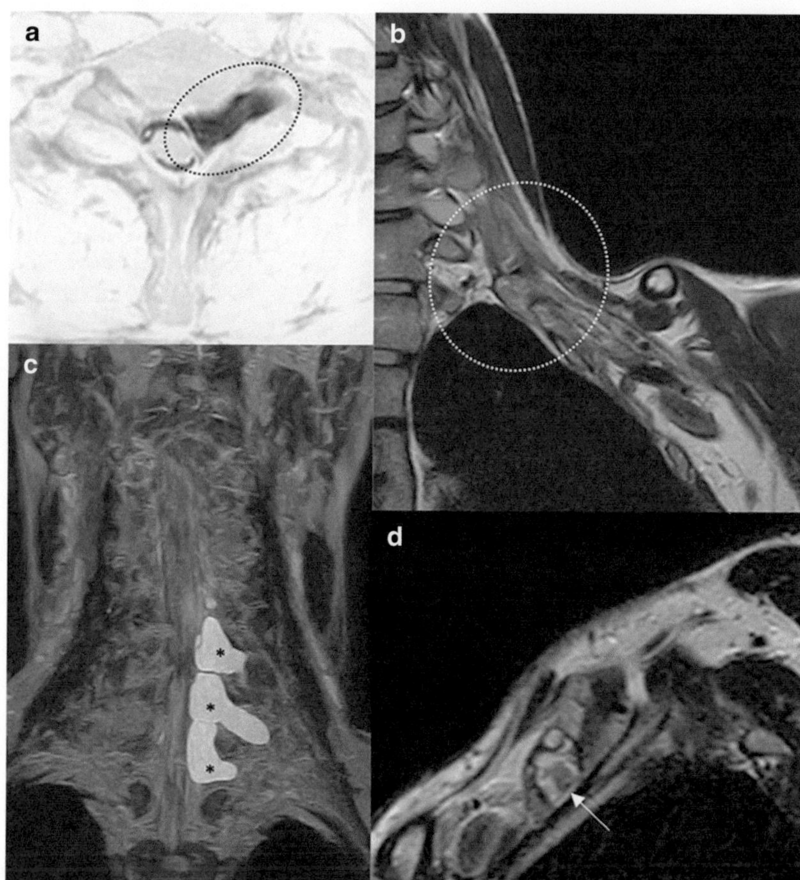

Fig. 5.26 Neurotmesis: Traumatic brachial plexus injury. Axial 3D-DRIVE (**a**) and coronal Myelographic Reconstruction (**b**) show pseudomeningocele formation (dotted circle and asterisks) associated with rupture of the trunks (Coronal T2—**c**). Sagittal T2 (**d**) demonstrates a terminal neuroma of the inferior trunk (arrow)

Preganglionic nerve lesions—findings:

- Direct signs ➔ Partial or complete root avulsion

  Indirect signs ➔

  - Muscle denervation, edema (within the first 24 h)
  - Pseudomeningocele (within the first 3–4 weeks)
  - Intradural fibrosis and scarring, spinal cord displacement (chronic stage)

Postganglionic nerve lesions—findings:

- Loss of fat planes
- Focal or diffuse nerve enlargement, enhanced signal intensity, diminished fascicular pattern, changes in the trajectory of the nerve
- Muscle denervation

Regarding the structure of the muscles, edema is seen in acute injury, whereas fatty infiltration and atrophy represents a sign of chronic injury (Fig. 5.27).

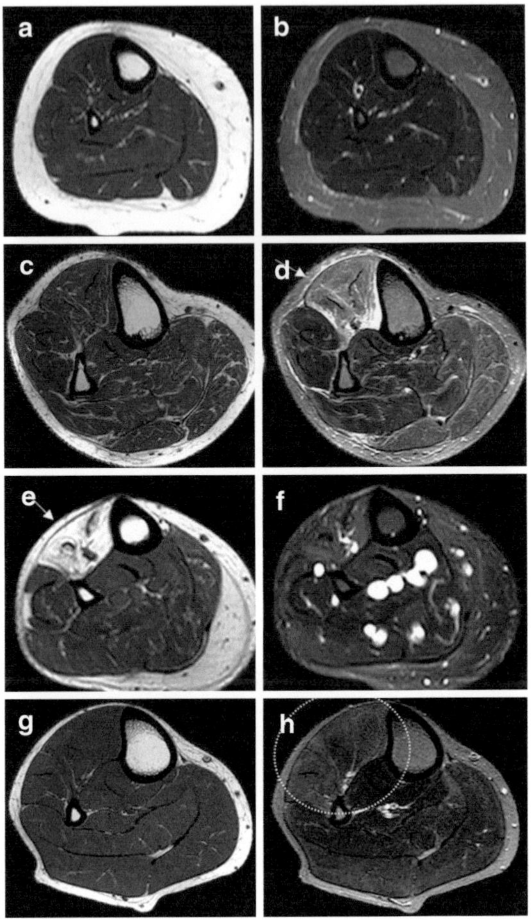

Fig. 5.27 Muscle-MRI: Normal skeletal muscle typically demonstrates intermediate to low signal intensity on T1 sequences (**a**) and low signal intensity on STIR (**b**) sequences. (**c**, **d**) show acute dennervation, (**e**, **f**) chronic dennervation, and (**g**, **h**) reinnervation. Note the changes in signal intensity, initially the muscle shows increased signal intensity on STIR, the mechanism is not completely understood but appears likely to reflect shifting of water from intracellular to extracellular spaces. If innervation is restored, the MR imaging findings slowly return to normal (**g**, **h**). If reinnervation does not take place fatty infiltration develops and is seen as increased signal on T1 sequences. Axial T1 (**a**, **c**, **e**, **g**) and axial STIR (**b**, **d**, **f**, **h**). PD-SPAIR: Proton Density Spectral Adiabatic Inversion Recovery

5.5 Intraoperative Diagnostic Tools

- **Direct nerve stimulation** provides information regarding both the anatomical location and the structural integrity of the nerve (e.g. determining whether the nerve is in continuity). It also serves as valuable intraoperative mapping tool.
- The assessment of **nerve action potentials (NAP)** can confirm nerve continuity. Stimulation is applied proximal to the lesion, with recording obtained distally.
  A measurable NAP indicates favorable prognosis for regeneration. Conversely, absence of a NAP at 3–4 months post trauma suggests poor recovery potential, and surgical intervention such as resection or reconstruction is generally indicated [40].
- **Motor evoked potentials (MEP)** allow differentiation between motor and sensitive fascicles and, in some cases, between individual fascicles within a nerve. This is particularly relevant during reconstructive procedures such as the Oberlin transfer, where accurate identification of fascicles within the ulnar nerve innervating the flexor carpi ulnaris muscle is critical.
- **Intraoperative electromyography (EMG)** involves placing recording needles into the target muscle while stimulating the nerve. The fascicle producing the highest amplitude response in the monitored muscle can be identified. This technique is frequently applied in surgical procedures such as the C7 nerve transfer.

5.6 Overview of the Diagnostic Tools

EMG

Denervation is characterized by pathological spontaneous activity on the EMG in the absence of voluntary motor activity.

Regarding advanced muscle atrophy, in cases where regeneration is no longer possible, spontaneous pathological activity is absent.

An early baseline EMG should be performed with follow-up studies recommended at four-week intervals.

Reinnervation can be detected electrophysiologically before clinical improvement becomes apparent.

Electromyography (EMG) or Conduction Velocity (CV)?

- Nerve entrapment syndrome ➔ CV
- Extend of injury ➔ CV/EMG
- Are other nerves involved? ➔ CV (EMG)
- Isolated or generalized nerve injury? ➔ CV (EMG)
- Acute versus chronic ➔ EMG
- Prognostic assessment ➔ CV/EMG
- Injured structure (axon versus myelin sheath) ➔ EMG (CV)
- Localization (plexus injury versus root avulsion injury) ➔ EMG/CV

MRI

Nerve imaging can detect intrinsic changes such as edema, loss of continuity, and neuroma formation; as well as secondary findings including denervation edema and muscle atrophy. It is particularly advantageous for visualization deeper nerves, surpassing the capabilities of other imaging modalities.

Sonography

High resolution sonography is capable of detecting even intradural changes, and has the advantage of not projecting artefacts due to metal implants, unlike MRI.

Mild injury (neurapraxia): No or minimal sonographic abnormalities

Moderate injury (axonotmesis): Diffuse nerve injury, intact but edematous fascicles, and partial fascicular discontinuity, which may manifest as a continuity neuroma

Severe injury (neurotmesis): Complete fascicular discontinuity, often associated with the formation of a stump neuroma

The ultrasound as well as the MRI both constitute a reliable diagnostic tool in depicting peripheral nerves.

Due to its accessibility, dynamic image display, its high spatial resolution and cost effectivity, the ultrasound should be used as a primary diagnostic device.

The MRI can be applied additionally as it is superior regarding deep located structures and contrast resolution. It furthermore gives more detailed information about the adjacent structures.

Further Reading

1. Novello BJ, Pobre T. Electrodiagnostic evaluation of peripheral neuropathy. In: StatPearls. StatPearls Publishing; 2023.
2. Oh SJ. Electromyographic studies in peripheral nerve injuries. South Med J. 1976;69(2):177–82. https://doi.org/10.1097/00007611-197602000-00015.
3. Jürgens TP, Puchner C, Schulte-Mattler WJ. Discharge rates in electromyography distinguish early between peripheral and central paresis. Muscle Nerve. 2012;46(4):591–3. https://doi.org/10.1002/mus.23453.
4. Chaudhry V, Cornblath DR. Wallerian degeneration in human nerves: serial electrophysiological studies. Muscle Nerve. 1992;15(6):687–93. https://doi.org/10.1002/mus.880150610.
5. Chung T, Prasad K, Lloyd TE. Peripheral neuropathy: clinical and electrophysiological considerations. Neuroimaging Clin N Am. 2014;24(1):49–65. https://doi.org/10.1016/j.nic.2013.03.023.
6. Kretschmer T, editor. Nervenchirurgie: trauma, tumor, kompression. Berlin: Springer; 2014.
7. Shanina E, Smith RG. Electrodiagnostic evaluation of myopathy. In: StatPearls. StatPearls Publishing; 2022.
8. Aminoff MJ. Chapter 11 – Clinical electromyography. In: Aminoff MJ, editor. Aminoff's electrodiagnosis in clinical neurology. 6th ed. W.B. Saunders; 2012. p. 233–59. https://doi.org/10.1016/B978-1-4557-0308-1.00011-X.
9. Pillen S, van Alfen N, Zwarts MJ. Chapter 3 – Ultrasound of muscle. In: Walker FO, Cartwright MS, editors. Neuromuscular ultrasound. W.B. Saunders; 2011. p. 37–56. https://doi.org/10.1016/B978-1-4377-1527-9.10003-8.
10. Müller-Vahl H, et al. Läsionen peripherer Nerven und radikuläre Syndrome. 2014. https://doi.org/10.1055/b-0034-97220.
11. Dy CJ, Colorado BS, Landau AJ, Brogan DM. Interpretation of electrodiagnostic studies: how to apply it to the practice of orthopaedic surgery. J Am Acad Orthop Surg. 2021;29(13):e646–54. https://doi.org/10.5435/JAAOS-D-20-00322.
12. Walsh ME, Sloane LB, Fischer KE, Austad SN, Richardson A, Van Remmen H. Use of nerve conduction velocity to assess peripheral nerve health in aging mice. J Gerontol A Biol Sci Med Sci. 2015;70(11):1312–9. https://doi.org/10.1093/gerona/glu208.
13. Tavee J. Chapter 14 – Nerve conduction studies: basic concepts. In: Levin KH, Chauvel P, editors. Handbook of clinical neurology, vol. 160. Elsevier; 2019. p. 217–24. https://doi.org/10.1016/B978-0-444-64032-1.00014-X.
14. Sorenson EJ. Sensory nerve conduction studies: sensory nerve action potentials. In: Clinical neurophysiology, Contemporary neurology series. 4th ed. Oxford Academic; 2016. https://doi.org/10.1093/med/9780190259631.003.0018.
15. Bischoff C, Schulte-Mattler W. Methodik der Neurografie – motorische und sensible Neurografie. Neurol Up2date. 2019;2(2):115–24. https://doi.org/10.1055/a-0881-6592.
16. Synek VM, Cowan JC. Somatosensory evoked potentials in patients with supraclavicular brachial plexus injuries. Neurology. 1982;32(12):1347–52. https://doi.org/10.1212/wnl.32.12.1347.
17. Bischoff C, et al. Referenz-Reihe Neurologie: Methoden: EMG NLG. 2008. p. 15–7. https://doi.org/10.1055/b-0034-32459.
18. Sugioka H. Evoked potentials in the investigation of traumatic lesions of the peripheral nerve and the brachial plexus. Clin Orthop Relat Res. 1984;(184):85–92.
19. Buchner H, Noth J, editors. Evozierte Potenziale, Neurovegetative Diagnostik, Okulographie: Methodik und klinische Anwendungen. Georg Thieme Verlag; 2005. https://doi.org/10.1055/b-0034-25648.
20. Calma AD, Triplett J, Vucic S, Yiannikas C. Somatosensory evoked potentials: technique, interpretation and clinical applications. Pract Neurol. Advance online publication. 2024. https://doi.org/10.1136/pn-2024-004179.
21. Gonzalez NL, Hobson-Webb LD. Neuromuscular ultrasound in clinical practice: a review. Clin Neurophysiol Pract. 2019;4:148–63. https://doi.org/10.1016/j.cnp.2019.04.006.
22. Lawande AD, Warrier SS, Joshi MS. Role of ultrasound in evaluation of peripheral nerves. Indian J Radiol Imaging. 2014;24(3):254–8. https://doi.org/10.4103/0971-3026.137037.
23. Fowler JR, Munsch M, Tosti R, Hagberg WC, Imbriglia JE. Comparison of ultrasound and electrodiagnostic testing for diagnosis of carpal tunnel syndrome: study using a validated clinical tool as the reference standard. J Bone Joint Surg. 2014;96(17):e148. https://doi.org/10.2106/JBJS.M.01250.
24. Mallouhi A, Pülzl P, Trieb T, Piza H, Bodner G. Predictors of carpal tunnel syndrome: accuracy of gray-scale and color Doppler sonography. AJR

Am J Roentgenol. 2006;186(5):1240–5. https://doi.org/10.2214/AJR.04.1715.
25. Nakamichi K, Tachibana S. Restricted motion of the median nerve in carpal tunnel syndrome. J Hand Surg Br. 1995;20(4):460–4. https://doi.org/10.1016/s0266-7681(05)80153-6.
26. Padua L, Di Pasquale A, Liotta G, Granata G, Pazzaglia C, Erra C, Briani C, Coraci D, De Franco P, Antonini G, Martinoli C. Ultrasound as a useful tool in the diagnosis and management of traumatic nerve lesions. Clin Neurophysiol. 2013;124(6):1237–43. https://doi.org/10.1016/j.clinph.2012.10.024.
27. Kerasnoudis A, Pitarokoili K, Behrendt V, Gold R, Yoon MS. Cross sectional area reference values for sonography of peripheral nerves and brachial plexus. Clin Neurophysiol. 2013;124(9):1881–8. https://doi.org/10.1016/j.clinph.2013.03.007.
28. Tagliafico A, Altafini L, Garello I, Marchetti A, Gennaro S, Martinoli C. Traumatic neuropathies: spectrum of imaging findings and postoperative assessment. Semin Musculoskelet Radiol. 2010;14(5):512–22. https://doi.org/10.1055/s-0030-1268071.
29. Demondion X, Herbinet P, Boutry N, Fontaine C, Francke JP, Cotten A. Sonographic mapping of the normal brachial plexus. AJNR Am J Neuroradiol. 2003;24(7):1303–9.
30. Gruber H, Loizides A, Moriggl B. Nervensonografie kompakt: Anatomie der peripheren Nerven mit Landmarks. Springer; 2018. https://doi.org/10.1007/978-3-662-56754-8.
31. Suk JI, Walker FO, Cartwright MS. Ultrasonography of peripheral nerves. Curr Neurol Neurosci Rep. 2013;13(2):328. https://doi.org/10.1007/s11910-012-0328-x.
32. Peer S, Kovacs P, Harpf C, Bodner G. High-resolution sonography of lower extremity peripheral nerves: anatomic correlation and spectrum of disease. J Ultrasound Med. 2002;21(3):315–22. https://doi.org/10.7863/jum.2002.21.3.315.
33. Kele H. Ultrasonography of the peripheral nervous system. Pers Med. 2012;1:417–21.
34. Howe FA, Filler AG, Bell BA, Griffiths JR. Magnetic resonance neurography. Magn Reson Med. 1992;28(2):328–38. https://doi.org/10.1002/mrm.1910280215.
35. Chhabra A, Andreisek G, Soldatos T, Wang KC, Flammang AJ, Belzberg AJ, Carrino JA. MR neurography: past, present, and future. AJR Am J Roentgenol. 2011;197(3):583–91. https://doi.org/10.2214/AJR.10.6012.
36. Binaghi D. MR imaging of the elbow. Magn Reson Imaging Clin N Am. 2015;23(3):427–40. https://doi.org/10.1016/j.mric.2015.04.005.
37. Wein S, Ashraf A, Patel M, et al. Schwannoma. Radiopaedia.org; 2012. https://doi.org/10.53347/rID-19575.
38. Nelson KR. Use of peripheral nerve action potentials for intraoperative monitoring. Neurol Clin. 1988;6(4):917–33. https://doi.org/10.1016/S0733-8619(18)30850-8.
39. Burg D, Infanger M, Meuli-Simmen C, et al. Methods, indications and validation of intraoperative nerve conductivity testing. Handchir Mikrochir Plast Chir. 2002;34(1):3–16. Georg Thieme Verlag Stuttgart, New York. ISSN 0722-1819.
40. Robert EG, Happel LT, Kline DG. Intraoperative nerve action potential recordings: technical considerations, problems, and pitfalls. Neurosurgery. 2009;65(4 Suppl):A97–A104. https://doi.org/10.1227/01.NEU.0000347473.67188.75.

6 Surgery (Techniques, Spasticity and Neuroplasticity)

Peripheral nerve surgery offers a broad and effective array of techniques to restore motor and sensory function following nerve injury, based on the regenerative potential of axons. Unlike central nervous system injuries such as spinal cord lesions, peripheral nerve injuries—particularly postganglionic lesions—can benefit from spontaneous regeneration or postsurgical recovery. This chapter outlines essential surgical strategies, ranging from decompression and neurolysis to neurorrhaphy and nerve grafting, with an emphasis on anatomical precision and functional recovery.

Advanced techniques such as nerve transfers (neurotization) are pivotal when primary repair or grafting is unfeasible, especially in cases of root avulsion or extensive lesion involving all spinal nerves of the brachial plexus. These procedures rely on selecting functional redundant donor nerves to reinnervate vital distal targets, guided by principles of axonal sprouting, cortical plasticity, and functional compatibility. Complementary approaches, including tendon and muscle transfers, serve as effective alternatives when nerve reconstruction is delayed or non-viable. Regarding spasticity management, selective peripheral denervation, and contralateral C7 transfers represent promising surgical interventions to relieve pain and improve mobility.

Crucially, the success of these interventions hinges not only on surgical technique but also on the capacity of the central nervous system for neuroplastic reorganization. Factors influencing neuroplasticity—such as timing, age, cortical representation, and rehabilitation—play a decisive role in functional outcomes. This chapter underscores the necessity of a tailored, multimodal approach in peripheral nerve surgery, balancing anatomical, functional, and neurophysiological insights to achieve optimal patient recovery.

The ability to receive functional recovery in peripheral nerve surgery, even after complete lesion, as opposed to spinal cord injury, is due to the fact that regeneration occurs at the level of axons rather than the neurons.

Differentiation in Nerve Injury

- *Preganglionic injury (root avulsion):*
  No spontaneous recovery, surgery is always indicated

- *Postganglionic injury:*
  Axonotmesis ➔
  In brachial plexus lesions especially by traction injury
  In lumbar plexus lesions especially by compression injury (bone displacement)

Neurotmesis ➔ Commonly seen in sharp wounds

K. Hobitsch, *Peripheral Nerve Surgery - A Compendium*,
https://doi.org/10.1007/978-3-032-03409-0_6

Clinical Significance of Preganglionic Lesions:

- Disturbances in the vasomotor and sudomotor systems (interruption of the sympathetic fibers)
- Horner syndrome (interruption of the sympathetic fibers)
- Diaphragmatic lesions (phrenic nerve palsy)
- Scapular winging (weakness of serratus anterior or rhomboid muscles)
- Scoliosis (cervical muscle weakness)

> In patients with chronic brachial plexus injury, it is essential to assess both passive joint mobility and the condition of the overlying skin, including any defects or impaired wound healing.

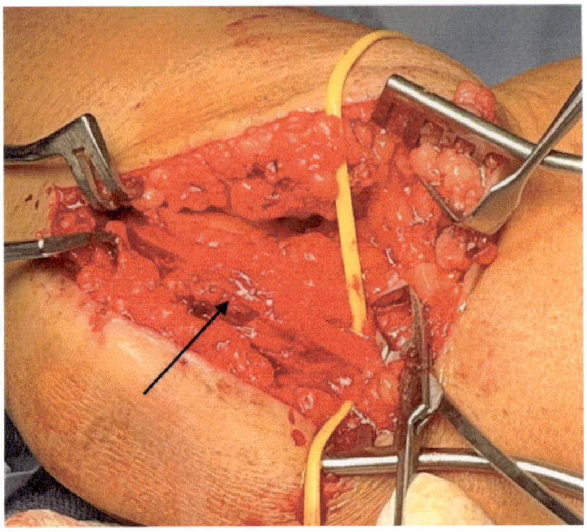

Fig. 6.1 Intraoperative picture showing the ulnar nerve (arrow) after decompression at the cubital tunnel

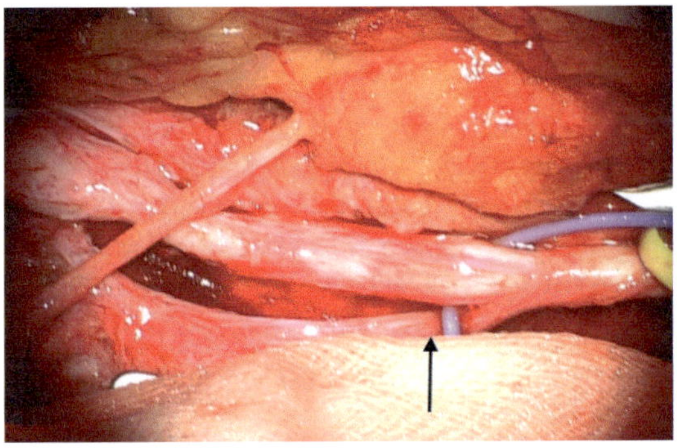

Fig. 6.2 Intraoperative picture showing interfascicular neurolyisis of the ulnar nerve (arrow). The fascicles are separated by a loop

6.1 Surgical Techniques

Note, that peripheral nerve surgery requires anesthesia without muscle relaxants, typically achieved with **total intravenous anesthesia** (**TIVA**), to allow for intraoperative monitoring and/or stimulation.

Decompression

Decompression refers to the surgical release of pressure on a nerve. The compressive structures may include bone (e.g. post-fracture), hypertrophied muscles, vessels, implants, or scar tissue. In nerve entrapment pathologies, this surgical technique is typically sufficient to alleviate symptoms (Fig. 6.1).

Neurolysis

Freeing a nerve from fibrosis and scar tissue along its entire circumference represents a surgical technique known as neurolysis.

Neurolysis can be performed either externally—at the level of the epineurium—or internally, in case of intraneural scarring, partial injuries, tumors, and spasticity.

An example of external neurolysis is the management of perineuriomas, where opening of the epineurium for decompression without resection may be sufficient to preserve nerve function.

Internal neurolysis, also referred to as endoneurolysis or interfascicular neurolysis, involves surgical exposure of individual fascicles through careful opening of the epineurium (Fig. 6.2).

Neurorrhaphy

Neurorrhaphy is defined as the direct repair of a transected nerve via suturing the severed ends, also knows as nerve coaptation.

> Anastomosis is the direct suture of vessels, not of nerves!

Direct nerve repair can be achieved either by end-to-end or end-to-side coaptation.

End-to-end coaptation is performed in cases of nerve lacerations or following neuroma resection. This technique is feasible when a tension-free suture can be achieved, typically in short gaps, provided that a healthy proximal stump is available and the two nerve ends are properly aligned (Fig. 6.3).

> **Moderate nerve tension** is beneficial for axonal regeneration as it promotes nerve growth. **Insufficient tension** may delay regeneration as axonal sprouting must traverse a longer distance. **Excessive tension**, however, increases the risk of suture rupture.

In blunt injuries, neuroma formation typically occurs within approximately three weeks. Neuromas are commonly a consequence of trauma and are more frequently observed in small cutaneous nerves.

The end-to-side suture represents an alternative technique for intraoperative situations in which the proximal stump of the lesioned nerve is not available or the gap between the proximal and the distal stump is too large. Clinical outcomes with this technique have been shown to be comparable to those achieved with end-to-end nerve coaptation [4].

The mechanism of regeneration is based on collateral sprouting.

A key advantage of this approach is that the donor nerve retains its original function, avoiding any functional sacrifice [3].

Epineural nerve coaptation involves suturing only the epineurium, typically requiring 4–6 stitches, whereas fascicular nerve coaptation entails repair of the individual fascicles with precise suture placement.

The Concept of Axonal Sprouting

Even after sacrificing a nerve branch to serve as a donor for transfer, collateral sprouting from the remaining branches can occur. Through this process, new fascicles may assume the function of the sacrificed branch, allowing nerve transfer to be performed without resulting in weakness or functional loss.

The precise mechanisms underlying axonal collateral sprouting are not yet fully understood; however, it is known to be induced by the uninjured axons in response to Wallerian degeneration [7, 8].

Under normal conditions, Schwann cells and myelin-associated proteins inhibit axonal growth by forming a physical and molecular barrier. Following end-to-side coaptation, this inhibitatory barrier can be disrupted, thereby enabling collateral sprouting [9].

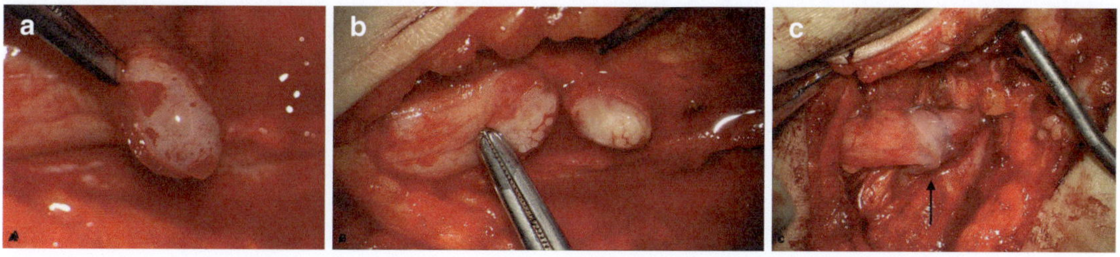

Fig. 6.3 Nerve stump with indistinct nerve fascicles due to scar tissue (**a**) after iatrogenic transection of the peroneal nerve during vein stripping. (**b**) shows the two nerve stumps with the nerve fascicle being clearly visible after cutting back the nerve to remove the scar tissue. A direct end-to-end coaptation is then performed (**c**) and fibrin glue is applied on the aligned nerve stumps for further support (arrow)

Nerve Repair Via Graft

Autologous nerve grafts harvested from sensory nerves are used to bridge large nerve gaps when direct coaptation is not feasible. This technique requires the presence of both proximal and distal stumps. The graft serves as a conduit, guiding axonal sprouting from the proximal stump toward the distal target. It is essential, that neither stump contains residual neuroma or fibrotic tissue, as these can impede direct axonal regeneration.

> It is preferable to use a nerve graft rather than performing direct coaptation under tension. Clinical outcomes with nerve reconstruction with grafts are comparable to those of neurorrhaphy performed under tension.

When the distal nerve stump is already divided into its terminal branches, multiple grafts are required for reconstruction of each branch. This technique is referred to as *cable grafting* [14]. The number of grafts that can be used to bridge the different terminal branches is limited by the diameter of the proximal nerve. Cable grafting is a widely used surgical technique in facial nerve lesion, where multiple nerve branches need to be reconstructed.

In theory, vascularized nerve grafts provide superior outcomes; [15] however, their use is generally not feasible in clinical practice.

Various graft types are available including autografts, allografts (cadaver nerves), and nerve conduits (biological or synthetic). Allografts are generally limited to gaps of less than 5 cm, due to their restrictive regenerative potential, whereas nerve conduits are suitable only for gaps shorter than 3 cm [16, 17].

Autografts remain the standard choice, as they are readily available and do not require extensive processing.

Harvesting sensitive nerves for grafting does not cause motor deficits, and the resulting sensory loss is typically minor because of the nerve's segmental distribution and overlapping innervation (Fig. 6.4).

Frequently Used Transplants:

- **Sural nerve**: This nerve contains a large number of fascicles, making it a reliable option for grafting. With a length of approximately 30–40 cm, it can be used to bridge multiple nerve gaps or it can be taken double to match the diameter of the injured nerve.
- Saphenous nerve
- Medial and lateral cutaneous antebrachial nerves
- Lateral cutaneous nerve of the thigh
- Femoral nerve branches
- Greater auricular nerve

Harvesting a nerve graft can be done either digitally or with the assistance of a nerve-stripper. After extirpation, the proximal stump is commonly infiltrated with ropivacaine to reduce the risk of postoperative neuropathic pain.

The graft is then secured to the proximal and distal nerve stumps using minimal microsutures, typically taking 10–0 suture, and may be supplemented with fibrin glue. Alternatively, fixation with fibrin glue alone is possible.

Contrary to previous assumptions, there is no need to orient the graft in an antidromic fashion to prevent misrouting of axonal sprouts. Recent studies indicate that nerve regeneration outcomes do not differ significantly between antidromic and orthodromic orientation [21].

Split Repair

In certain cases, only specific fascicles within a lesioned nerve are affected by neuroma or scar tissue. Prior to resecting the nerve—for example, to remove a neuroma—it is essential to identify functioning fascicles, using intraoperative direct stimulation, and preserve them. These intact fascicles continue to propagate action potentials distally. Only the nonfunctional, affected fascicles are resected and bridged with a nerve graft. This surgical technique is referred to as split repair (Fig. 6.5).

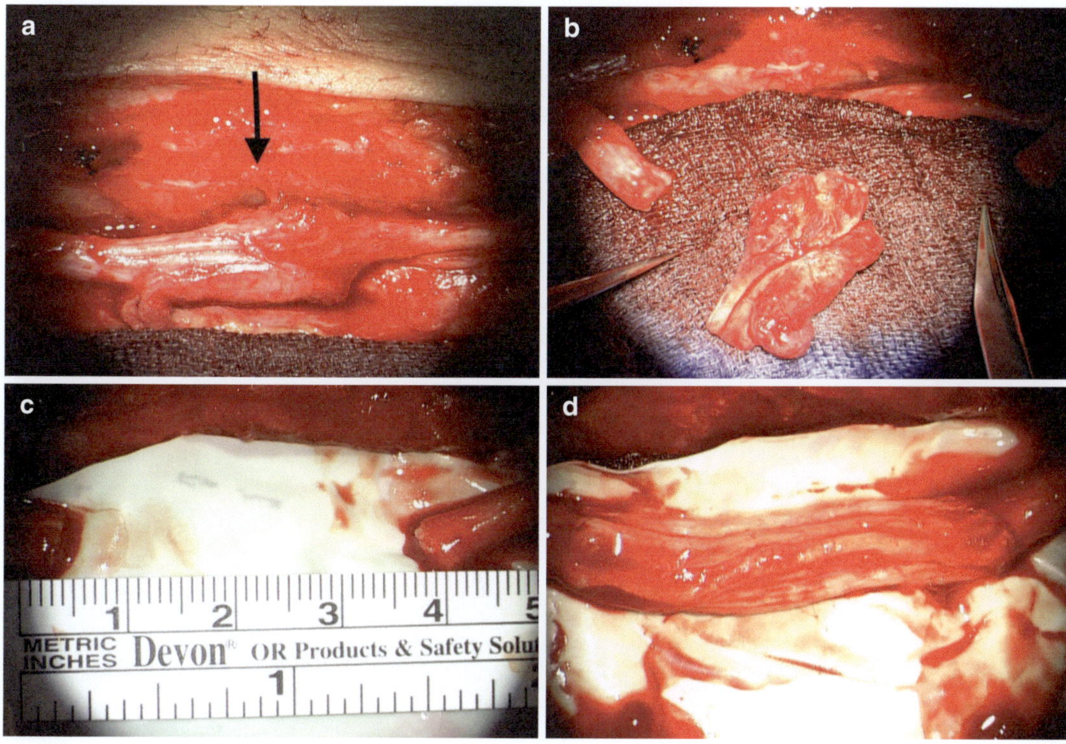

Fig. 6.4 Neuroma of the ulnar nerve (**a**, arrow) after trauma. (**b**) shows the resected neuroma with the two nerve stumps. As the resulting gap (**c**) is too big for direct nerve repair, nerve grafting via sural nerve transplant (**d**) is performed

> Split repair is a technique employed when only partial reconstruction of a nerve is required

Nerve Transfer/Neurotization/Nerve Crossing
Nerve transfers have proven to be an effective method for restoring both motor and sensory function in severe nerve injuries where direct neurorrhaphy or nerve grafting is not feasible.

Indications include situations in which the proximal nerve stump cannot be used due to their far too proximal lesion, as seen in nerve root avulsion or intraforaminal lesions. In those cases, there is no possibility to surgically reach the proximal stump.

Other indications comprise long distance nerve defects, significant bony or vascular injuries in the brachial plexus region, or previously failed nerve reconstructions.

Nerve transfers are frequently employed in complete brachial plexus injuries, but can also be indicated in non-traumatic conditions such as chronic nerve compression with functional loss, in paralytic complications following myelitis, spinal cord injuries involving brachial plexus avulsion, or post-stroke paralysis [27].

The surgical principle involves sacrificing a functioning, uninjured donor nerve to reinnervate the distal targets of a lesioned nerve. The donor nerve thereby assumes the role of the non-usable proximal stump, and is sutured to the distal stump of the uninjured nerve.

This approach requires precise anatomical knowledge and a careful selection of the donor nerve, as its original function will be lost while it assumes the function of the recipient nerve. Surgical planning prioritizes the restoration of specific functions based on clinical goals.

While theoretically every nerve can serve as an axon donor, optimal candidates possess cer-

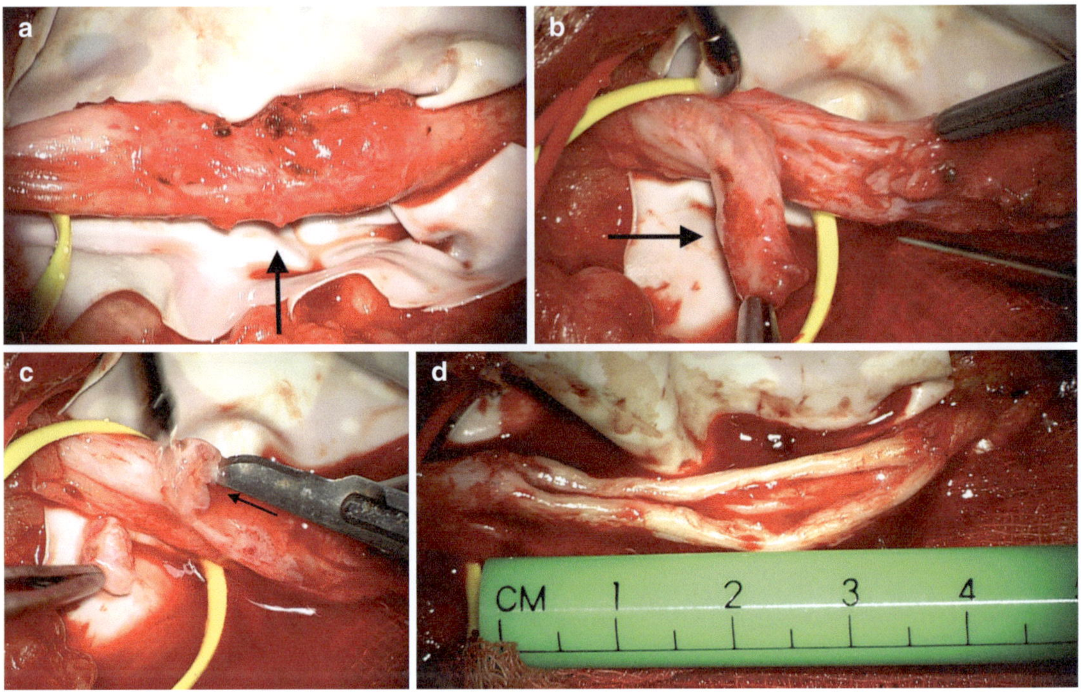

Fig. 6.5 Surgical technique presenting split repair: (**a**) shows a partial neuroma (arrow) within the tibial nerve. As some fascicles of the nerve are still functioning, only the neuroma is resected (arrow, **b**) leaving the remaining intact fascicles in situ. The affected nerve fascicle is cut back until healthy fascicular tissue (arrow, **c**) is visible. The resulting gap is then interposed via sural nerve graft (**d**)

tain characteristics: a high axonal count, suitable diameter, close proximity to the recipient nerve to avoid the use of additional grafts, and functional combatibility with the recipient nerve.

When appropriately selected, **cortical plasticity** allows the brain to voluntarily control the transferred nerve for its new function [28, 31].

Avoiding the use of nerve grafts may further improve outcomes. Clinical evidence suggests that tension-free nerve transfers yield superior results compared with direct coaptation under tension, as excessive tension may compromise blood flow and promote scar tissue formation [37].

> Outcomes also depend on several other factors, including the interval between injury and surgery, the patient's age, the localization of nerve injury and the surgeon's expertise.

Distal nerve transfers, performed close to the target muscle, generally achieve faster regeneration compared with proximal transfers, as misrouting of the axons and unintended innervation of less critical muscles can be prevented.

These considerations are important when planning surgical strategies involving short versus long (>10 cm) nerve grafts. The fundamental objective is: the shorter the graft, the better, while still accounting for potential axonal misrouting [39].

And with respect to the assumption that distal nerve transfers may be more effective in certain cases, longer nerve grafts should be accepted. For example a phrenic nerve transfer to the anterior division of the upper trunk (ADUT) of the brachial plexus results in a shorter graft but may produce weaker elbow flexion and additional contraction of the pectoral muscles, compared with direct transfer to the musculocutaneous nerve, where elbow flexion remains the sole function [40, 41].

Nerve transfers aimed at restoring sensory function are particularly important in cases of sciatic or tibial nerve injury, which can lead to loss of plantar sensation, impaired proprioception, and severe gait disturbances (may also be seen in diabetic polyneuropathy). The saphenous nerve is often used as donor to restore plantar sensitivity.

Axonal donors can be either intraplexal or extraplexal. The following nerve transfer combinations are frequently employed:

Intraplexal Nerve Transfers

Oberlin transfer:

The Oberlin transfer, first described by Christophe Oberlin in 1992, involves transferring a fascicle of the ulnar nerve—typically the fascicle innervating the flexor carpi ulnaris muscle (FCU)—to the biceps branch of the musculocutaneous nerve. The appropriate fascicle is identified using direct nerve stimulation.

The double Oberlin includes the additional transfer of a median nerve fascicle to the brachial branch of the musculocutaneous nerve. As with the ulnar nerve, it is crucial to select a fascicle that innervates wrist function, avoiding fascicles supplying the intrinsic hand muscles to preserve fine motor function.

The primary objective of this nerve transfer is the restoration of elbow function.

The Oberlin transfer is considered a save and effective procedure, providing excellent functional outcomes, due to the close anatomical proximity of donor and recipient nerves and the functional similarity among the involved nerves [44] (Fig. 6.6).

Note, that the Oberlin procedure is not a classical nerve transfer as only selected fascicles are used as a donor, resulting in minimal or no loss of original nerve function.

Somsak's procedure:

Another intrabrachial reconstructive technique involves the transfer of the motor branch to the long head of the triceps to the anterior branch of the axillary nerve, performed via a posterior surgical approach, to reinnervate the deltoid muscle. The anterior branch is preferentially utilized, as it provides innervation not only to the anterior but also to the posterior portion of the deltoid muscle, thereby serving as a more robust donor target compared to the posterior branch [48].

This procedure facilitates shoulder stability, as well as improvement in arm abduction and external rotation.

Contralateral C7 (CC7)/Hemi-C7 transfer:

The contralateral C7 nerve transfer (CC7) is an established technique for the management of brachial plexus avulsion injuries preferentially performed in Asian surgical practice. Given that the C7 root comprises multiple nerve fascicles, it serves as a suitable donor for axonal transfer,

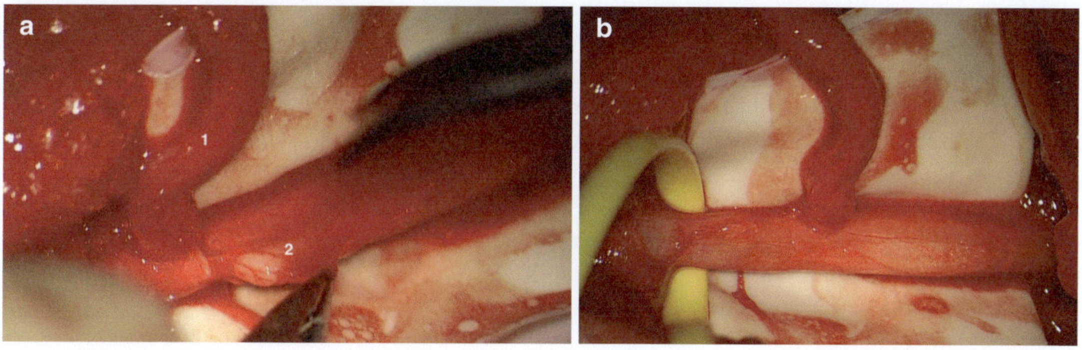

Fig. 6.6 Oberlin transfer: The biceps branch of the musculocutaneous branch is already prepared (**a1**) while a fascicle of the ulnar nerve (**a2**) is carefully dissected for transfer. The biceps branch is then sutured via an end-to-side-anastomosis to the dissected fascicle of the ulnar nerve (**b**)

enabling the restoration of various motor functions and, in some cases, reconstitution of sensory function.

Due to its overlapping innervation and compensatory contributions from the remaining ipsilateral brachial plexus roots, functional deficits in the donor upper extremity following C7 transection are generally limited and complete recovery may be possible [55]. Nonetheless, donor-site morbidity has been documented in clinical studies [56].

Despite the fact that the CC7 transfer can theoretically target any muscle group in the upper extremity, clinical experience has demonstrated that proximal targets such as shoulder (for elevation) and elbow (for flexion) yield suboptimal outcomes. Consequently, CC7 transfer is primarily employed for the restoration of hand function [57].

> Independent voluntary movement following CC7 transfer is not achievable, primarily due to the limited capacity of cortical plasticity. The motor cortical representations of the donor and recipient functions are located in separate hemispheres, and the interhemispheric distance and complexity of reorganization exceed the brain's adaptive potential.

The most compelling indication for contralateral C7 (CC7) transfer is the alleviation of phantom limb pain, attributable to the substantial proportion of sensory fibers contained within the C7 root [58].

From a surgical standpoint, the procedure involves proximal transection of the C7 nerve, typically performed anterior to its division. The nerve is then transferred to a graft—most commonly utilizing the nonfunctional ulnar or median nerve from the affected limb. The distal end of the graft is subsequently sutured to the recipient median and radial nerves [59].

Extraplexal Nerve Transfers

- Accessory nerve to the suprascapular or axillary nerve (Fig. 6.7)
- Axillary branch to the suprascapular nerve
- Intercostal nerve to the suprascapular or musculocutaneous nerve: As the intercostal nerves are very small in caliber, harvesting a minimum of three intercostal nerves is generally required to achieve sufficient axonal input for effective reinnervation and meaningful clinical recovery (Fig. 6.8)
- Phrenic nerve to musculocutanous nerve: In complete brachial plexus injury, the lower trunks are typically affected, rendering procedures such as the Oberlin transfer infeasible. The phrenic nerve originating from spinal roots C3–C5, and primarily responsible for diaphragmatic innervation, is considered an

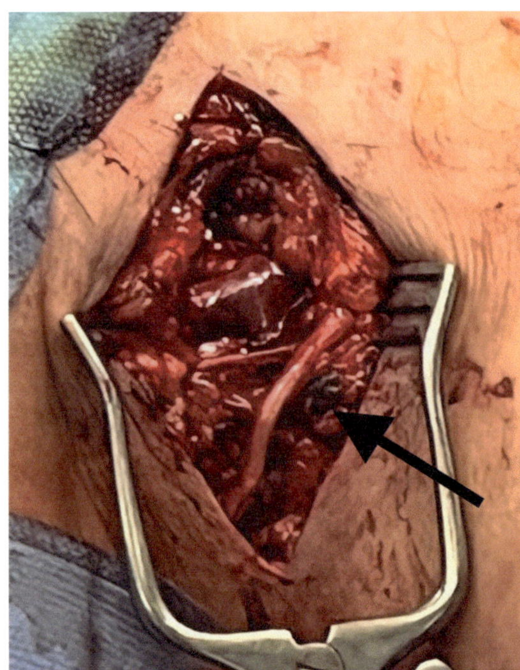

Fig. 6.7 Intraoperative picture showing an accessory-to-axillary nerve transfer (arrow) via sural nerve graft in a patient with axillary nerve lesion. This transfer is performed with the goal to restore shoulder stability

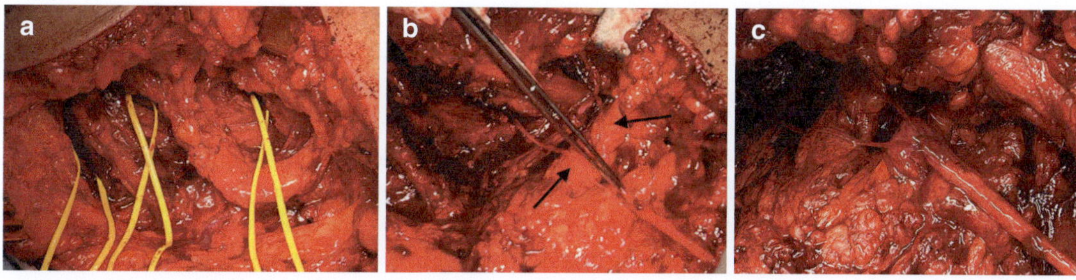

Fig. 6.8 Three-panel surgical photo showing an intercostal nerve transfer to the musculocutaneous nerve: The three yellow loops entail dissected intercostal nerves (**a**). They are then arranged to increase the diameter of the donor nerve (**b**, arrows), before being coaptated to the recipient musculocutaneous nerve (**c**). Fibrin glue is applied for fixation as suturingis not recommended in this case

extrabrachial plexus donor nerve and may therefore be utilized. With more than 800 axons, the phrenic nerve represents a robust motor donor, offering reliable outcomes in terms of functional reinnervation [40].

Multiple studies have demonstrated that unilateral sacrifice of the phrenic nerve does not generally result in clinically significant respiratory compromise. However, two major contraindications exist: pediatric patients and individuals with obesity. Standard preoperative evaluation as pulmonary function tests should be performed [63].

The preferred surgical technique involves transection of the phrenic nerve at the supraclavicular level, followed by interposition of a sural nerve graft directed toward a distal target, such as the musculocutaneous nerve. This approach helps to reduce the risk of axonal misrouting.

- Branch of the hypoglossal nerve (ansa cervicalis) to the inferior recurrent laryngeal nerve: Injury to the recurrent laryngeal nerve occurs most commonly by iatrogenic means or by trauma. Clinical signs are vocal cord paralysis and dysphagia. Reinnervation, using a branch of the hypoglossal nerve, can restore function of the laryngeal adductor muscles, leading to improvements in phonation and swallowing.
- Median pectoral nerve to the suprascapular nerve.
- Ulnar fascicle to the suprascapular nerve.

Supercharge nerve transfers are performed to enhance motor recovery in patients with motor weakness without complete paralysis following nerve injury. It is indicated when spontaneous or surgically induced regeneration is insufficient to achieve a functionally satisfactory outcome.

The surgical procedure involves coaptation of a donor nerve or selected fascicles to the recipient nerve using an end-to-side neurorrhaphy [67].

A representative example is the Oberlin transfer, in which fascicles of the ulnar and/or median nerve are sutured end-to-side to the musculocutaneous nerve in order to reinforce weak biceps function.

The principle advantage of this method is to preserve the integrity and the regeneration process of the recipient nerve.

Nerve bypass is another reconstructive technique primarily applied in spinal cord lesion. Basically, it describes connecting a donor nerve proximal (superior) to the spinal cord lesion to a recipient nerve located distal (inferior) to the lesion, thereby bypassing the site of injury and restoring function.

Tendon Transfer

In cases where nerve reconstruction is not possible, tendon or tendon-muscle transfers provide a surgical option to restore essential motor function with minimal donor side morbidity. This can be achieved by rerouting intact tendons and suturing them to the tendons of the affected muscle.

The surgical procedure of tendon transfers is not new, indeed, it has been done for more than a century with Codivilla first describing this procedure in 1899 [69].

The transfer of synergistic tendons, such as employing a wrist extensor to restore finger flexion, has demonstrated favorable outcomes, as patients can more readily adapt to the new function.

Several principles are critical for successful tendon transfer. The donor tendon should possess sufficient muscle strength, ideally graded at least M4 on the Medical Research Council (MRC) scale, as tendon transfer typically results in the loss of approximately one grade of muscle power. Additionally, the target joint should have an adequate range of motion (ROM) to allow proper function of the transfer [71]. A smooth, scar-free soft tissue bed will provide gliding of the tendon.

This method is applied after failed nerve reconstruction procedures or long-standing lesions (>1 year) where regeneration of the nerve is not possible anymore. Other indications besides traumatic injury of the nerves are poliomyelitis, cerebral palsy, stroke, injury to the musculotendinous unit itself, or rheumatoid arthritis [72].

Commonly performed tendon transfers include those aimed at restoring wrist and finger flexion or extension, as well as dorsiflexion of the foot.

Example of Tendon Transfers

Radial nerve palsy:

The goal of this tendon transfer is to restore active extension of the wrist, thumb, and fingers. The frequently preformed procedure is the triple tendon transfer, which typically implies following components [73]:

Wrist extension: Transfer of the pronator teres to the extensor carpi radialis brevis tendon.

Thumb extension and abduction: Transfer of the palmaris longus or the flexor digitorum superficialis to the extensor pollicis longus tendon.

Finger extension: Transfer of either the flexor carpi radialis or the flexor carpi ulnaris to the extensor digitorum communis, or alternatively, the flexor digitorum superficialis of the long finger to the extensor digitorum communis tendon.

Peroneal nerve palsy:

The peroneal nerve is among the most commonly injured peripheral nerve after the median and ulnar nerves. Compression, traction, and laceration are frequently encountered mechanisms of injury. Although lesions may occur along the entire course of the nerve, the fibular head represents the most common site of injury.

The resulting muscular imbalance following peroneal nerve lesion typically manifests as a pathognomic steppage gait, often accompanied by an increased risk of falls. Over time, progressive plantar flexion and shortening of the gastrocnemius muscle may lead to fixed foot deformity.

The goal of treatment is a normalization of the gait pattern, thereby reducing fall risk.

In cases of chronic peroneal nerve lesions, where peripheral nerve reconstruction is no longer feasible, tendon transfer provides a reliable surgical alternative.

Two essential prerequisites should be met prior to surgery: The joints must demonstrate full passive mobility—which requires preoperative passive movement of the joints—and the donor muscle should exhibit a strength of at least grade 4 on the Medical Research Council scale, as tendon transfer typically results in loss of approximately one grade of muscle strength.

With respect to the surgical technique, the posterior tibial tendon is transected at its distal insertion, pulled through the interosseus membrane to reach the anterior compartment of the distal leg. Depending on the chosen method, it can then be secured to various recipient structures:

- *Cuneiform bone II or III*: Sole transfer of the posterior tibial tendon to the cuneiform bone restoring dorsiflexion by elevating the longitudinal arch of the foot [75].
- *Bridle transfer*: A tri-tendon anastomosis involving the posterior tibial tendon, the anterior tibial tendon (dorsiflexion), and the peroneus longus tendon (strongest pronator and plantar flexor) [76].

- *Total Split Posterior Tibial Tendon Transfer (T-SPOTT)*: The posterior tibial tendon is split and anastomosis is performed with 50% to the peroneus brevis tendon (plantar flexion and pronation) and 50% to the anterior tibial tendon [77].
- *Carayon transfer*: Transposition of the posterior tibial tendon to the cuneiform bone, combined with transfer of the flexor digitorum longus to the extensor digitorum longus and the flexor hallucis longus to the extensor hallucis longus to restore dorsiflexion of the toe [78].

The Bridle procedure is the most frequently employed technique to re-establish active dorsiflexion of the foot by transferring the tendon of the posterior tibial muscle to the dorsal side of the foot via the interosseus membrane. The posterior tibial tendon is then sutured to the tendons of the anterior tibial and the peroneus longus muscles.

Postoperatively, the foot should be immobilized in a cast for six weeks, positioned at 90° dorsiflexion.

Following cast removal, intense physiotherapy is essential to achieve optimal functional outcomes.

Although complete restoration of the peroneal nerve-innervated muscle function cannot be achieved, this procedure re-establishes physical muscular balance, enabling a stable gait pattern and thereby reducing the risk of falling. High patient satisfaction rates have been reported.

In selected cases, a combined approach of nerve repair and tendon transfer has shown to be superior versus tendon transfer alone. These results are based on the theory of better nerve regeneration due to active dorsiflexion of the foot following tendon transfer, thereby preventing muscle atrophy. Furthermore, improved gait stability allows earlier mobilization which may also positively influence the regeneration process (Fig. 6.9).

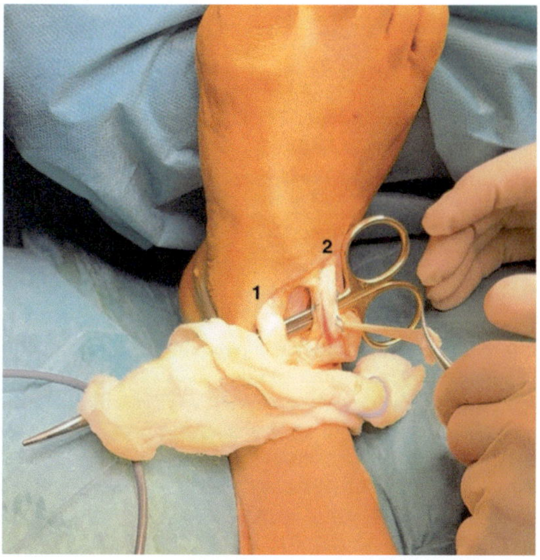

Fig. 6.9 Tendon transfer in Peroneal nerve transfer—Bridle technique: The posterior tibial tendon is grasped with the surgical clamp, mobilized, and subsequently interwoven with the tibialis anterior tendon (1) and the peroneus longus tendon (2) in a process called "tri-tendon-anastomosis

Muscle Transfer

Muscle transfer represents a supplementary surgical option—similar to the tendon transfer—for restoring movement when delayed presentation precludes nerve reconstruction. In this procedure, a redundant muscle and its vascular pedicle are harvested as a free flap to replace the non-functioning muscle. Nervous innervation is enabled by coaptation of a nearby motor nerve to the donor nerve.

Commonly used donor muscles include the gracilis or the rectus femoris from the thigh, as they provide good motor function, have a reliable vascular supply, and do not result in significant donor-site morbidity.

Other donor muscles with proven functional outcomes in cases of severe brachial plexus injury include the latissimus dorsi, pectoralis major, or the tensor fascia lata [83].

Regarding the gracilis muscle as an example for restoring elbow flexion—it substitutes for an atrophied biceps muscle. The spinal accessory nerve is typically used as the donor nerve and sutured to the obturator nerve of the transferred muscle flap to provide innervation.

Given the critical importance of vascular supply in free muscle transfers, meticulous postoperative monitoring—including Doppler

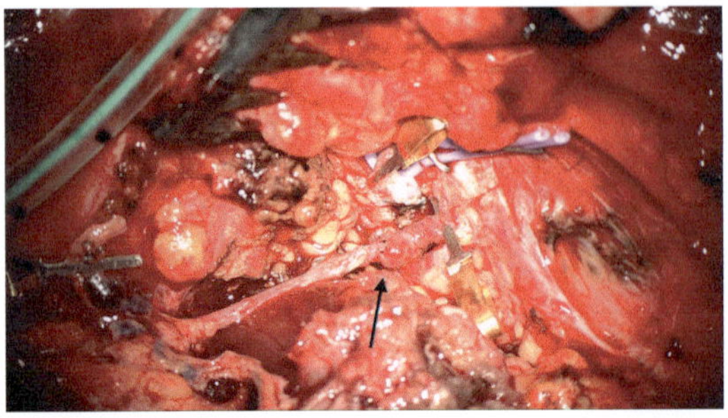

Fig. 6.10 Surgical image in a patient with complete brachial plexus lesion after skiing accident: Free muscle transfer with the gracilis combined with vascular anastomosis is performed to compensate the non-functioning deltoid muscle. Direct nerve transfer of the donor obturator nerve to a branch of the accessory nerve was possible (arrow)

ultrasound assessment, evaluation of skin color, and capillary refill – is essential to ensure flap viability (Fig. 6.10).

For tendon and/or muscle transfer procedures, standard general anesthesia is typically employed, as intraoperative nerve stimulation is not required.

Arthrodesis

In chronic brachial plexus injuries or long-standing peroneal nerve lesions, the affected joints often remain in an unfavorable position thereby reducing the patient's quality of life.

Classically, the shoulder may present in subluxation, while peroneal nerve lesions result foot drop. Beyond the functional limitations—such as an increased risk of tripping due to impaired dorsiflexion—these positions frequently cause pain, for example, shoulder discomfort associated with internal rotation of the girdle.

The concept of arthrodesis suggests a stable joint position that does not impede the residual or paralyzed function of the extremities.

Bioelectrical Orthoses

Bioelectrical orthoses receive signals from the nerve or directly from the target muscle and transmit them to actuators thereby amplifying voluntary muscle contractions and facilitating functional movement [85]. These devices are primarily designed to assist the patients during rehabilitation phase and to support activities of daily living, promoting greater independence.

An essential requirement for their use is the presence of a functional nerve confirmed electrophysiologically (i.e. detectable action potentials) even if clinical function is absent, as well as a non-degenerated target muscle.

6.2 Spasticity

Spasticity refers to an increase in muscle tone resulting from upper motor neuron lesions, as seen after cerebral stroke, intracerebral hemorrhage, or spinal cord injury [87]. Lesions to the pyramidal tract disrupt the balance between excitatory and inhibitory inputs, leading to muscle overactivity and hyperexcitable tonic stretch reflexes.

The resultant muscle hypertonia is typically velocity-dependent, restricts passive movement of the affected limb, and is often accompanied by muscle weakness. Patients frequently experience significant pain due to the persistently increased muscle tone.

In cases of chronic spasticity, passive movement of the affected limb may become impossible despite intensive physio- and ergotherapy.

The *Ashworth-scale* represents a frequently used to classify the severity of muscle tone [88] (Table 6.1):

Table 6.1 Ashworth scale to measure resistance during passive stretching as a measure for spasticity

Ashworth scale	
Grade	Clinical manifestation
0	No muscle tone increase
1	Slight increase in muscle tone (catch and release at the end of the ROM movement)
1+	Slight increase in muscle tone (catch and release followed by minimal resistance throughout ROM)
2	Moderate increase in muscle tone
3	Marked increase in muscle tone throughout ROM
4	Rigid in flexion/extension

ROM Range of motion

Therapeutic modalities for the management of spasticity include physiotherapy, massages, acupuncture, and electric stimulation. Cold therapy has also been described as a therapeutic approach, based on the hypothesis that it reduces nerve conduction velocity and decreases the amplitude of the motor action potential, thereby diminishing excessive muscle activity.

First-line pharmacological treatments include Botulinum type A toxin (Botox) and baclofen injections, which can provide temporarily relief of spasticity and associated pain; however, their effects may diminish over time [91].

Selective peripheral nerve denervation defines a surgical technique designed to reduce spasticity by transecting selected fascicles innervating the affected muscle, thereby decreasing muscle overactivity [92] (Fig. 6.11).

The procedure involves exposure of the target nerve, direct stimulation, identification of individual fascicles, and selective transection of fascicles.

A concentric bipolar stimulation probe is typically used to achieve precise fascicular stimulation.

This technique can be applied to any peripheral nerve of the extremities and is often performed in a staged manner, with repeated interventions to progressively reduce spasticity.

Although selective denervation is not curative and the immediate treatment postoperative clinical picture may appear unsatisfying, patients frequently experience significant relief from pain.

Intensive ergo- and physiotherapy remain essential components regarding the treatment of spasticity.

The *contralateral C7 transfer* is a specialized surgical approach for the management of spasticity.

In patients with spasticity and partial motor loss following cerebral lesions, the uninjured contralateral C7 nerve root—either partial or in its entirety—can serve as a donor for reinnervation of the affected extremity. This technique seems to work due to the functional redundancy of the C7 spinal nerve, which receives contributions from the C6, C8, and Th1 spinal nerves. By establishing voluntary control of the affected limb via the non-lesioned cerebral hemisphere, this procedure can reduce spasticity and improve motor function [101].

6.3 Neuroplasticity

Neuroplasticity—also referred to as brain plasticity or cortical plasticity—describes a complex mechanism of the central nervous system of being capable to undergo adaptive functional and structural modifications, in response to external and internal stimuli. Within the white matter, activity-dependent modulation has been

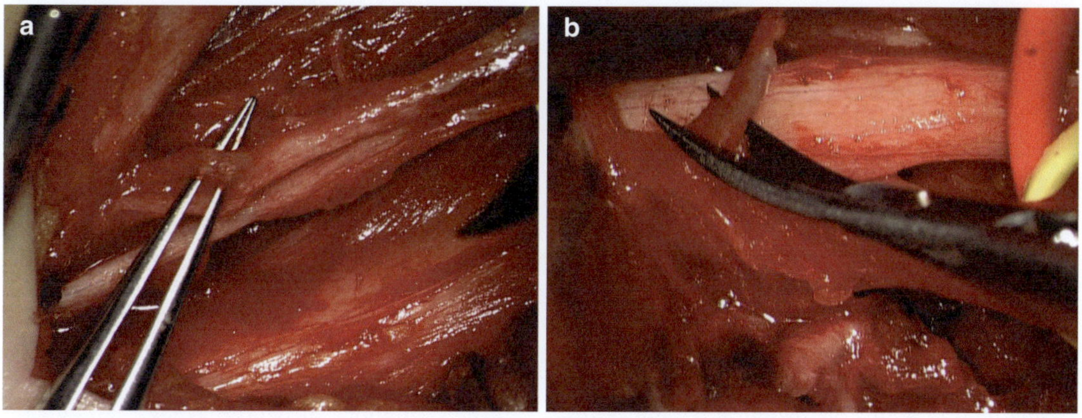

Fig. 6.11 Selective peripheral nerve denervation in a patient with spasticity following diffuse after cerebral edema during heart surgery: Fascicles of the median, ulnar and musculocutaneous nerve are selected (**a**) and cut (**b**) to reduce overactivity of the target muscle

observed, including the formation of new myelin sheaths and the thickening of preexisting myelin in areas of increased activity. In the gray matter of the cerebral cortex, synaptic plasticity and axonal sprouting has also been detected [103].

This phenomenon plays a pivotal role in the planning of nerve transfers, as different donor-recipient nerve combinations result in distinct clinical outcomes. Changes in neurotransmitter and synaptic activation that are controlled by pre-existing but low active connections within the brain may play a role in the mediation of brain plasticity [105].

The extent of neuroplastic adaptation is further influenced by various factors including the interval between trauma and surgical intervention, the patient's age and body mass index (BMI), the axonal count within nerve grafts, and the degree of postoperative rehabilitation and physiotherapy [106].

The cortical distance between functional representations, as depicted in the motor homunculus, also exerts a significant impact on regeneration. This explains why some nerve transfers achieve superior outcomes compared to others—for example, facial-to-hypoglossal transfer tends to yield better clinical results than hypoglossal-to-musculocutaneous nerve transfer [105].

Another interesting aspect represents the surface area of cortical representation, as it influences the regenerative capacity. For instance, the face and hand occupy disproportionately large regions of the motor cortex relative to the upper arm, reflecting the complexity of fine motor control in these areas. This contributes to the greater difficulty encountered in restoring function of the hand or face compared to proximal muscles.

Optimal outcomes are achieved when nerve transfers follow the principle of preexisting cortical connections, particularly where donor and recipient regions share overlapping motor control pathways.

Finally, neuroplastic capacity is higher in infants than in adults, as pediatric patients demonstrate superior adaptive capacity to process functional changes induced by peripheral nerve transfers.

A well documented example of neuroplasticity represents the frequently performed phrenic-to-musculocutaneous nerve transfer to restore elbow flexion. During the early stages of reinnervation, voluntary elbow flexion is not yet feasible; however, arm movement can already be elicited during forced inspiration. Eventually, patients develop awareness of this simultaneous activation, an with repeated training, elbow flexion becomes gradually increasingly independent from respiratory effort. Complete independence from inspiratory activity, however, will not be achieved. Nevertheless, certain functional tasks—as lifting heavy objects—do require active inspiration, hence, this simultaneous movement is generally well tolerated and is not perceived as significantly impairing by the patients.

The hypoglossal-to-musculocutaneous nerve transfer represents a rather unfavorable approach, underscoring the importance of pre-existing cortical connections and common motor pathways. Unlike the hypoglossal-to-facial transfer, where cortical representations are anatomically proximate, the cortical areas controlling tongue movement and the biceps contraction are spatially distant. Consequently, patients undergoing hypoglossal-to-musculocutaneous transfer often experience maladaptive outcomes, such as the need to press the tongue to the palate in order to initiate elbow flexion. Speech or mastication will induce contractions of the biceps muscle.

Another debated procedure is the contralateral C7 transfer, utilized in complete brachial plexus injury. Concerns have been raised regarding the lack of independent control, as patients may require activation of the unaffected limb to facilitate movement of the reinnervated arm. Some reports suggest that this dependency can be more disadvantageous than the original state of paralysis [56].

It has been suggested that harvesting the C7 root very proximally—prior to receiving contributions from the C8 branch—does not result in development of new motor deficits.

The limitations of neuroplasticity are evident in patients with severe traumatic brain injury, where concomitant white matter lesions impair the structural integrity required for plastic regeneration.

Similarily, reinnervation of two antagonistic recipient muscles from a single donor nerve (e.g., use of the phrenic nerve for elbow flexion and extension) does typically not lead to satisfying outcomes.

Surprisingly, however, favorable results have been reported when an antagonist donor is used to reinnervate an agonist muscle. A notable example is the medial pectoral nerve transfer (responsible for shoulder adduction) to the axillary nerve (responsible for shoulder abduction), which has demonstrated good functional recovery in selected cases [104].

In the context of hand reinnervation, the generally poor outcomes observed following nerve grafting may be explained by two principle factors: the long distance between cortical initiation and the distal hand muscles, and the large cortical representation area of the hand, which appears to have limited capacity for functional recovery after injury [106, 107].

Neuroplasticity of the lower limb seems to work differently from that of the upper limb, with nerve transfers demonstrating lower rates of success. One hypothesis might be the more automatically induced lower-limb movements (walking, running etc.), requiring less complex cortical wiring than upper-limb movements [108].

Another important aspect to consider in surgical planning is the **muscular fatigue** that differs in the donor nerves. In comparative studies of phrenic versus spinal accessory nerve transfers to the musculocutaneous nerve, the phrenic-to-musculocutaneous transfer was associated with greater muscule fatigue [106]. By contrast, the spinal accessory-to-musculocutaneous transfer provided more endurance in strength. These findings can be attributed to the physiological role of the respective nerves: the spinal accessory nerve innervates muscles essential for continuous contraction to maintain posture (trapezius and sternocleidomastoid), whereas the phrenic nerve drives rhythmic, short, and partially involuntary contractions during inspiration.

Finally, neuroplasticity is not exclusively beneficial. Maladaptive plastic changes are implicated in conditions such as phantom limb pain, where the same mechanisms that promote functional recovery also contribute to persistent maladaptive cortical regeneration.

Further Reading

1. Burchiel KJ. Surgical management of pain. In: Surgical procedures; 2002. https://doi.org/10.1055/b-0034-45956.
2. Price BA, Miller G. Internal neurolysis. J Foot Surg. 1992;31(3):250–9.
3. Rovak JM, Cederna PS, Kuzon WM Jr. Terminolateral neurorrhaphy: a review of the literature. J Reconstr Microsurg. 2001;17(8):615–24. https://doi.org/10.1055/s-2001-18817.
4. Kalliainen LK, Cederna PS, Kuzon WM Jr. Mechanical function of muscle reinnervated by end-to-side neurorrhaphy. Plast Reconstr Surg. 1999;103(7):1919–27. https://doi.org/10.1097/00006534-199906000-00017.
5. Yu Q, Zhang SH, Wang T, Peng F, Han D, Gu YD. End-to-side neurorrhaphy repairs peripheral nerve injury: sensory nerve induces motor nerve regeneration. Neural Regen Res. 2017;12(10):1703–7. https://doi.org/10.4103/1673-5374.217350.
6. Marshall KL, Farah MH. Axonal regeneration and sprouting as a potential therapeutic target for nervous system disorders. Neural Regen Res. 2021;16(10):1901–10. https://doi.org/10.4103/1673-5374.308077. PMID: 33642358; PMCID: PMC8343323.
7. Bao Q, Xiao C, Wang T, Gu Y. Novel atraumatic end-to-side repair model exhibits robust collateral sprouting independent of donor fiber injury. Plast Reconstr Surg. 2016;137(2):523–33. https://doi.org/10.1097/01.prs.0000475764.76278.eb.
8. Collyer E, Catenaccio A, Lemaitre D, Diaz P, Valenzuela V, Bronfman F, Court FA. Sprouting of axonal collaterals after spinal cord injury is prevented by delayed axonal degeneration. Exp Neurol. 2014;261:451–61. https://doi.org/10.1016/j.expneurol.2014.07.014.
9. Matsumoto M, Hirata H, Nishiyama M, Morita A, Sasaki H, Uchida A. Schwann cells can induce collateral sprouting from intact axons: experimental study of end-to-side neurorrhaphy using a Y-chamber model. J Reconstr Microsurg. 1999;15(4):281–6. https://doi.org/10.1055/s-2007-1000102.
10. Kline DG. Surgical repair of peripheral nerve injury. Muscle Nerve. 1990;13(9):843–52. https://doi.org/10.1002/mus.880130911.
11. Becker M, Lassner F, Fansa H, Mawrin C, Pallua N. Refinements in nerve to muscle neurotization. Muscle Nerve. 2002;26(3):362–6. https://doi.org/10.1002/mus.10205.

12. Kretschmer T, Birch R. Management of acute peripheral nerve injuries. In: Winn R, editor. Youmans neurological surgery. 6th ed. Saunders; 2011. p. 2465–83.
13. Kakibuchi M, Tuji K, Fukuda K, Terada T, Yamada N, Matsuda K, Kawai K, Sakagami M. End-to-side nerve graft for facial nerve reconstruction. Ann Plast Surg. 2004;53(5):496–500. https://doi.org/10.1097/01.sap.0000116283.76872.de.
14. Samardzić MM, Rasulić LG, Grujicić DM. Results of cable graft technique in repair of large nerve trunk lesions. Acta Neurochir. 1998;140(11):1177–82. https://doi.org/10.1007/s007010050234.
15. Breidenbach WC. Vascularized nerve grafts. A practical approach. Orthop Clin North Am. 1988;19(1):81–9.
16. Saheb-Al-Zamani M, Yan Y, Farber SJ, Hunter DA, Newton P, Wood MD, Stewart SA, Johnson PJ, Mackinnon SE. Limited regeneration in long acellular nerve allografts is associated with increased Schwann cell senescence. Exp Neurol. 2013;247:165–77. https://doi.org/10.1016/j.expneurol.2013.04.003.
17. Deal DN, Griffin JW, Hogan MV. Nerve conduits for nerve repair or reconstruction. J Am Acad Orthop Surg. 2012;20(2):63–8. https://doi.org/10.5435/JAAOS-20-02-063.
18. Assmus H. Nervus-suralis-Entnahme mit Hilfe eines Nervstrippers [Sural nerve removal using a nerve stripper]. Neurochirurgia (Stuttg). 1983;26(2):51–2. https://doi.org/10.1055/s-2008-1053611.
19. Hill HL, Vasconez LO, Jurkiewicz MJ. Method for obtaining a sural nerve graft. Plast Reconstr Surg. 1978;61(2):177–9. https://doi.org/10.1097/00006534-197802000-00003.
20. Griffin JW, Hogan MV, Chhabra AB, Deal DN. Peripheral nerve repair and reconstruction. J Bone Joint Surg Am. 2013;95(23):2144–51. https://doi.org/10.2106/JBJS.L.00704.
21. Kim J, Choi YE, Kim JH, Lee SH, Oh S, Kim SH. Nerve repair and orthodromic and antidromic nerve grafts: an experimental comparative study in rabbit. Biomed Res Int. 2020;2020:5046832. https://doi.org/10.1155/2020/5046832.
22. Kretschmer T, editor. Nervenchirurgie: trauma, tumor, kompression. Springer; 2014.
23. Grinsell D, Keating CP. Peripheral nerve reconstruction after injury: a review of clinical and experimental therapies. Biomed Res Int. 2014;2014:698256. https://doi.org/10.1155/2014/698256.
24. Werkmann DN, Bäzner UM, Petkov M, Minzenmay L, Durner G, Antoniadis G, Wirtz CR, Pedro MT, Knoll A, Pala A. Clinical outcome after surgical treatment of traumatic peroneal nerve injury: an analysis of risk factors after different surgical approaches. Neurol Int. 2025;17(1):7. https://doi.org/10.3390/neurolint17010007.
25. Glaser JJ, Aman M, Böcker AH, Thielen M, Harhaus L. Nerventransfers bei peripheren Nervenläsionen [nerve transfers in peripheral nerve lesions]. Handchirurgie Mikrochirurgie Plastische Chirurgie. 2024;56(1):49–54. https://doi.org/10.1055/a-2228-7062.
26. Tung TH, Mackinnon SE. Nerve transfers: indications, techniques, and outcomes. J Hand Surg Am. 2010;35(2):332–41. https://doi.org/10.1016/j.jhsa.2009.12.002.
27. Wilson TJ. Novel uses of nerve transfers. Neurotherapeutics. 2019;16(1):26–35. https://doi.org/10.1007/s13311-018-0664-x.
28. Sun G, Wu Z, Wang X, Tan X, Gu Y. Nerve transfer helps repair brachial plexus injury by increasing cerebral cortical plasticity. Neural Regen Res. 2014;9(23):2111–4. https://doi.org/10.4103/1673-5374.147939.
29. Bateman EA, Larocerie-Salgado J, Ross DC, Miller TA, Pripotnev S. Assessment, patient selection, and rehabilitation of nerve transfers. Front Rehabil Sci. 2023;4:1267433. https://doi.org/10.3389/fresc.2023.1267433.
30. Lin JS, Jain SA. Challenges in nerve repair and reconstruction. Hand Clin. 2023;39(3):403–15. https://doi.org/10.1016/j.hcl.2023.05.001.
31. Zhang D, Varadharajan V, Bhardwaj P, Venkatramani H, Sabapathy SR. Considerations in the selection of donor nerves for nerve transfer for reanimation of elbow and shoulder in traumatic brachial plexus injuries. J Hand Surg Asian Pac Vol. 2022;27(1):10–21. https://doi.org/10.1142/S242483552230002X.
32. Millesi H. Reappraisal of nerve repair. Surg Clin North Am. 1981;61(2):321–40. https://doi.org/10.1016/s0039-6109(16)42384-4.
33. Trehan SK, Model Z, Lee SK. Nerve repair and nerve grafting. Hand Clin. 2016;32(2):119–25. https://doi.org/10.1016/j.hcl.2015.12.002.
34. Ansselin AD, Davey DF. The regeneration of axons through normal and reversed peripheral nerve grafts. Restor Neurol Neurosci. 1993;5(3):225–40. https://doi.org/10.3233/RNN-1993-5307.
35. Millesi H. The nerve gap: theory and clinical practice. Hand Clin. 1986;2(4):651–63.
36. Flores AJ, Lavernia CJ, Owens PW. Anatomy and physiology of peripheral nerve injury and repair. Am J Orthop (Belle Mead NJ). 2000;29(3):167–73.
37. McDonald DS, Bell MS. Peripheral nerve gap repair facilitated by a dynamic tension device. Can J Plast Surg. 2010;18(1):e17–9.
38. Becker MHJ, Lassner F, Nolte KW, Brook GA, Weis J. The role of length of nerve grafts in combination with free functional muscle transplantation for brachial plexus injury: a single-center experience. J Pers Med. 2024;14(9):940. https://doi.org/10.3390/jpm14090940. PMID: 39338194; PMCID: PMC11433337.
39. Socolovsky M, Di Masi G, Battaglia D. Use of long autologous nerve grafts in brachial plexus reconstruction: factors that affect the outcome. Acta Neurochir. 2011;153(11):2231–40. https://doi.org/10.1007/s00701-011-1131-1.

40. Monreal R. Restoration of elbow flexion by transfer of the phrenic nerve to musculocutaneous nerve after brachial plexus injuries. Hand. 2007;2(4):206–11. https://doi.org/10.1007/s11552-007-9050-6.
41. Socolovsky M, Cardoso MM, Lovaglio A, di Masi G, Bonilla G, de Amoreira Gepp R. Comparison between supraclavicular versus video-assisted intrathoracic phrenic nerve section for transfer in patients with traumatic brachial plexus injuries: case series. Oper Neurosurg. 2020;19(3):249–54. https://doi.org/10.1093/ons/opaa163.
42. Siqueira MG, Socolovsky M, Heise CO, Martins RS, Di Masi G. Efficacy and safety of Oberlin's procedure in the treatment of brachial plexus birth palsy. Neurosurgery. 2012;71(6):1156–61. https://doi.org/10.1227/NEU.0b013e318271ee4a.
43. Moses MJ, Dai AZ, Lowe DT, Chu A, Protopsaltis TS. Case report: double Oberlin nerve transfer to restore elbow flexion following C5-C6 avulsion injury. Oper Neurosurg. 2019;16(1):23–6. https://doi.org/10.1093/ons/opy064.
44. Venkatramani H, Bhardwaj P, Faruquee SR, Sabapathy SR. Functional outcome of nerve transfer for restoration of shoulder and elbow function in upper brachial plexus injury. J Brachial Plex Peripher Nerve Inj. 2008;3:15. https://doi.org/10.1186/1749-7221-3-15.
45. Colbert SH, Mackinnon S. Posterior approach for double nerve transfer for restoration of shoulder function in upper brachial plexus palsy. Hand. 2006;1(2):71–7. https://doi.org/10.1007/s11552-006-9004-4. PMID: 18780028; PMCID: PMC2526027.
46. Tashjian RZ, Hutchinson DT, Wang AA. Management of the flail elbow. Hand Clin. 2008;24(1):113–24. https://doi.org/10.1016/j.hcl.2007.11.006.
47. Leechavengvongs S, Malungpaishorpe K, Uerpairojkit C, Ng CY, Witoonchart K. Nerve transfers to restore shoulder function. Hand Clin. 2016;32(2):153–64. https://doi.org/10.1016/j.hcl.2015.12.004.
48. Leechavengvongs S, Teerawutthichaikit T, Witoonchart K, Uerpairojkit C, Malungpaishrope K, Suppauksorn S, Chareonwat B. Surgical anatomy of the axillary nerve branches to the deltoid muscle. Clin Anat. 2015;28(1):118–22. https://doi.org/10.1002/ca.22352.
49. Thatte MR, Agashe M, Rathod C, Lad P, Mehta R. An approach to the supraclavicular and infraclavicular aspects of the brachial plexus. Tech Hand Up Extrem Surg. 2011;15(3):188–97. https://doi.org/10.1097/BTH.0b013e3182164b15.
50. Bhandari PS, Deb P. Posterior approach for both spinal accessory nerve to suprascapular nerve and triceps branch to axillary nerve for upper plexus injuries. J Hand Surg Am. 2013;38(1):168–72. https://doi.org/10.1016/j.jhsa.2012.10.024.
51. Kim SJ, Bang JH, Yang HJ, Moon SH, Choi YR, Lee HY. Anatomical considerations for nerve transfer in axillary nerve injury. Sci Rep. 2024;14(1):1262. https://doi.org/10.1038/s41598-024-51923-w. PMID: 38218996; PMCID: PMC10787799.
52. Klika BJ, Spinner RJ, Bishop AT, Kircher MF, Shin AY. Posterior branch of the axillary nerve transfer to the lateral triceps branch for restoration of elbow extension: case report. J Hand Surg Am. 2013;38(6):1145–9. https://doi.org/10.1016/j.jhsa.2013.03.044.
53. Zhang CG, Gu YD. Contralateral C7 nerve transfer—our experiences over past 25 years. J Brachial Plex Peripher Nerve Inj. 2011;6(1):10. https://doi.org/10.1186/1749-7221-6-10.
54. Li WJ, He LY, Chen SL, Lyu YW, Wang SF, Yong Y, Tian W, Tian GL, Gu YD. Contralateral C7 nerve root transfer for function recovery in adults: a meta-analysis. Chin Med J. 2017;130(24):2960–8. https://doi.org/10.4103/0366-6999.220316.
55. Bhagat ND, Gross JN, Adkinson JM, Borschel GH. Contralateral C7 nerve transfer for severe pediatric brachial plexus injuries: donor site morbidity. Child's Nerv Syst. 2023;39(8):1–4. https://doi.org/10.1007/s00381-023-05942-z.
56. Yang G, Chang KW, Chung KC. A systematic review of outcomes of contralateral C7 transfer for the treatment of traumatic brachial plexus injury: part 2. Donor-site morbidity. Plast Reconstr Surg. 2015;136(4):480e–9e. https://doi.org/10.1097/PRS.0000000000001616.
57. Chen X, Guo J, Zhou Y, Lao J, Zhao X, Rui J. Modified contralateral C7 transfer to restore ulnar nerve function without sacrificing median nerve recovery: an experimental study. J Hand Surg Eur Vol. 2023;48(8):731–7. https://doi.org/10.1177/17531934231170103.
58. Monsivais JJ. Contralateral C7 transfers: an innovative approach to improving peripheral neuropathic pain after traumatic brachial plexus injury with C5 rupture and avulsion of C6, C7, C8 and T1. A case series study. Clin Neurol Neurosurg. 2020;191:105693. https://doi.org/10.1016/j.clineuro.2020.105693.
59. Songcharoen P, Wongtrakul S, Mahaisavariya B, Spinner RJ. Hemi-contralateral C7 transfer to median nerve in the treatment of root avulsion brachial plexus injury. J Hand Surg Am. 2001;26(6):1058–64. https://doi.org/10.1053/jhsu.2001.27764.
60. Robla-Costales J, Socolovsky M, Di Masi G, Domitrovic A, Campero J, Fernández-Fernández J, Ibáñez-Plágaro J, García-Cosamalón L. Técnicas de reconstrucción nerviosa en cirugía del plexo braquial traumatizado. Parte 1: Transferencias nerviosas extraplexuales [Nerve reconstruction techniques in traumatic brachial plexus surgery. Part 1: extraplexal nerve transfers]. Neurocirugía (Asturias). 2011;22(6):507–20. https://pubmed.ncbi.nlm.nih.gov/22167281/
61. Midha R. Nerve transfers for severe brachial plexus injuries: a review. Neurosurg Focus. 2004;16(5):E5. https://doi.org/10.3171/foc.2004.16.5.6.

62. Socolovsky M, di Masi G, Bonilla G, Domínguez Paez M, Robla J, Calvache Cabrera C. The phrenic nerve as a donor for brachial plexus injuries: is it safe and effective? Case series and literature analysis. Acta Neurochir. 2015;157(6):1077–86. https://doi.org/10.1007/s00701-015-2387-7.
63. Socolovsky M, Malessy M, Bonilla G, Di Masi G, Conti ME, Lovaglio A. Phrenic to musculocutaneous nerve transfer for traumatic brachial plexus injuries: analyzing respiratory effects on elbow flexion control. J Neurosurg. 2019;131(1):165–74. https://doi.org/10.3171/2018.4.JNS173248.
64. Standring S, editor. Gray's anatomy: the anatomical basis of clinical practice. 39th ed, Chapters 31 & 64. London: Elsevier Churchill Livingstone; 2004. p. 554–1084.
65. Luedemann W, Hamm M, Blömer U, Samii M, Tatagiba M. Brachial plexus neurotization with donor phrenic nerves and its effect on pulmonary function. J Neurosurg. 2002;96(3):523–6. https://doi.org/10.3171/jns.2002.96.3.0523.
66. Khalifeh JM, Dibble CF, Van Voorhis A, Doering M, Boyer MI, Mahan MA, Wilson TJ, Midha R, Yang LJS, Ray WZ. Nerve transfers in the upper extremity following cervical spinal cord injury. Part 2: preliminary results of a prospective clinical trial. J Neurosurg Spine. 2019;31(5):641–53. https://doi.org/10.3171/2019.4.SPINE19399.
67. Farber SJ, Glaus SW, Moore AM, Hunter DA, Mackinnon SE, Johnson PJ. Supercharge nerve transfer to enhance motor recovery: a laboratory study. J Hand Surg Am. 2013;38(3):466–77. https://doi.org/10.1016/j.jhsa.2012.12.020.
68. von Guionneau N, Sarhane KA, Brandacher G, Hettiaratchy S, Belzberg AJ, Tuffaha S. Mechanisms and outcomes of the supercharged end-to-side nerve transfer: a review of preclinical and clinical studies. J Neurosurg. 2020;134(5):1590–8. https://doi.org/10.3171/2020.3.JNS191429.
69. Codavilla A. The classic: tendon transplants in orthopedic practice by a Codvilla. Clin Orthop Relat Res. 1976;118:2–6.
70. Sharma YK, Saini N, Khurana D, Meena DS, Gautam V. Tendon transfer for persistent radial nerve palsy using single-split FCU technique and re-routing of extensor pollicis longus: a prospective study of 25 cases. Indian J Orthop. 2019;53(5):607–12. https://doi.org/10.4103/ortho.IJOrtho_9_18. PMID: 31488927; PMCID: PMC6699211.
71. Vigasio A, Marcoccio I, Patelli A, Mattiuzzo V, Prestini G. New tendon transfer for correction of drop-foot in common peroneal nerve palsy. Clin Orthop Relat Res. 2008;466(6):1454–66. https://doi.org/10.1007/s11999-008-0249-9.
72. Wilbur D, Hammert WC. Principles of tendon transfer. Hand Clin. 2016;32(3):283–9. https://doi.org/10.1016/j.hcl.2016.03.001.
73. Tordjman D, d'Utruy A, Bauer B, Bellemère P, Pierrart J, Masmejean E. Tendon transfer surgery for radial nerve palsy. Hand Surg Rehabil. 2022;41S:S90–7. https://doi.org/10.1016/j.hansur.2018.09.009.
74. Lauer H, Heinzel JC, Vasselli B, Farzaliyev F, Ritter J, Kolbenschlag J, Daigeler A, Prahm C. Tendon transfer procedures for correction of foot drop due to injury to the peripheral nerves or muscles. J Brachial Plex Peripher Nerve Inj. 2025;20(1):e1–8. https://doi.org/10.1055/s-0044-.
75. Ponseti IV, Smoley EN. The classic: congenital club foot: the results of treatment. Clin Orthop Relat Res. 2009;467(5):1133–45. https://doi.org/10.1007/s11999-009-0720-2.
76. Dy CJ, Inclan PM, Matava MJ, Mackinnon SE, Johnson JE. Current concepts review: common peroneal nerve palsy after knee dislocations. Foot Ankle Int. 2021;42(5):658–68. https://doi.org/10.1177/1071100721995421.
77. Scheepers F, Bhatnagar T, Davies K, Wickenheiser D, Black A, Mulpuri K, Alvarez CM, Leveille L. Split tendon transfer of the posterior tibialis for spastic equinovarus foot deformity: does tendon routing impact post-operative ankle kinematics? Gait Posture. 2025;117:268–72. https://doi.org/10.1016/j.gaitpost.2025.01.003.
78. Movahedi YM. Triple tendon transfer for correction of foot deformity in common peroneal nerve palsy. Foot Ankle Int. 2016;37(6):665–9. https://doi.org/10.1177/1071100716629779.
79. Garozzo D, Ferraresi S, Buffatti P. Surgical treatment of common peroneal nerve injuries: indications and results. A series of 62 cases. J Neurosurg Sci. 2004;48(3):105–12.
80. Ho B, Khan Z, Switaj PJ, Ochenjele G, Fuchs D, Dahl W, Cederna P, Kung TA, Kadakia AR. Treatment of peroneal nerve injuries with simultaneous tendon transfer and nerve exploration. J Orthop Surg Res. 2014;9:67. https://doi.org/10.1186/s13018-014-0067-6.
81. Barrie KA, Steinmann SP, Shin AY, Spinner RJ, Bishop AT. Gracilis free muscle transfer for restoration of function after complete brachial plexus avulsion. Neurosurg Focus. 2004;16(5):E8. https://doi.org/10.3171/foc.2004.16.5.9.
82. Berger A, Flory PJ, Schaller E. Muscle transfers in brachial plexus lesions. J Reconstr Microsurg. 1990;6(2):113–6. https://doi.org/10.1055/s-2007-1006809.
83. Bishop AT. Functioning free-muscle transfer for brachial plexus injury. Hand Clin. 2005;21(1):91–102. https://doi.org/10.1016/j.hcl.2004.10.005.
84. Li X, Galvin JW, Zalneraitis BH, Gasbarro G, Parada SA, Eichinger JK, Boileau P, Warner JJP, Elhassan BT. Muscle tendon transfers around the shoulder: diagnosis, treatment, surgical techniques, and outcomes. J Bone Joint Surg. 2022;104(9):833–50. https://doi.org/10.2106/JBJS.21.00398.
85. Webber CM, Egginton JS, Shin AY, Kaufman KR. Application of a myoelectric elbow flexion assist orthosis in adult traumatic brachial plexus

injury: patient perspectives. Prosthetics Orthot Int. 2021;45(6):526–31. https://doi.org/10.1097/PXR.0000000000000047.
86. Sheean G. The pathophysiology of spasticity. Eur J Neurol. 2002;9(Suppl 1):3–61. https://doi.org/10.1046/j.1468-1331.2002.0090s1003.x.
87. Trompetto C, Marinelli L, Mori L, Pelosin E, Currà A, Molfetta L, Abbruzzese G. Pathophysiology of spasticity: implications for neurorehabilitation. Biomed Res Int. 2014;2014:354906. https://doi.org/10.1155/2014/354906.
88. Meseguer-Henarejos AB, Sánchez-Meca J, López-Pina JA, Carles-Hernández R. Inter- and intra-rater reliability of the modified Ashworth scale: a systematic review and meta-analysis. Eur J Phys Rehabil Med. 2018;54(4):576–90. https://doi.org/10.23736/S1973-9087.17.04796-7.
89. Harb A, Margetis K, Kishner S. Modified Ashworth scale. In: StatPearls. StatPearls Publishing; 2025.
90. Watanabe T. The role of therapy in spasticity management. Am J Phys Med Rehabil. 2004;83(10 Suppl):S45–9. https://doi.org/10.1097/01.phm.0000141130.58285.da.
91. Marsden J, Stevenson V, Jarrett L. Treatment of spasticity. Handb Clin Neurol. 2023;196:497–521. https://doi.org/10.1016/B978-0-323-98817-9.00010-7.
92. Sindou M, Mertens P. Selective neurotomy of the tibial nerve for treatment of the spastic foot. Neurosurgery. 1988;23(6):738–44. https://doi.org/10.1227/00006123-198812000-00009.
93. Sindou M. Historique du traitement neurochirurgical de la spasticité [History of neurosurgical treatment of spasticity]. Neuro-Chirurgie. 2003;49(2–3 Pt 2):137–43.
94. Braun V, Richter HP. Selective peripheral denervation for the treatment of spasmodic torticollis. Neurosurgery. 1994;35(1):58–63. https://doi.org/10.1227/00006123-199407000-00009.
95. Maarrawi J, Mertens P, Luaute J, Vial C, Chardonnet N, Cosson M, Sindou M. Long-term functional results of selective peripheral neurotomy for the treatment of spastic upper limb: prospective study in 31 patients. J Neurosurg. 2006;104(2):215–25. https://doi.org/10.3171/jns.2006.104.2.215.
96. Thum J, Bazarek S, Sten M, Friedman G, Mandeville R, Brown JM. Selective tibial neurotomy for spastic equinovarus foot: operative technique. Oper Neurosurg. 2023;25(5):e267–71. https://doi.org/10.1227/ons.0000000000000863.
97. Leclercq C. Selective neurectomy for the spastic upper extremity. Hand Clin. 2018;34(4):537–45. https://doi.org/10.1016/j.hcl.2018.06.010.
98. Xu WD, Hua XY, Zheng MX, Xu JG, Gu YD. Contralateral C7 nerve root transfer in treatment of cerebral palsy in a child: case report. Microsurgery. 2011;31(5):404–8. https://doi.org/10.1002/micr.20877.
99. Zheng MX, Hua XY, Feng JT, Li T, Lu YC, Shen YD, Cao XH, Zhao NQ, Lyu JY, Xu JG, Gu YD, Xu WD. Trial of contralateral seventh cervical nerve transfer for spastic arm paralysis. N Engl J Med. 2018;378(1):22–34. https://doi.org/10.1056/NEJMoa1615208.
100. Hua XY, Qiu YQ, Li T, Zheng MX, Shen YD, Jiang S, Xu JG, Gu YD, Xu WD. Contralateral peripheral neurotization for hemiplegic upper extremity after central neurologic injury. Neurosurgery. 2015;76(2):187–95. https://doi.org/10.1227/NEU.0000000000000590.
101. Xu W. Harnessing the uninjured hemisphere for treatment of the stroke or brain-injured patient–evolution of the contralateral C7 transfer. J Hand Surg Eur Vol. 2025;50:796–806. Advance online publication. https://doi.org/10.1177/17531934251314640.
102. Puderbaugh M, Emmady PD. Neuroplasticity. In StatPearls: StatPearls Publishing; 2023.
103. Xin W, Chan JR. Myelin plasticity: sculpting circuits in learning and memory. Nat Rev Neurosci. 2020;21(12):682–94. https://doi.org/10.1038/s41583-020-00379-8.
104. Socolovsky M, di Masi G, Bonilla G, Lovaglio A, Battaglia D, Rosler R, Malessy M. Brain plasticity in neonatal brachial plexus palsies: quantification and comparison with adults' brachial plexus injuries. Child's Nerv Syst. 2024;40(2):479–86.
105. Socolovsky M, Malessy M, Lopez D, Guedes F, Flores L. Current concepts in plasticity and nerve transfers: relationship between surgical techniques and outcomes. Neurosurg Focus. 2017;42(3):E13. https://doi.org/10.3171/2016.12.FOCUS16431.
106. Socolovsky M, Malessy M. Brain changes after peripheral nerve repair: limitations of neuroplasticity. J Neurosurg Sci. 2021;65(4):421–30. https://doi.org/10.23736/S0390-5616.21.05298-X.
107. Navarro X. Chapter 27: Neural plasticity after nerve injury and regeneration. Int Rev Neurobiol. 2009;87:483–505. https://doi.org/10.1016/S0074-7742(09)87027-X.
108. Forrester LW, Wheaton LA, Luft AR. Exercise-mediated locomotor recovery and lower-limb neuroplasticity after stroke. J Rehabil Res Dev. 2008;45(2):205–20. https://doi.org/10.1682/jrrd.2007.02.0034.

7 Pathologies

Nerve entrapment syndromes encompass a wide spectrum of clinical entities characterized by the compression, irritation, or injury of peripheral nerves, often within anatomical bottlenecks or due to external influences. The following chapter delineates the anatomical, pathophysiological, clinical, and diagnostic aspects of common and rare entrapment neuropathies affecting both the upper and lower extremities. Different other pathologies of peripheral nerves such as the Parsonage-Turner syndrome and traumatic nerve injuries—including obstetric and traumatic brachial plexus palsies—and iatrogenic nerve lesions are elaborated.

Special attention is given to peripheral nerve tumors. Diagnostic strategies including MRI, ultrasonography, and electrophysiological studies are emphasized, alongside therapeutic approaches ranging from conservative management to microsurgical decompression and nerve transfer techniques. This chapter aims to provide a detailed reference for clinicians and surgeons managing peripheral nerve pathologies, highlighting the importance of accurate diagnosis, individualized treatment, and awareness of rare but significant etiologies.

7.1 Nerve Entrapment Syndromes

Nerve entrapment syndromes typically occur at anatomical sites where the nerve is vulnerable to external compression, where it traverses a fibrous, muscular, or osseus canal, or at points where it alters its course and is thereby more prone to mechanical irritation.

Any peripheral nerve can be affected being compressive pathology, with the clinical presentation varying according to the specific nerve involved.

The following represent the most commonly encountered nerve entrapments:

7.1.1 Occipital Neuralgia

Occipital neuralgia typically presents with sudden paroxysmal pain localized in the posterior part of the skull base. It is expressed as a sharp and stabbing sensation radiating cranially toward the parietal and frontal regions of the head. Diagnostic and therapeutic nerve blockade may be employed to both confirm the diagnosis and

K. Hobitsch, *Peripheral Nerve Surgery - A Compendium*,
https://doi.org/10.1007/978-3-032-03409-0_7

relief the symptoms. The afflicted nerve can generally be identified between the mastoid process and the occipital protuberance.

If the characteristic pain can be elicited, surgical decompression of the nerve can be considered.

If pain can be reliably reproduced through palpation or manipulation, microsurgical decompression of the occipital nerve may be indicated.

Classically, the greater occipital nerve (GON), the lesser occipital nerve (LON) or the third occipital nerve (TON) are involved in occipital neuralgia (Fig. 7.1).

The **greater occipital nerve**, the largest of these, represents an afferent nerve originating from the C2 spinal nerve. During its course towards the superior nuchal line of the skull it perforates the semispinalis capitis muscle and, occasionally, the trapezius and the inferior oblique muscles, rendering susceptible to compression or irritation.

The **lower occipital nerve** —arising from spinal nerves C2 and C3—follows a course similar to the GON toward the occipital region, eventually communicating with it. The LON divides into three branches—the auricular, the mastoid, and the occipital branch.

The **third occipital nerve**, a superficial medial branch of the C3 spinal nerve may likewise be subject to compression. It pierces the splenius capitis, semispinalis capitis, and the trapezius muscles. The TON communicates with the GON and, in most individuals, with the contralateral TON [2].

7.1.2 Neurogenic Thoracic Outlet Syndrome (TOS)

The **thoracic outlet syndrome (TOS)** refers to a disorder caused by compression of the neurovascular structures as they traverse the thoracic outlet. The **neurogenic** form classically involves compression of the inferior trunk of the brachial plexus, whereas **vascular** TOS results from compression of the subclavian or axillary artery (Fig. 7.2). Several anatomical structures may

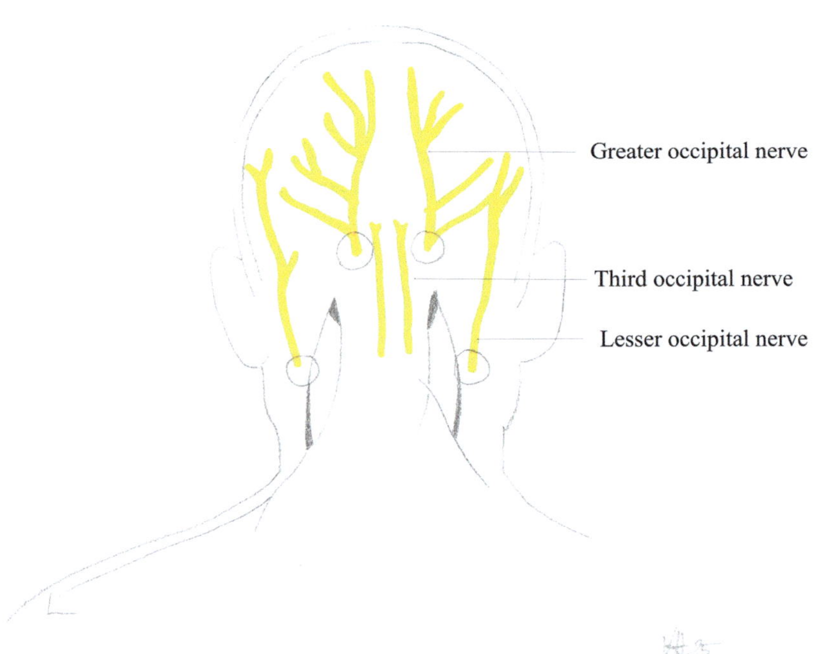

Fig. 7.1 Schematic drawing of the anatomy of the three occipital nerves showing furthermore the points for the occipital nerve block (circles)

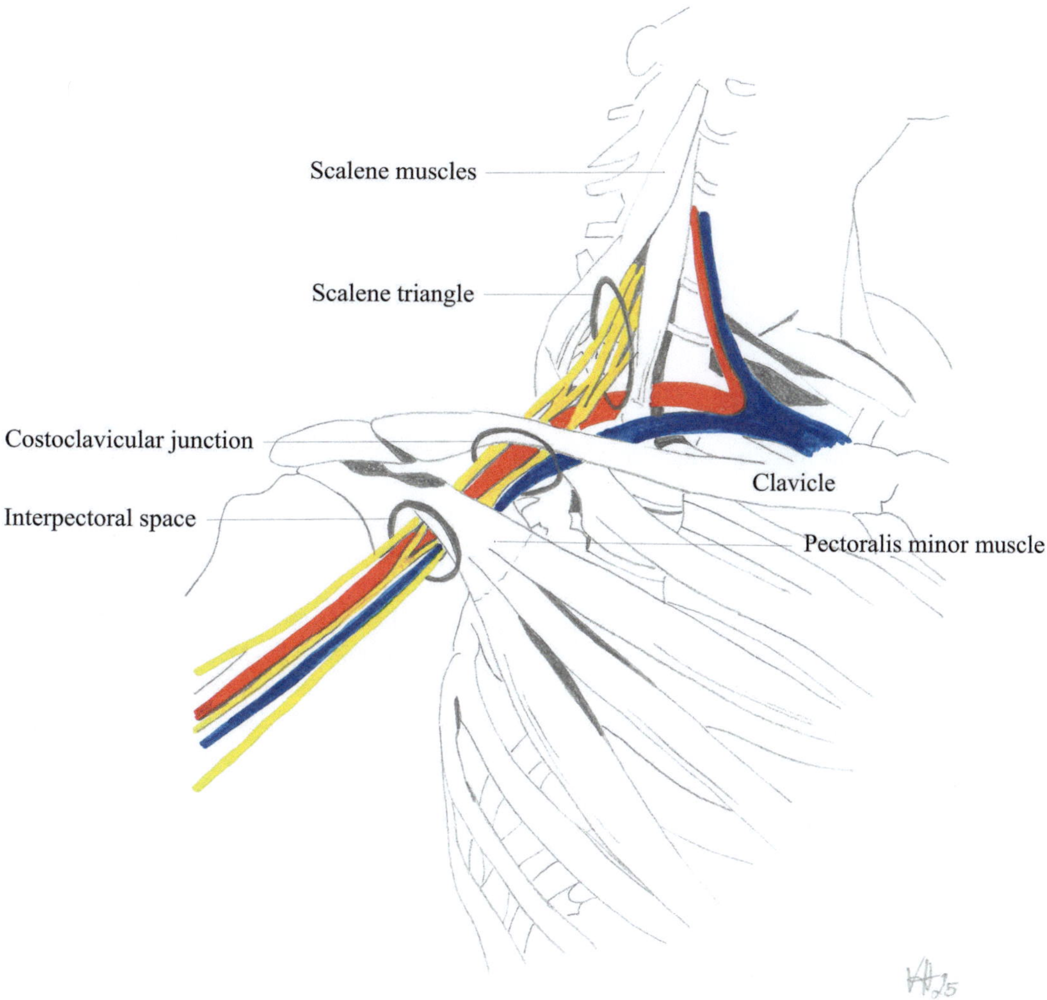

Fig. 7.2 Schematic drawing of the anatomy in thoracic outlet syndrome (TOS): Common sites of compression are the scalene triangle, the costoclavicular junction and the interpectoral space

contribute to this compression with the most common being:

> The anterior scalene muscle is usually not the cause of compression

- The medial scalene muscle and the first rib ➔ **Scalene syndrome**
- The first rib and/or the clavicule (commonly due to fractures) ➔ **Costoclavicular syndrome**
- The pectoral muscle and the coracoid process (e.g., through elevation and retroversion of the arm) ➔ **Minor pectoral syndrome** (Hyperabduction syndrome)
- Others (tumors, anatomical changes, e.g., after trauma)

> A thickened fascia of the middle scalene muscle represents the most common cause of TOS.

Patients with thoracic outlet syndrome are usually presenting with a dull pain in the shoulder and axillary region. Neuological manifestations may include paresthesia, weakness, or atrophy of the thenar and hypothenar musculature (innervated by the median and ulnar nerves)—a finding sometimes referred to as the "Gilliat-Sumner hand".

TOS occurs more frequently in women aged between 20 and 50 years [5, 6].

Identified risk factors include occupations or activities that place stress on the thoracic outlet (e.g. violinists or flutists), traumatic injuries such as heavy weight falling on the shoulder, or following cervical spine surgery which may alter regional biomechanics [4].

The diagnosis of TOS is typically one of exclusion, requiring careful differentiation from other causes of shoulder and upper extremity symptoms, such as nerve entrapment syndromes (particularly pectoralis minor syndrome or scalene syndrome), neoplasms, rotator cuff pathology, shoulder impingement or arthrosis, cervical disc protrusion, CRPS, and fibromyalgia.

A positive Tinel sign at the scalene triangle may indicate neural compression or injury of the nerve.

Several provocative maneuvers have been describes, including:

Adson test: With the patient seated and the affected shoulder placed in retroversion, the patient is asked to rotate the head to the ipsilateral side. While palpating the radial pulse, the patient is then instructed to take a deep inspiratory breath—a reduction in pulse amplitude is considered a positive test.

Roos test (elevated arm stress test)

Wright's test

Costoclavicular maneuver [8].

However, none of them are regarded as reliable tests to establish the diagnosis of TOS.

Symptoms are often position-dependent, but provocative maneuvers are often false positive. Therefore, the conditions remains a diagnosis of exclusion after ruling out more common underlying causes.

> Two quite simple test's that can be applied in cases whether the differential diagnosis may be a spinal root compression are the Spurling's test and the shoulder abduction sign. The Spurling's test involves passive lateral flexion of the head thereby compressing the ipsilateral nerve root to elicit radiating pain along the corresponding dermatome. Shoulder abduction or elevating the arm above the head will widen the neuroforamen thus relieving the pain. Patients with TOS will not tolerate this maneuver as it tends to reproduce or aggravate pain [9].

Physical examnation should be complemented with electrodiagnostic studies (EMG) and magnetic resonance imaging (MRI) of the brachial plexus. MRI of the sagittal plane provides the best visualization for TOS. A frequent finding is straightening of the cervical spine secondary to loss of the normal lordotic curvature (Fig. 7.3).

Because TOS represents a dynamic rather than a fixed nerve entrapment syndrome, intrinsic nerve changes are not typically observed. However, radiological indicators may include loss of perineural fat tissue or adjacent gliding tissue, as well as the presence of a compressive structure. In chronic or longstanding cases, alterations in nerve signal intensity or deviations in the course of a nerve may become apparent.

The ultrasound represents another valuable diagnostic modality in the assessment of TOS. It allows for differentiation between a supraclavicular compression—classically caused by hypertrophy of the medial scalene muscle—and costoclavicular narrowing. The latter is particularly evident during dynamic ultrasonography with the arm placed in hyperabduction, and often involves compression of the subclavian artery by a cervical rib.

Clinical differentiation of TOS from cervical discopathy can be challenging. Magnetic resonance imaging may demonstrate characteristic nerve changes, thereby aiding in diagnosis.

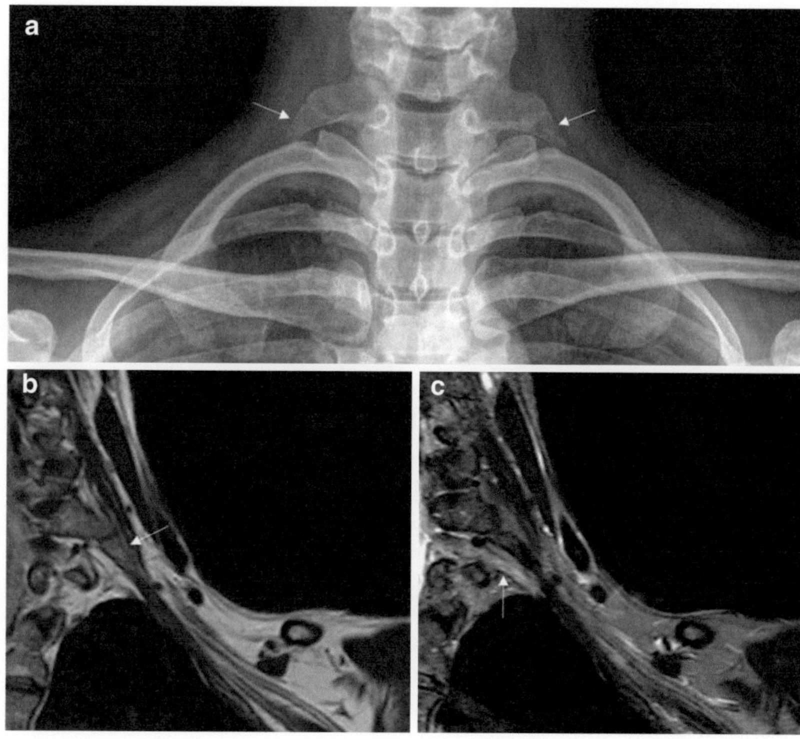

Fig. 7.3 X-ray and MRI images of the upper chest and neck region. Demonstration characteristic imaging findings in Thoracic Outlet Syndrome: Bilateral cervical ribs (arrows) visualized on (**a**) anteroposterior plain radiograph of the upper thorax and (**b**) coronal T2 MRI, associated with increased signal intensity of the C8 nerve root, as seen on (**c**) coronal STIR sequence (arrow)

Additionally, sensory nerve action potential (SNAP) can be useful in differentiating TOS from cervical spine pathology, specifically in localizing preganglionic versus postganglionic lesions.

Close attention should be paid on the patient's history, especially regarding the characteristic pain. Patients with cervical nerve root compression often report pain relief when elevating the arm above shoulder level, which may serve as a distinguishing clinical feature.

Regarding treatment, initial treatment should be conservative consisting of analgesic therapy and physiotherapy. Surgical intervention is reserved for cases refractory to conservative treatment, and is aimed at decompression of the involved neural structures, and if indicated, the vascular structures.

With respect to the surgical technique, the three brachial plexus trunks are typically approached via a supraclavicular incision or a combined supra- and infraclavicular in cases when a first rib anomaly constitutes the compressive etiology. Decompression of the inferior trunk is most commonly achieved through resection of the compressive structure.

Potential complications include fibrous adhesions, lymphatic fistula, hematoma, surgical site infection, pneumothorax and iatrogenic injury to the C7 spinal root, long thoracic nerve, or the adjacent artery. Persistent postoperative pain most frequently arises from inappropriate patient selection or incomplete resection of the compressive structure.

7.1.3 Suprascapular Nerve Entrapment Syndrome (SNES)

The **suprascapular nerve entrapment syndrome** (**SNES**)—although rare—should be considered in patients presenting with shoulder pain in the posterior-lateral region as the predominant symptom. Clinical manifestations may include muscular weakness secondary to atrophy of the supraspinatus and infraspinatus muscles. Given that the suprascapular nerve is a purely motor nerve, sensory deficits are not observed.

The most common etiologies of SNES are either the compressing superior transverse scapular ligament at the suprascapular notch or the inferior transverse scapular ligament at the spinoglenoid notch (Fig. 7.4).

Athletes participating in sports such as volleyball, tennis and swimming, exhibit a higher predisposition to suprascapular nerve entrapment syndrome. Ganglion cysts are also frequently observed. Additionally, injuries to the rotator cuff muscles serve as another etiological factor.

Clinically, patients typically complain about shoulder pain secondary to shoulder girdle-disbalance. In cases of chronic lesions, associated muscle atrophy—particularly of the supraspinatus and infraspinatus muscles—may be evident [10].

The MRI may reveal denervation edema of the infraspinatus muscle. Furthermore, the suprascapular nerve can be visualized and traced using ultrasonography.

Surgical treatment generally implies microsurgical or arthroscopic decompression of the suprascapular nerve [11].

7.1.4 Parsonage-Turner Syndrome (Neuralgic Shoulder Amyotrophy)

The **Parsonage-Turner Syndrome**—also referred as **brachial plexus neuritis**—is, in fact, not classified as a nerve entrapment syndrome but is important to consider as a differential diagnosis.

It is characterized by the acute onset of severe nocturnal shoulder pain. Within hours to days, patients may develop paresis of the shoulder and

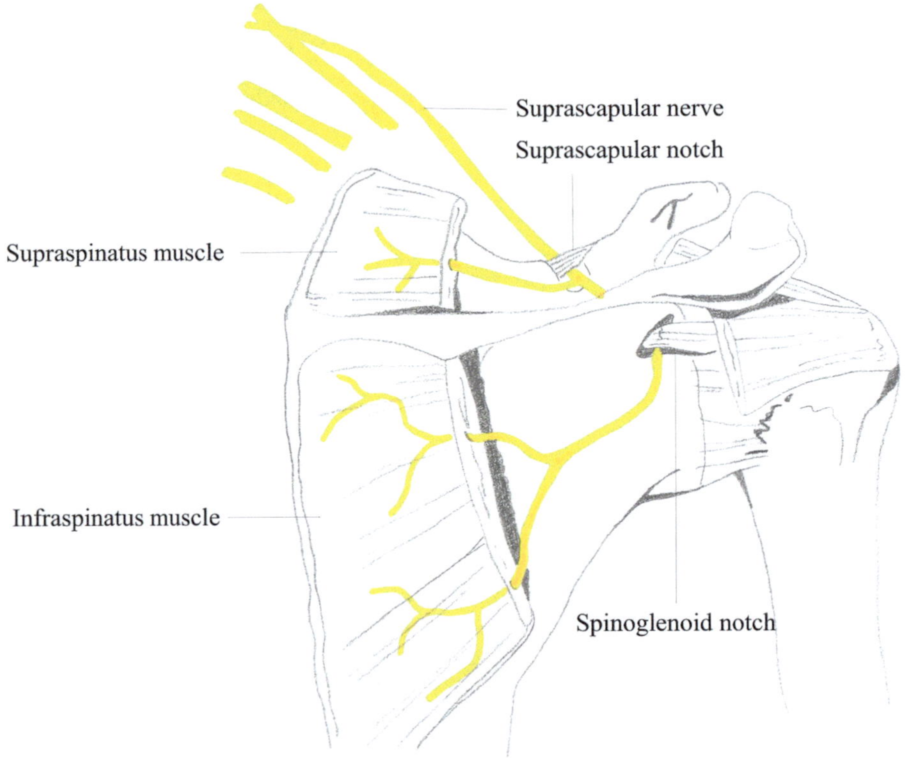

Fig. 7.4 An anatomical diagram of the shoulder region highlighting the suprascapular nerve and its pathway

upper arm, classically affecting the deltoid and serratus anterior muscles.

The exact pathophysiology remains unclear, however, an autoimmune etiology is suspected.

Electrophysiological studies typically demonstrate a decreased nerve conduction velocity and denervation signs in the deltoid muscle.

Denervation of the deltoid muscle initially is expressed by edema on imaging, progressing to atrophy over time. The affected nerve may appear normal or exhibit varying degrees of swelling, with or without focal constriction [14] (Fig. 7.5).

Neurological deficits usually manifest within 24 hours to 2 weeks following the onset of pain, and and sensorimotor deficits [15].

Historically, treatment has been entirely conservative, including glucocorticoids, analgetic medication, and physiotherapy.

Surgical interventions, typically involving primarily nerve reconstruction or nerve transfer techniques, is indicated in cases where no functional recovery is observed.

Another rare neurological condition, primarily characterized by its morphological appearance on ultrasound and magnetic resonance neurography (MRN), is the *hourglass-like constriction (HGC)* of a peripheral nerve. This finding has been observed in patients with neuralgic amyotrophy, Lyme borreliosis, postinfectious neuropathies, or trauma.

Specifically, HGC constitutes a severe focal constriction affecting either the entire nerve or fascicles with or without additional torsion [17] (Fig. 7.6).

The precise pathomechanism is not clearly understood yet, as this phenomenon is not attributable to external compression, despite its morphological appearance. An inflammatory response involving the extrinsic vascular system may contribute to the development of this disorder [18–20].

On imaging, fascicular constriction with or without torsion can be identified. These changes may occur in multiple nerves simultaneously, at multiple sites along a single nerve, or in several fascicles within the nerve.

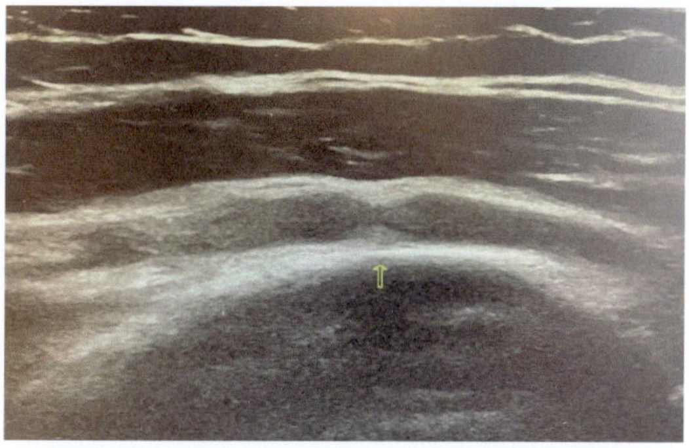

Fig. 7.6 Ultrasound image showing a cross-sectional view of an hour-glass formation of the radial nerve (arrow) in a patient who suffered from neuralgic shoulder amyotrophy

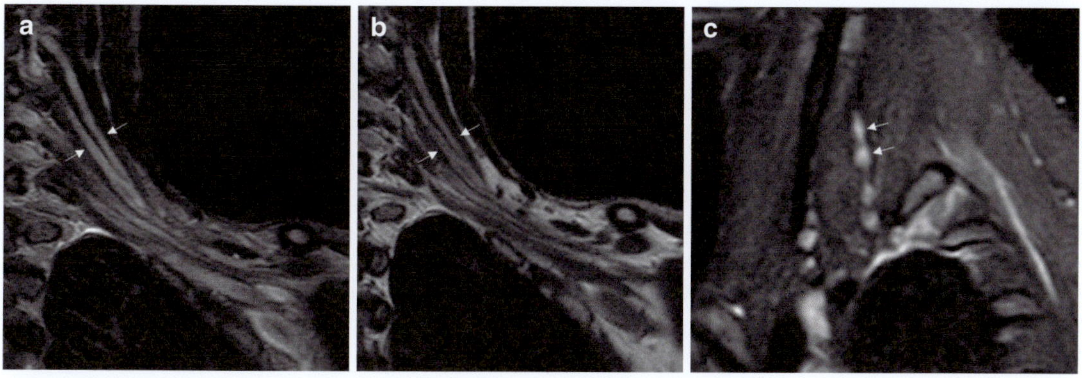

Fig. 7.5 Magnetic resonance imaging demonstrating characteristic sings of Parsonage-Turner Syndrome: C5 and C6 nerve roots are affected (arrows) and exhibit increased signal intensity on coronal STIR (**a**), coronal T2 (**b**), and sagittal STIR (**c**)

> In fact, the hourglass-like constriction represents a highly challenging morphological finding that is frequently overlooked on magnetic resonance neurography and ultrasonography.

The hourglass-like constriction predominantly affects nerves of the upper extremities, particularly the radial, the median, and the anterior interosseus nerves, with the notable exception of the ulnar nerve [23]. A potential explanation is that torsion is associated with nerve motion. The ulnar nerve follows a relatively straight course through the arm, whereas the medial and the radial nerves—especially the anterior and posterior interosseous nerves—exhibit multiple curves along their path to the target muscle.

HGC has not been observed in the lower extremities.

Clinically, a sudden onset of symptoms with pain, sensitive disturbances, and motor weakness is typical.

The prognosis of an hourglass-like constriction is generally poor. Regarding treatment options, there is no consensus yet, due to the rarity of this condition.

In cases without spontaneous recovery, surgical intervention—ranging from interfascicular neurolysis to nerve grafting, depending on the severity—may provide functional benefit [24].

7.1.5 Compression of the Axillary Nerve/Quadrilateral Space Syndrome (QSS)

The **quadrilateral space** describes an anatomical quadrangular space within the axillary region that encompasses the axillary nerve and the posterior humeral circumflex artery together with its accompanying vein. Its borders are mainly defined by the surrounding musculature of the shoulder region. Compression of either the neural or vascular structures within this space constitutes a form of neurovascular compression syndrome, termed quadrilateral space syndrome (QSS).

Compression my result from fibrous ligaments, muscular hypertrophy, paralabral or ganglion cysts, or space occupying lesions such as tumors [25].

QSS is more frequently seen in male patients and in individuals engaged in overhead or throwing activities such as volleyball which may predispose to localized impingement.

The predominant clinical manifestation is posterior shoulder pain, typically aggravated by abduction, anteversion, or external rotation of the arm. Paresthesias in the distribution of the axillary nerve may also occur.

The diagnosis of QSS is primarily clinical and requires the exclusion of other etiologies of shoulder pain and neuromuscular compromise.

Magnetic resonance imaging (MRI) may show denervation edema of the deltoid and teres minor muscles in chronic stages, whereas magnetic resonance angiography (MRA) may reveal compression of the posterior humeral circumflex artery.

Conservative management is the first-line approach consisting of physiotherapy, therapeutic massage, and analgetic medication. Surgery is indicated rarely.

7.1.6 Holstein-Lewis Fracture

Fractures involving the middle and distal third of the humeral shaft are associated with a risk of **radial nerve entrapment injury** in approximately 2–17% of patients [28]. The clinical presentation corresponds to a radial nerve palsy typically manifesting as wrist drop and sensory deficits over the dorsal aspect of the hand.

In the absence of spontaneous neurological recovery within 3 months, surgical exploration and intervention is indicated.

7.1.7 Lesion of the Musculocutaneous Nerve

Isolated **musculocutaneous nerve (MCN) injuries** are exceedingly rare. They may occur secondary to shoulder dislocation or direct trauma, or iatrogenic causes following surgical procedures [29].

Clinically, patients typically present with hypesthesia over the antero-lateral aspect of the forearm and weakness in elbow flexion due to impaired biceps brachii and brachial function.

Two important differential diagnoses must be considered:

The C6 radiculopathy, which is a condition characterized by pain and paresthesia radiating into the thumb and index finger, which is not observed in isolated MCN lesions as the lateral antebrachial cutaneous nerve does not supply sensory innervation distal to the wrist. Additionally, motor deficits extend beyond musculocutaneous-innervated muscles, distinguishing it from a pure MCN lesion.

Rupture of the biceps tendon represents with acute pain and characteristic "Popeye sign" in which the retracted biceps muscle can be palpated or visualized proximally after contraction [30]. It should be considered as a differential diagnosis too.

7.1.8 Compression of the Median Nerve

Compression of the Median Nerve in the Upper Arm—Complete Lesion

Patients typically present with hypesthesia involving the thenar eminence, the palmar surface of the hand, the thumb and middle and fingers as well as the radial aspect of the ring finger.

In terms of motor deficit, affected individuals demonstrate an inability to pronate the forearm—either against resistance or, in severe cases, even against gravity.

Weak pronation of the forearm is possible because of the preserved function of the brachioradialis muscle.

Flexion of the hand is markedly weakened, still partially preserved owing to the contribution of the ulnar-nerve innervated flexor carpi ulnas muscle. In contrast, abduction and opposition of the thumb are absent due to median nerve dysfunction.

In cases of chronic median nerve palsy, characteristic deformities may develop, including the "ape hand" deformity and the or "benediction sign", the latter resulting from an inability the flex the thumb, index and middle fingers [31] (Fig. 7.7).

The "bottle sign" serves as a clinical test of abductor pollicis brevis and opponens pollicis weakness. Affected patients are unable to grasp and enclose a cylindrical object, such as a bottle, with all fingers.

Ultrasound and electrophysiological studies are valuable diagnostic tools to confirm median nerve compression and to evaluate the extent of functional impairment.

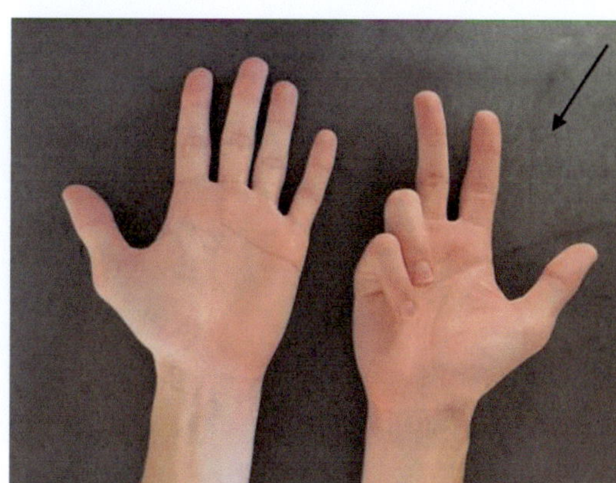

Fig. 7.7 "Benediction sign" seen in the right hand, due to the inability to flex the thumb, index and middle fingers (arrow) in individuals with prolonged median nerve injury. Flexion of digits IV and V is still possible due to preserved ulnar nerve function

When the median nerve injury arises in the context of trauma or a humeral fracture, concomitant injury to the brachial artery must also be considered.

Supracondylar fractures of the humerus are frequently displaced or complicated by excessive callus formation. These fractures often involve injury to the anterior interosseus nerve, which is particularly vulnerable due to its fixed course in the posterior tissues. Such injuries occur more commonly in children [32].

Compression of the Median Nerve at the Struthers Ligament

The **Struthers ligament** represents an additional structure extending between the supracondylar process and the medial epicondyle of the humerus. It was first described by John Struthers in 1848 and may become thickened, either congenitally or as a result of inflammatory processes [35].

The median nerve, accompanied by the brachial artery, traverses the space between the Struthers ligament and the humeral shaft.

The predominant clinical manifestation is pain in the median-nerve innervated dermatome which is typically aggravated by elbow flexion. Occasionally, a palpable bony prominence proximal to the elbow can be identified. Motor and sensory deficits are uncommon [37, 38].

> In some cases, a branch to the pronator teres muscle arises proximal the Struthers ligament, resulting in preservation of this muscle function.

Compression of the Median Nerve by the Bicipital Aponeurosis (Lacertus Syndrome)

This represents a rare site of median nerve compression typically caused by a thickened bicipital aponeurosis (lacertus fibrosis) or by a hypertrophic or hypertonic biceps brachii muscle, most often associated with repetitive movements of the arm [41] (Fig. 7.8).

Clinically, patients present with a persistent forearm pain and localized tenderness on palpation over the lacertus fibrosus, situated a few centimeters distal to the elbow joint. In addition, motor deficits may occur, particularly involving the flexor pollicis longus, flexor carpi radialis, and flexor digitorum profundus muscles [43, 44].

Anterior Interosseus Nerve Syndrome

The most common etiologies of **anterior interosseus nerve (AIN) syndrome** include idiopathic inflammatory processes, trauma (such as penetrating injuries), fracture, or compression by adjacent muscular or tendinous structures.

The anterior interosseus nerve provides motor innervation to three muscles: the flexor pollicis longus, the pronator quadratus, and the radial portion of the flexor digitorum profundus. Consequently, motor deficits predominantly affect the thumb and the index finger. A classical clinical maneuver is the "pinch test", in which the patient is asked to hold a sheet of paper between thumb and index finger. Inability to approximate the fingertips, resulting instead in a pulp-to-pulp pinch, represents a positive sign of AIN weakness [45, 47] (Fig. 7.9).

Conservative treatment—including analgesic therapy and physiotherapy—represents the first-line approach, as this condition is classically self-limiting. Surgical decompression may be considered if pain persists beyond six months or if there is evidence of progressive motor deficit [46].

Pronator-Teres Syndrome

Pronator teres syndrome is a proximal median nerve compression neuropathy, most commonly caused by hypertrophy of the pronator teres muscle secondary to repetitive pronation or grasping movements. Other etiologies include peripheral nerve sheath tumors or direct trauma [49]. Gradual onset of pain in the proximal arm, which may be aggravated by pronation and localized tenderness over the pronator teres muscle are the leading symptoms of this compression neuropathy.

Hypoesthesia or motor weakness are uncommon, but when present, weakness of flexion in the second and third fingers can be observed.

Pronator teres muscle strength is classically preserved, as the nerve branches supplying this muscle originate more proximally.

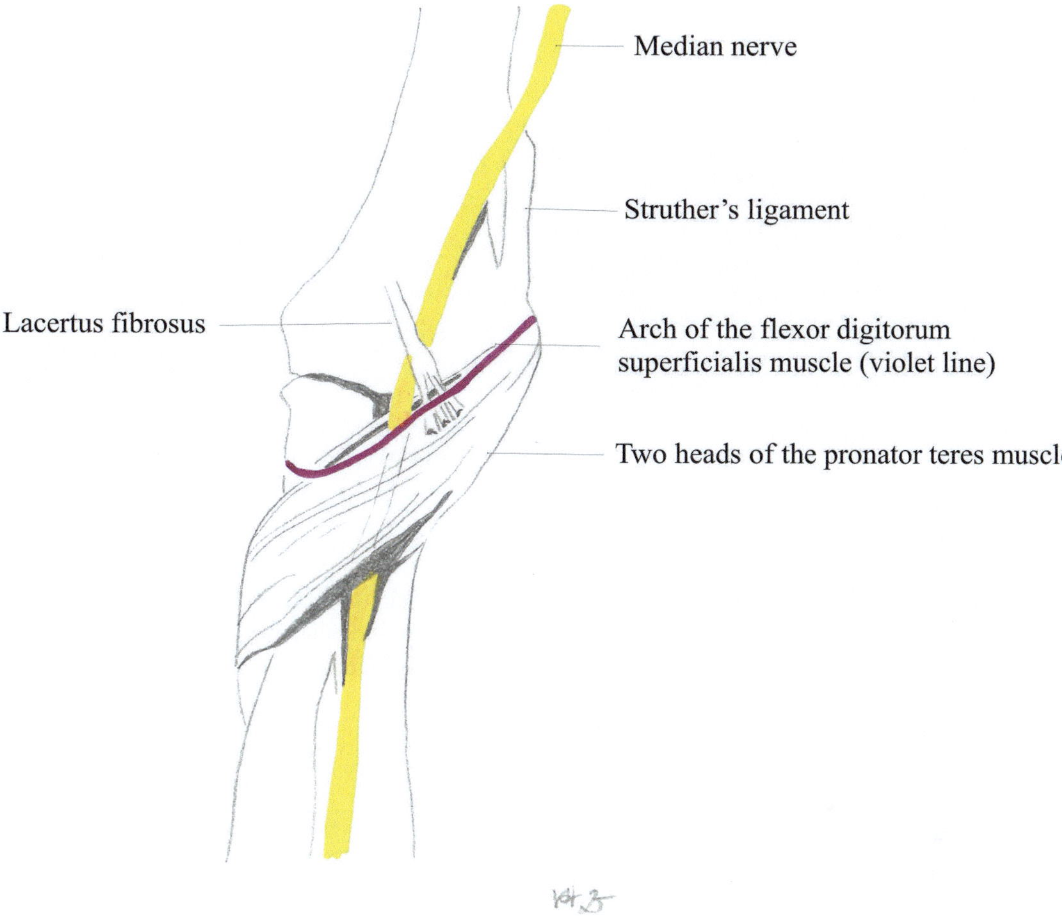

Fig. 7.8 Anatomical drawing showing the course of the median nerve in the elbow region with possible sites of compression

The absence of nocturnal pain and sensory deficits differentiates the pronator-teres syndrome from the carpal tunnel syndrome [53].

Carpal-Tunnel Syndrome (CTS)

Carpal tunnel syndrome (**CTS**) is the most common entrapment neuropathy resulting from compression of the median nerve beneath the flexor retinaculum at the palmar aspect of the wrist.

Systemic predisposing factors include diabetes mellitus, chronic renal insufficiency with dialysis, rheumatoid arthritis, adipositas, acromegaly, hypothyroidism, and pregnancy [54, 55].

Patients typically report electric shock-like pain and paresthesia radiating from the wrist to the thumb, index and middle fingers, and the radial aspect side of the ring finger, often worse at night.

Hypoesthesia is usually mild, as the palmar cutaneous branch of the median nerve, which supplies most of the palmar sensation, courses superficially over the flexor retinaculum of the hand and is therefore spared [58].

In severe or chronic cases, thenar muscle atrophy can be observed.

Clinical examination may reveal positive Hofmann-Tinel's, Phalen's and Flick sign. The

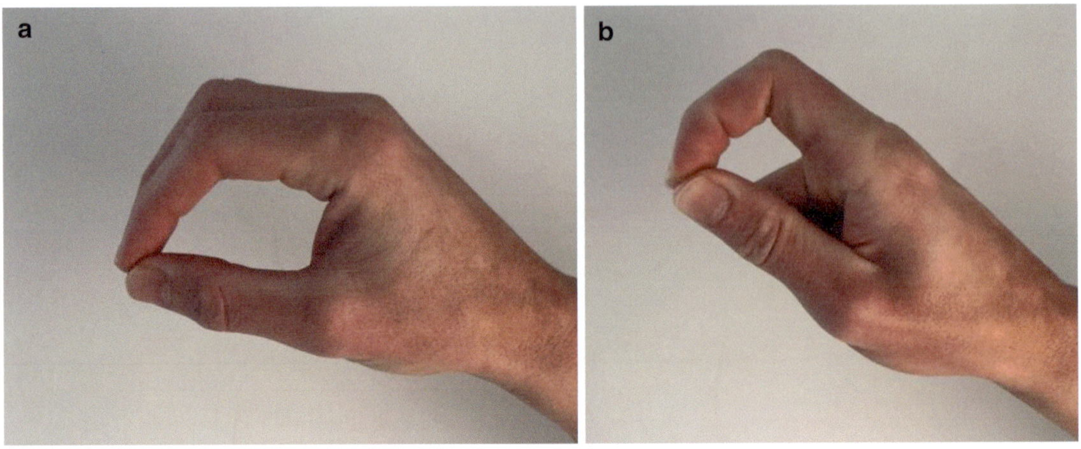

Fig. 7.9 Two-panel image demonstrating anterior interosseus syndrome: (**a**) shows the "OK-sign" in an unaffected hand. Hand posture due to paresis of the flexor digitorum profundus and the flexor pollicis brevis muscles is demonstrated in (**b**)

Durkan test is another commonly used maneuver, considered positive when pain or paresthesia in the median nerve innervated-digits is elicited after pressing over the carpal tunnel for approximately 30 seconds.

Electrophysiological studies are recommended to determine the severity of nerve compression, while ultrasonography can be particularly useful for preoperative evaluation.

Conservative treatment includes analgesics, local corticosteroid injections, physiotherapy, and wrist splinting. In cases refractory to conservative therapy or in the presence of progressive muscle weakness, surgery is indicated.

7.1.9 Compression of the Ulnar Nerve

Compression of the Ulnar Nerve at the Upper Arm—Complete Ulnar Lesion

Due to its anatomical proximity, an ulnar nerve injury at this level may also involve the median nerve and the brachial artery, particularly in the setting of trauma [59].

A variety of signs and symptoms may be evident, the most common ones are listed below:

<u>Hypoesthesia in following locations:</u>

- At the hypothenar eminence (palmar cutaneous branch of the ulnar nerve)
- Along the ulnar side of fourth and fifth digits (superficial sensory division)
- At the dorsomedial third of the hand and fingers (dorsal cutaneous branch of the ulnar nerve)

> If hypoesthesia extends more than 2 cm proximal to the wrist (territory of the medial cutaneous antebrachial nerve), a proximal lesion should be suspected, particularly involving the medial fascicle of the brachial plexus or the C8/T1 nerve roots.

<u>Motor weakness in the following:</u>

- Ulnar abduction of the wrist (flexor carpi ulnaris and extensor carpi ulnaris muscles)
- Flexion of the distal interphalangeal (DIP) joint of digits IV + V (flexor digitorum profundus muscle)
- Intrinsic muscles of the hand
- Abduction (dorsal interossei muscles) and adduction of the fingers (palmar interossei muscles)

Muscular atrophy is most evident at the hypothenar eminence and the dorsal interosseous I muscles.

The classically seen "claw hand" in individuals with chronic ulnar nerve injury, results from hyperextension of metacarpophalangeal (MCP) joints of digits IV–V accompanied by the partial flexion of the proximal and the distal interphalangeal (PIP and DIP) joints (Fig. 7.10).

Due to loss of lumbrical and interossei muscle function, flexion of the affected fingers is only possible at the distal segments.

The Wartenberg sign represents the unvoluntary abduction of digit V—due to weakness of the palmar interosseus muscle being responsible for the adduction movement—caused by the unopposed action of the extensor digiti minimi muscle (Fig. 7.11).

The Froment-sign is a clinical indicator, characterized by compensatory flexion of the DIP joint of the thumb. This occurs when the patient is asked to grasp a piece of paper firmly between the thumb and index finger, reflecting loss of function of the abductor pollicis muscle [62] (Fig. 7.12).

As already mentioned in median nerve compression syndromes, additional sonographic and electrophysiological studies should be performed prior to surgery.

Compression of the Ulnar Nerve at the Cubita

At that level of the elbow, the ulnar nerve is susceptible to compression to multiple sites, with the **cubital tunnel syndrome** being the most frequent (Fig. 7.13).

Compression by the arcade of Struther's:

The arcade of Struther's is an aponeurotic band spanning from the supracondylar process to the medial epicondyle of the humerus in the distal third of the humeral bone, thereby forming a

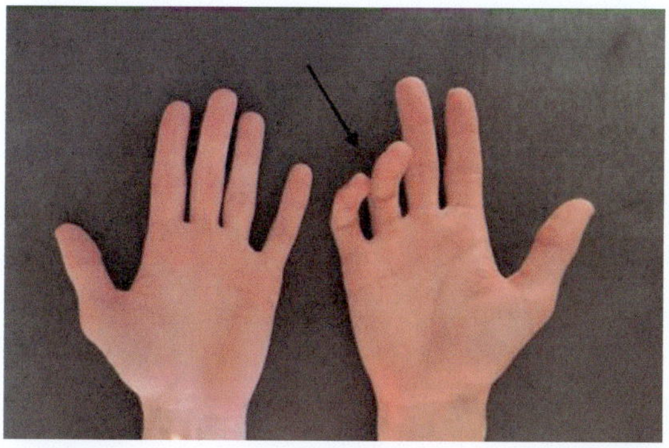

Fig. 7.10 The right hand demonstrates the characteristic claw hand: Hyperextension of the metacarpophalangeal joints and flexion of the proximal and distal interphalangeal joints (arrow) in chronic ulnar nerve injury

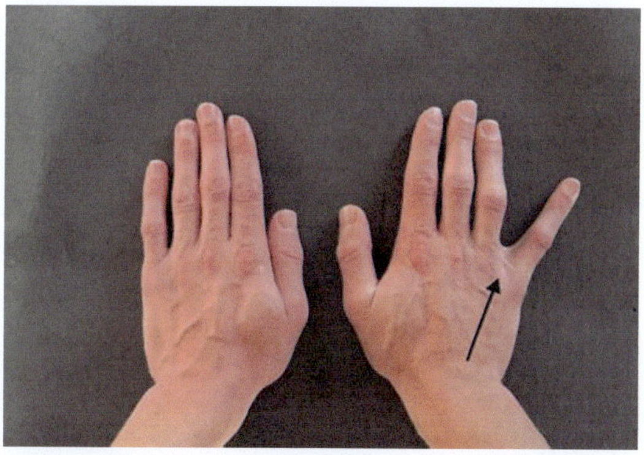

Fig. 7.11 The right hand demonstrates Wartenberg-sign: Involuntary abduction of the fifth finger (arrow) due to weakness of the adducting palmar interosseus III muscle

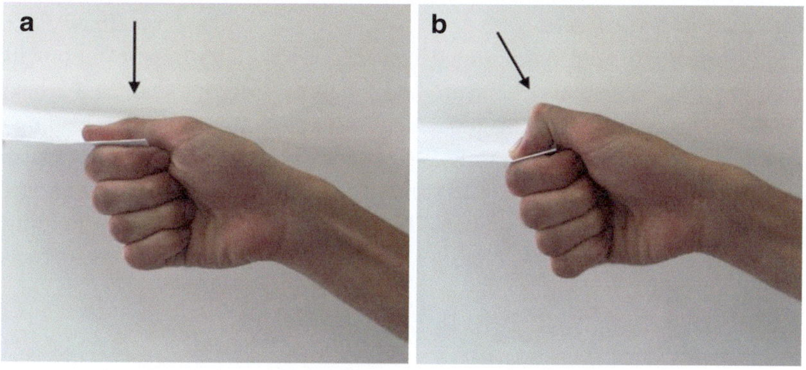

Fig. 7.12 Two-panel image showing. Froment sign in (**b**) due to weakness of the abductor policies muscle. (**a**) Demonstrates the unaffected thumb

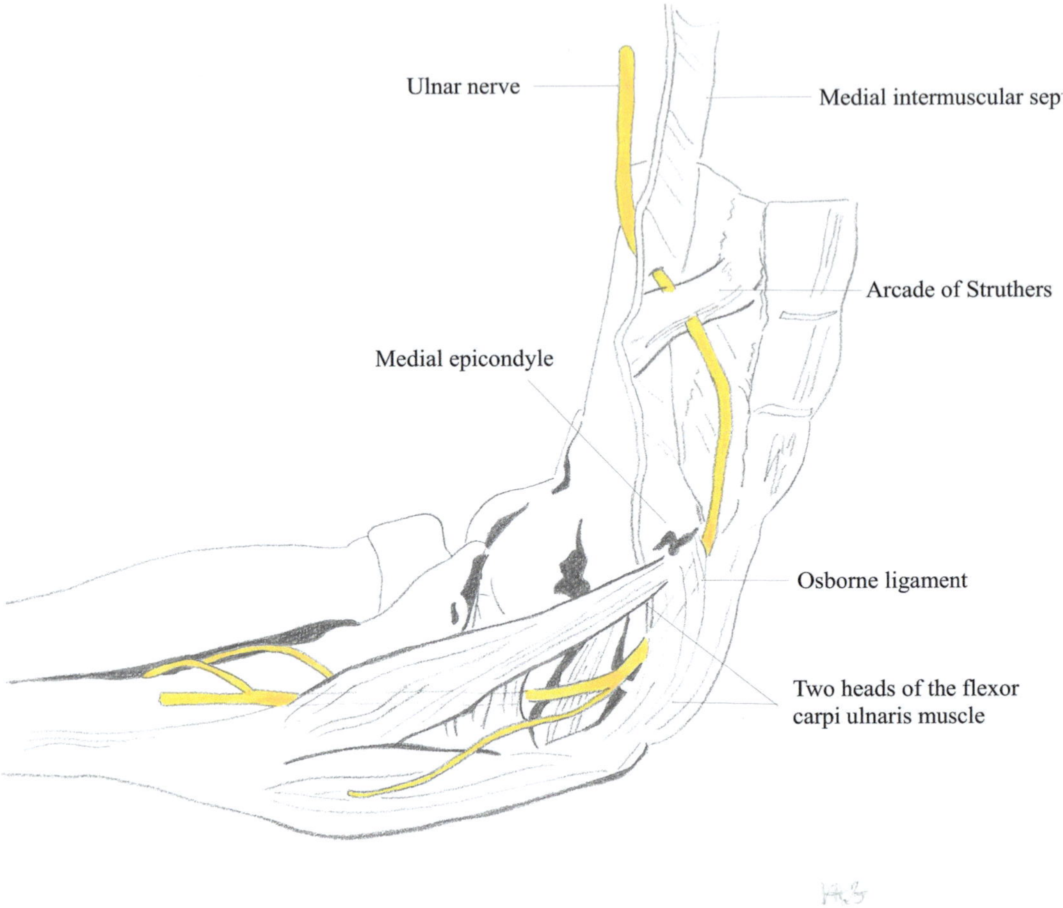

Fig. 7.13 Course of the ulnar nerve in the distal upper arm and proximal forearm with its possible sites of compression

fibro-osseus tunnel (Struther's arcade) through which the ulnar nerve passes [64].

Neuropathy at this site is most commonly observed following surgical transposition of the ulnar nerve, if the compressing arcade of Struther's is not released.

Cubital tunnel syndrome:

The **cubital tunnel syndrome** describes compression of the ulnar nerve beneath the aponeurosis between the humeral and ulnar heads of the flexor carpi ulnaris (FCU) muscle, also known as the humeroulnar arcade or Osborne ligament [66]. The ulnar nerve— accompanied by the posterior ulnar recurrent artery— passes beneath this band, and thickening of the Osborne ligament may lead to nerve compression.

Sonography may reveal a flattened nerve beneath the arcade with proximal edema.

Early symptoms may include hypoesthesia of the fifth digit and the ulnar side of the fourth digit, elicited by elbow flexion or direct compression. Later manifestations include pain along the ulnar dermatome, and weakness of the intrinsic hand muscles, often leading to difficulty holding a pen.

The **Dellon classification** categorizes ulnar nerve compression at the elbow based on symptom severity, providing a useful classification for guiding treatment decisions [71] (Table 7.1):

Table 7.1 Dellon classification for ulnar nerve lesion in the cubital tunnel

Dellon classification			
Grade	Mild	Moderate	Severe
Sensitivity	Intermittent paresthesia	Intermittent paresthesia	Persistent paresthesia
Motor	Subjective weakness	Measurable weakness	Palsy with muscle atrophy (Claw hand)
EMG	>40 m/s	40–30 m/s	<30 m/s
Treatment	Conservative	Decompression	Decompression ± anterior transposition

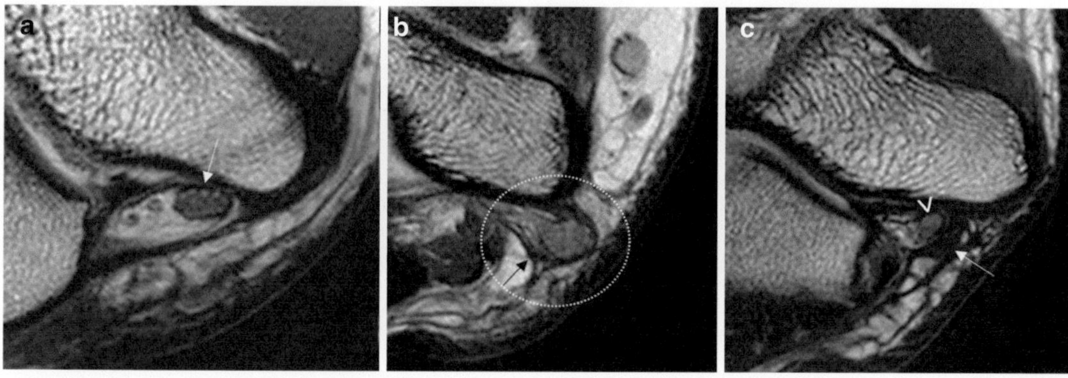

Fig. 7.14 Ulnar nerve within the ulnar tunnel on axial MRI images: (**a**) shows a normal ulnar nerve, while in (**b**) the nerve is subluxated, and in (**c**) it is compressed by a thickened Osborne ligament (arrow)

Subluxation of the ulnar nerve at the ulnar sulcus:

The "snapping ulnar nerve" is typically caused by anatomical variations, such as the presence of a shallow groove or weakness of the ligaments [72].

Aquired factors include arthritic changes of the elbow cartilage and repetitive elbow-flexion movements, for example during throwing activities [75].

Patients commonly report tingling or paresthesia, and occasionally pain in the ulnar nerve distribution of the hand.

Diagnosis can be made clinically by palpating the snapping nerve at the medial epicondyle during elbow flexion and extension, with the ultrasound or MRI serving as adjunctive imaging modalities (Figs. 7.14 and 7.15).

Treatment implies the surgical transposition of the ulnar nerve to a more medial subcutaneous position [74]. Care must be taken to avoid excessive tension, as overly tight fixation may result in postoperative compression of the ulnar nerve.

> Snapping triceps syndrome is characterized by dislocation of the distal part of the triceps tendon over the medial epicondyle during elbow flexion or extension.

Ulnar Nerve Entrapment at the Level of the Forearm and Hand

Compression by a thickened fascia of the flexor carpi ulnaris (FCU) and flexor digitorum profundus muscle (FDP):

Typically located approximately 5 cm distal to the medial epicondyle, this is a rare site of ulnar nerve entrapment syndrome [77]. Symptoms are nonspecific and may be provoked by repeated pronation and wrist flexion.

Compression of the dorsal cutaneous branch of the ulnar nerve at the level of the wrist between the FCU and the ulnar bone:

Causes include carpal ganglion, ulnar bone fracture, or iatrogenic injury. Patients typically perceive hypoesthesia at the dorsomedial third of the hand [78].

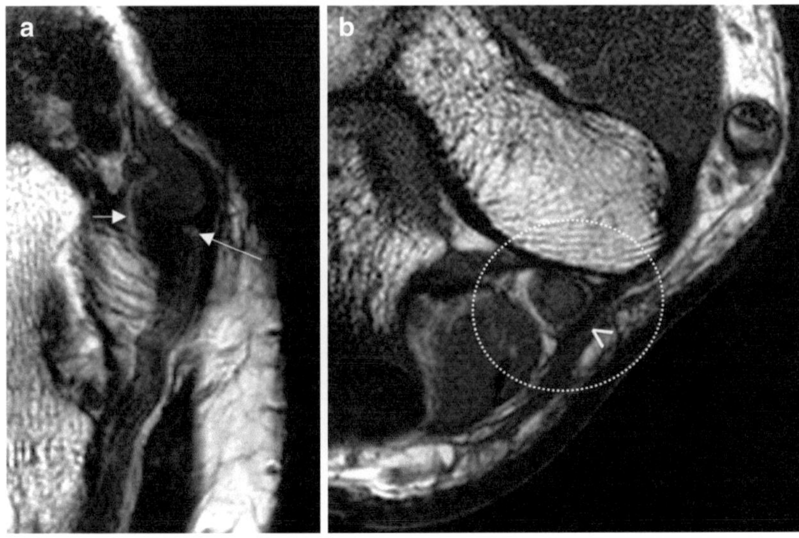

Fig. 7.15 Compression of the ulnar nerve (dotted circle in **b**—axial MRI) caused by fibrotic bands (arrows in **a**—coronal T2 and arrowhead in **b**). Note the abrupt change in the nerve trajectory visible in (**a**) (arrows)

Guyon canal syndrome:

The **Guyon canal** is defined by following borders [81, 83]:

Pisiform bone = ulnar border

Hamate bone = radial border

Palmar or volar carpal ligament = roof (stabilizes wrist motion)

Transverse carpal ligament = floor

Both the ulnar nerve and ulnar artery traverse the Guyon canal with the ulnar artery positioned radially. Within the canal, the ulnar nerve bifurcates into its superficial and deep branches, as does the artery.

The Guyon canal syndrome is classically caused by prolonged compression of the hypothenar eminence, as seen in cyclists, extensive computer workers or writers. Other possible causes are ganglion cysts, fractures (more proximally located in the canal), or ulnar artery aneurysm/thrombosis (more distally located in the canal).

Based on the segment of the ulnar nerve, Guyon canal syndrome can be divided into three zones [85]:

Zone I: Proximal ulnar nerve injury prior to its bifurcation leads to hypesthesia of the fifth digit and the ulnar side of the fourth digit, as well as weakness of the intrinsic muscles. Pain at the palmar aspect of the wrist and hypothenar region due to compression, is present.

Zone II: Affects the deep ulnar branch. No sensitive deficits are present. If the site of compression affects the proximal part of the ulnar nerve, the deep ulnar branch—as well as the muscular branches— are lesioned resulting in weakness of the hypothenar muscles (abductor digiti minimi, opponens digiti minimi, and flexor digiti minimi brevis) with an evident claw hand in chronic injury. In cases of distal compression (distal to the hamate bone), the hypothenar muscle is preserved and only the dorsal interossei muscles are weakened thus having a patient presenting with difficulties in finger spreading, but without the presence of a claw hand.

> Presence of a palmar brevis muscle contraction indicates a more proximal lesion, as this muscle is innervated by the superficial ulnar branch.

Zone III: Compression of the superficial branch of the ulnar nerve results in hypesthesia of the ulnar-nerve innervated sensitive dermatome and weakness of the palmar brevis muscle (Fig. 7.16).

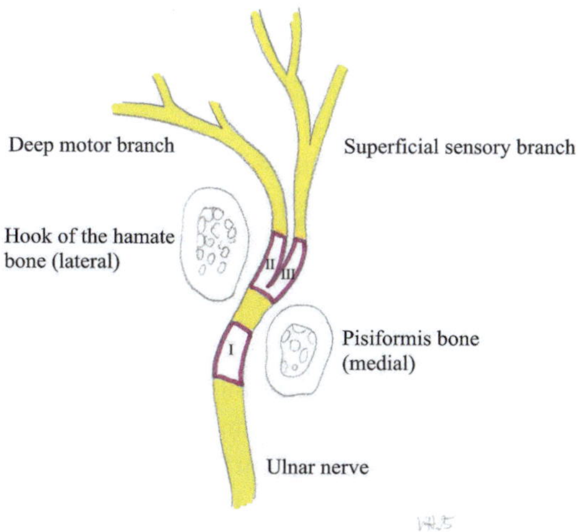

Fig. 7.16 Schematic drawing of the ulnar nerve in the Guyon canal with its 3 zones (I–III)

7.1.10 Compression of the Radial Nerve

Paresis of the Triceps Muscle

Paresis of the triceps muscle represents a very rare condition, usually occuring after trauma—affecting the branch to the triceps muscle located proximally in the axilla [87].

If present, it leads to only minimal functional restriction, as gravity assists elbow extension.

Reinnervation after radial nerve injury is generally successful as the radial nerve does not heavily contribute to fine motor movements. Recovery of the finger extensor muscles is often poor and may require tendon transfer.

> Proximal radial nerve lesions preserve function of the deltoid (axillary branch) and the latissimus dorsi muscle (thoracodorsal branch), in contrast to posterior cord lesions. In proximal radial versus posterior cord versus C7 lesions, hypoesthesia of palmar and dorsal digit III as well as weakness of the pronator teres and flexor carpi radialis longus muscles (median nerve) may occur.

Complete Radial Nerve Lesion at the Axilla (Park Bench/Saturday Night Palsy or Honeymoon Palsy)

Trauma, compression or iatrogenic causes—as infiltration of the deltoid muscle—represent the classical etiologies leading to **complete radial nerve lesion in the axillary region**.

Clinically, a motor deficit with paralysis of all extensor muscles may be evident, leading to wrist drop [90]. As the brachioradial muscle is affected too, a weaker elbow flexion due to involvement of the brachioradialis muscle can be observed. Additionally, supination weakness due to only residual function of the biceps brachii muscle, is present. Extension of the distal finger is preserved by the function of the lumbrical and interossei muscles.

Sensory loss can be evident in the posterior aspect of the forearm, the dorsal side of the hand and digits II (radial side) to V. Sensation in the posterior upper arm is preserved.

Compression of the Radial Nerve by the Lateral Intermuscular Septum

The **lateral intermuscular septum**— extending from the greater tubercle to the medial epicondyle—represents a fascia that forms a compartment enclosing neurovascular structures. It is perforated by the radial nerve and the deep branch of the brachial artery, which represents a possible site of compression [92, 93].

Clinically, muscle weakness—especially of the extensor digitorum minimi muscle—and paresthesia in the radial nerve innervated aspect of the forearm and the dorsum of the hand, is observed. The occurrence of pain is usually not seen.

Lesion of the Radial Nerve in the Radial Groove/Sulcus

This location represents the most common traumatic radial lesion, either by direct contusion or by fracture of the humeral shaft [86].

Other causes may be secondary to fracture, during surgery or following callus formation. More rarely described etiologies include prolonged compression, hypertrophy of the lateral head of the biceps muscle, blood pressure cuff, or tumors.

A motor deficit can be observed in all radial nerve innervated muscles distal to the elbow, including the brachioradial muscle. However, this muscle is classically the first muscle to be reinnervated in case of recovery.

The triceps muscle is usually not affected by radial injury located in the radial groove, but minor weakness may be present in individuals having additional branches to the triceps.

Hypoesthesia is present in the radial nerve innervated dermatomes except for the posterolateral aspect of the arm, as the posterior cutaneous branch of the radial nerve is not affected.

Radial Tunnel Syndrome and Posterior Interosseus Nerve Entrapment

At the cubital fossa, the radial nerve bifurcates into a superficial and a deep branch (DBRN). The deep branch enters the radial tunnel as it passes beneath the arcade of Frohse, which represents the anterior edge of the superficial and deep head of the supinator. It represents the most common site of compression [96, 97].

The Leash of Henry—formed by branches of the recurrent radial artery and its accompanying vein [98]—represents a fibrous band anterior to the radiocapitellar joint, or the edge of the extensor carpi radialis muscle are amongst possible causes of compression. Rarely, ganglions or lipomas can be identified as compressive structures.

Compression to the DBRN in the radial tunnel is referred to *radial tunnel syndrome*.

Repetitive pronation-supination movements, leading to irritation of the nerve, favor this clinical syndrome.

The *posterior interosseus syndrome* represents another, highly controversial syndrome implicating the posterior interosseus nerve (PIN). The clinical presentation is similar to the above mentioned and the two conditions are often considered as one common syndrome. Nevertheless, they differ in their location.

The radial tunnel syndrome refers to a compression more proximally, close to the epicondyle, with the deep branch of the radial nerve being the affected structure. Patients primarily suffer from pain in the elbow region and the dorsal aspect of the forearm. Sensoric-motor deficits are not seen [102]. The more frequently observed epicondylitis ("tennis arm")—a condition that meliorates by corticosteroid therapy—represents a differential diagnosis.

The posterior interosseous nerve compression syndrome—as the name implies—involves the posterior interosseus nerve, which actually represents the continuation of the DBRN. The site of compression is located distally to the radial tunnel. Weakness in wrist and finger extension represents the leading symptom [105].

> The DBRN is located approximately 3.5 cm distal to the radial head, whereas the PIN lies around 7.5 cm distal. As the distal continuation of the DBRN, the PIN is usually smaller in diameter. In the literature, the DBRN and the PIN are often considered synonymous, although they differ slightly in anatomical course and distal innervation.

Sensory deficits are typically absent, as the posterior interosseus nerve is primarily a pure motor nerve with only a few sensory fibers innervating the wrist joint (Fig. 7.17).

Wartenberg Syndrome (Cheiralgia Paraesthesia)

The **Wartenberg syndrome** constitutes a rare nerve entrapment syndrome involving the superficial branch of the radial nerve (SBRN). Causes include prolonged compression by watches or hand cuffs [106].

As it is a pure sensory nerve, clinical symptoms comprise hypesthesia and pain in the dorsal radial aspect of the hand and thumb without the presence of muscle weakness. Pain can be elicited by palpating the area approximately 8–10 cm proximal to the styloid process, accompanied by a positive Tinel sign.

Besides the clinical presentation, a positive Finkelstein test may also be suggestive for Wartenberg syndrome: Sudden ulnar-abduction

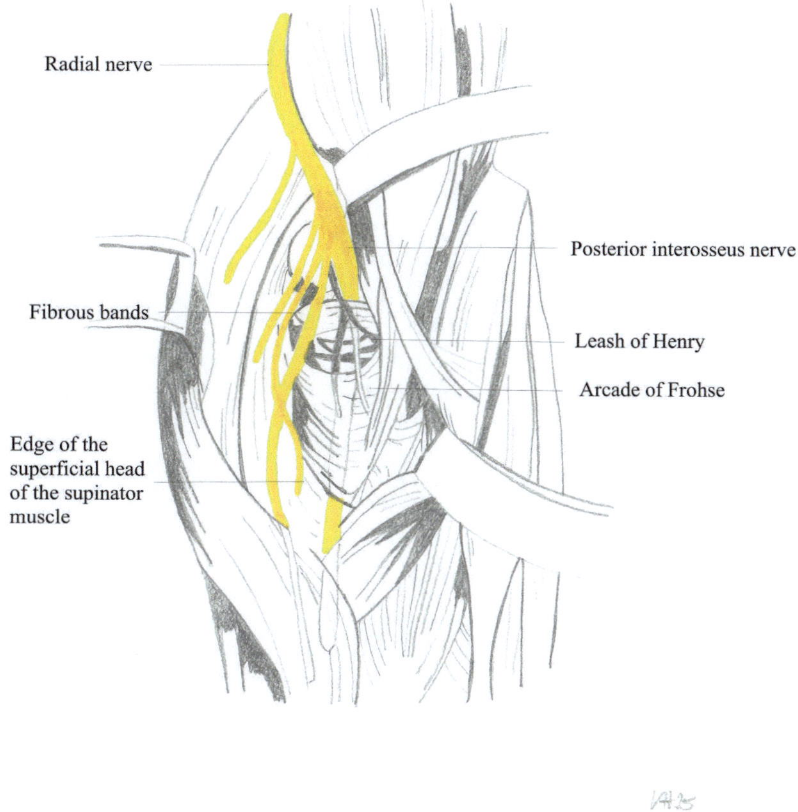

Fig. 7.17 Illustration of the course of the radial nerve in the proximal forearm

of the wrist while grasping the patients thumb provokes exaggerating pain at the styloid process.

Prior to treatment, the differential diagnosis of tendovaginitis stenosans de Quervain should be ruled out.

> In tendovaginitis stenosans de Quervain, Finkelstein test may be positive too, but hypesthesia is not observed.

7.1.11 Compression of the Sciatic Nerve

The **sciatic nerve compression** describes a lesion of the sciatic nerve located proximal to the leg, prior to exiting the subgluteal region (Fig. 7.18).

Compressing structures (disc herniation, hypertrophic muscles, fibrous bands, scar tissue) as well as trauma, tumors, or hematomas are the main causes for sciatic nerve lesion [109].

The Piriformis Syndrome

Being one of the most controversial nerve entrapment syndromes, the **piriformis syndrome** is described by irritation of the sciatic nerve at the level of the greater sciatic foramen by the piriformis muscle due to hypertrophy of the muscle. Secondary causes may imply edema, inflammation, or following trauma [112].

The most common clinical manifestation represents pain—with or without accompanying paresthesia—along the sciatic nerve distribution, especially during walking or prolonged sitting.

Piriformis syndrome is a diagnosis of exclusion with the lumbar disc herniation presenting the primarily differential diagnosis.

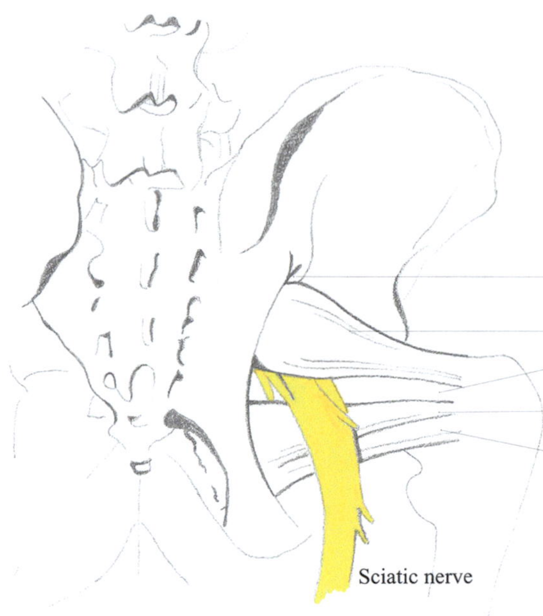

Fig. 7.18 Anatomic drawing of the pelvis with the sciatic nerve being depicted in yellow

Magnetic resonance imaging may reveal a hypertrophic prirformis muscle. The conduction of an additional electrophysiological examination may be helpful.

> The controversy surrounding pririformis syndrome stems from the anatomical consideration that a large nerve is compressed by a relatively small muscle. Furthermore, surgical outcomes are generally poor, with improvement primarily observed in patients who experience a placebo effect.

Management of the pririformis syndrome represents predominantly conservative therapy including physical therapy and analgetics, as well as corticosteroid injections and the use of botulinum toxin [113]. Some centers offer surgery to decompress the sciatic nerve in the grater sciatic foramen, although, only a small number of patients undergo the procedure.

Ischiofemoral Impingement

Ischiofemoral impingement may result in compression of sciatic nerve fibers traversing the ischiofemoral space. Anatomically, this space is bounded medially by the ischial tuberosity and laterally by the lesser trochanter of the femur, and it may be narrowed in patients with ischiofemoral impingement [115, 116].

Pain located in the hip region, followed by stiffness and weakness of the hip joint, are the presenting symptoms. Factors associated to ischiofemoral impingement, are patients following hip surgery or trauma. The diagnosis is mainly clinically based on exclusion of other causes. MRI can demostrate muscle edema or atrophy; depending on the stage and severity of compression (Fig. 7.19).

Conservative treatment, including physical therapy and analgetic therapy is recommended.

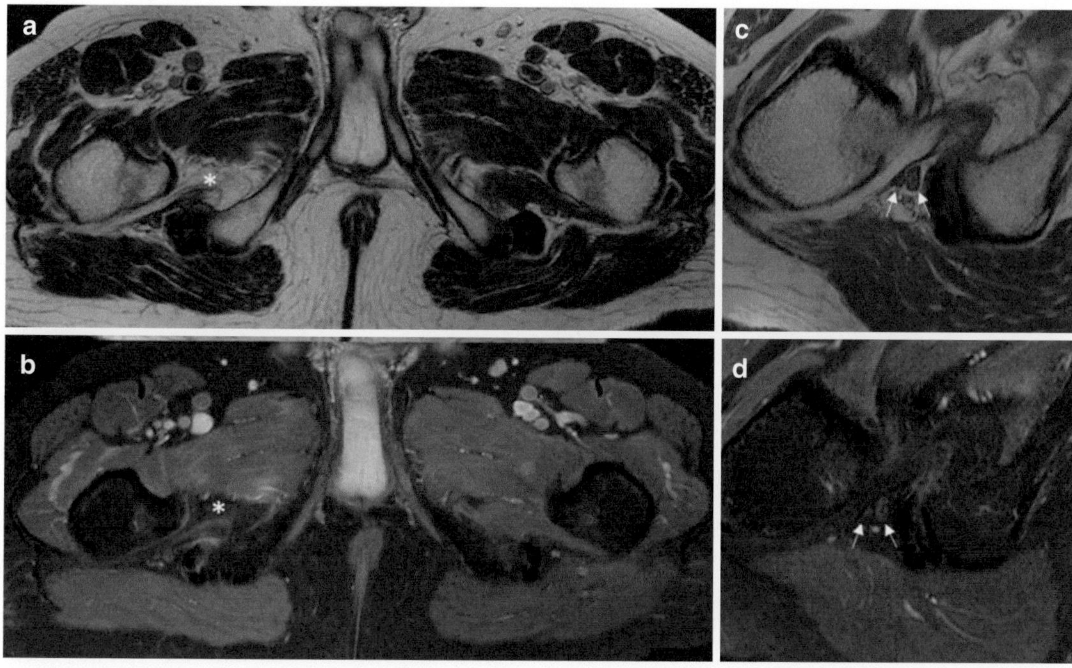

Fig. 7.19 Ischiofemoral syndrome: (**a**) axial T2 and (**b**) axial PD-SPAIR demonstrate narrowing of the right ischiofemoral space and atrophy of the quadratus femoris muscle with fatty replacement (asterisk). (**c, d**) Are high-resolution focused images depicting the regional anatomy and its relationship to the sciatic nerve (arrows)

7.1.12 Compression of the Obturator Nerve

Obturator nerve entrapment most commonly occurs at the level of the obturator canal and is typically observed in pregnancy, following hip surgery, or secondary to periarticular cysts. In athletes, an additional etiology may involve spams or weakness of the adductor muscles related to chronic tendinopathy [118].

Typical clinical manifestations include pain in the inguinal region and at the medial thigh, accompanied by weakness of the adductor muscles [119].

MRI may reveal changes within the nervous structure and diameter, compressing structures, or muscular abnormalities.

If conservative treatment is not effective, surgical decompression of the nerve can be offered to the patient.

7.1.13 Lateral Femoral Cutaneous Nerve Compression (Meralgia Paresthetica)

The **lateral femoral cutaneous nerve** (**LFCN**) is a purely sensory nerve; therefore, its compression results in pain and paresthesia localized to the anterolateral aspect of the thigh, without any associated motor deficits.

Through its course, the LFCN passes several potential bottleneck sites, predisposing it to compression syndromes. The most common site of entrapment is beneath the inguinal ligament.

Etiologies are diverse and include external compression from belts or waistbands, iatrogenic injury, trauma, or space-occupying lesions such as retroperitoneal tumors. Weight gain and pregnancy are recognized risk factors for the development of meralgia paresthetica.

The reported incidence is approximately 32 per 100,000 population, with a rising trend attributed both to the increasing prevalence of obesity and diabetes as well as improved diagnostic modalities [121].

Imaging with MRI or high-resolution ultrasound may reveal nerve thickening or demonstrate a compressive structure.

Management is primarily conservative, consisting of corticosteroid injections. In refractory cases, radiofrequency ablation or surgical neurolysis may be considered.

Surgical intervention is considered only after the patient has undergone three successful diagnostic and therapeutic nerve block injections. Surgical strategies include either **simple decompression** of the lateral femoral cutaneous nerve or **neurectomy**. Considerable debate exists regarding which approach provides superior outcome. To date, no level 1 evidence exists to demonstrate the superiority of one technique over the other.

7.1.14 Compression of the Saphenous Nerve

The **saphenous nerve**, a purely sensory branch of the posterior division of the femoral nerve, may be subject to entrapment during its course through the adductor (Hunter's) canal. Additional etiologies of saphenous neuropathy include direct trauma to the adductor canal, iatrogenic injury—most frequently in the context of knee surgeries—as well traction or stretch-related injuries [124].

The **Hunter's canal** is anatomically formed by the vastus medialis, the sartorius and the adductor muscles [122].

Patients typically present with pain and paresthesia localized to the distal medial leg with radiation to the great toe.

MRI may assist in diagnosis by revealing either a compressive structure or nerve thickening.

The differential diagnosis includes L4 radiculopathy as well as knee pathology such as synovitis or meniscal lesion.

Prior to considering surgical intervention—which implies nerve decompression or neurectomy—diagnostic and therapeutic anesthetic injections should be performed.

7.1.15 Compression of the Peroneal Nerve

Common Peroneal Nerve Compression

Before entering the peroneal tunnel, where it subsequently divides into the superficial and deep peroneal nerves, the **common peroneal nerve** courses superficially around the fibular neck, being exposed to lesioning [129] (Fig. 7.20).

Causes of nerve compression or injury are diverse and include direct trauma (e.g. fracture or dislocation of the knee), prolonged sitting or squatting, ganglion or synovial cysts, varicose veins, and hypertrophy of the short head of the biceps femoris muscle.

Clinical symptoms comprise pain with paresthesia, and motor weakness. The most prominent manifestation is foot drop which results in a steppage gait [127].

The clinical examination supported by sonography and electrophysiological studies is usually sufficient to establish the diagnosis. MRI may provide additional information.

Given, that the peroneal nerve demonstrates limited potential for spontaneous recovery, early surgical decompression is recommended in patients with a clear compressive etiology and no evidence of clinical improvement.

Anterior Tarsal Tunnel Syndrome

Deep peroneal nerve entrapment at the level of the anterior tarsal tunnel may result in pain paresthesia localized to the dorsal aspect of the foot and the first two toes, often accompanied by a positive Tinel sign. On clinical examination, weakness or even atrophy of the extensor hallucis

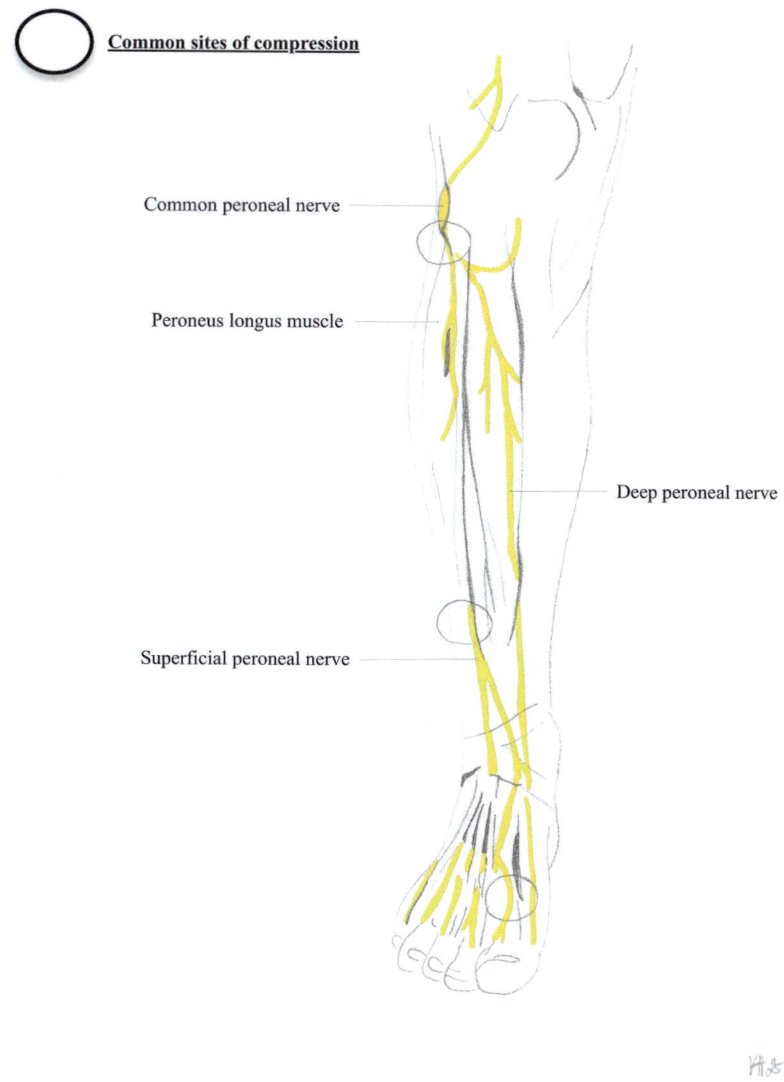

Fig. 7.20 Anatomical drawing presenting common sites of compression of the peroneal nerve (circles)

brevis and the extensor digitorum brevis muscles may be observed [131].

External causes include direct trauma or tight footwear, whereas internal compressive factors may involve bony deformities (e.g. osteophytes) or cystic lesions [132, 133].

Ultrasound is frequently sufficient for diagnosis, though MRI may provide additional information regarding space-occupying lesions.

In the presence of resectable compressive structures, surgical decompression is indicated.

Superficial Peroneal Nerve Entrapment

Superficial peroneal nerve entrapment may occur at the level where the nerve pierces the lateral deep fascia. This site is particularly vulnerable to dancers, in whom repetitive plantar flexion and inversion injuries can cause overstitching of the fascia. Additional causes include thickening of the lateral deep fascia, anatomical variations or cystic lesions [135].

Patients typically report paresthesia involving the lateral aspect of the lower leg and the dorsum of the foot, with sparing of the first interdigital space and the fifth digit.

A positive Tinel sign can be elicited over the site of entrapment. Motor weakness is uncommon.

Ultrasound and MRI are valuable in confirming the diagnosis and identifying compressive lesions. Treatment options include physical therapy, corticosteroid injection, and, in refractory cases surgical decompression of the nerve.

7.1.16 Compression of the Tibial Nerve

Tarsal Tunnel Syndrome

This syndrome refers to **entrapment of the posterior tibial nerve** at the level of the tarsal tunnel, a confined anatomical space bordered by the calcaneus, talus, and medial malleolus bones, and roofed by the flexor retinaculum (Fig. 7.21).

Within the tarsal tunnel, the tibial nerve is accompanied by the tibial artery and vein. Distally, the tibial nerve divides into the medial calcaneal nerve as well as the lateral and medial plantar nerves.

Etiological factors implicated in tarsal tunnel syndrome include hypertrophy of the abductor hallucis muscle, ganglion cysts, space-occupying lesions such as tumors, varicose veins and post-traumatic or post-inflammatory fibrosis [136, 137]. However, in a considerable number of patients, no definite cause can be identified.

Clinical signs encompass pain of burning character and paresthesia in the plantar aspect of the foot and toes, typically aggravated by physical activity. Tinel sign elicited over the tarsal tunnel is a common finding.

MRI may demonstrate the compressive pathology. Management is usually initiated with conservative measures such as analgesics and corticosteroid injections. In cases refractory to nonoperative treatment, surgical decompression of the tarsal tunnel is indicated.

Morton Metatarsalgia/Morton Neuroma

Entrapment of the digital nerves II and III, which arise from the lateral plantar nerve, within the intermetatarsal space may result in perineural fibrosis commonly referred to as **Morton's neuroma**.

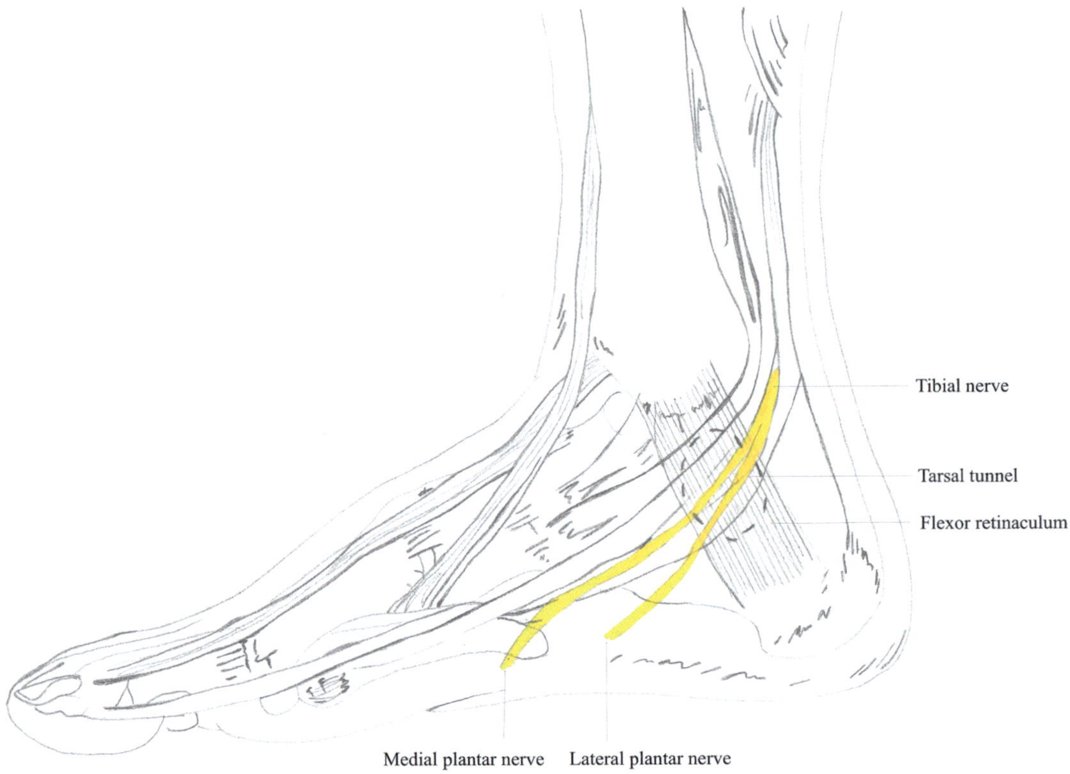

Fig. 7.21 Anatomical drawing to the tibial nerve entering the tarsal tunnel

The second and third intermetatarsal spaces are anatomically narrower compared to the first and fourth interspacing, predisposing them to Morton's neuroma formation.

Potential risk factors associated with the formation of Morton's neuroma include structural deformities of the forefoot and the use of high-heels [138, 139].

Histologically, Morton's neuroma represents a "partial neuroma". It is characterized being fibrotic thickening of perineurial tissue, with central regions showing evidence of axonal loss secondary to axonotmesis.

Patients typically report of localized pain, which can be aggravated by palpation of the intermetatarsal space from the plantar aspect. A positive Mulder's click test—elicited by compressing the first and fifth metatarsal heads while simultaneously palpating the plantar intermetatarsal space—produces pain and sometimes a palpable click, supporting the diagnosis.

Magnetic resonance imaging and ultrasonography may reveal a dumbbell-shaped enlargement within the intermetatarsal space, consistent with the lesion (Fig. 7.22). Initial treatment is conservative, but in refractory cases, surgical excision is indicated. This involves transection and removal the affected nerve proximal to the lesion.

7.2 Traumatic Nerve Lesions—Neuroma and Pain

Approximately 70% of patients with peripheral nerve injury develop neuropathic pain [140].

Neuropathic pain may arise from two principle mechanisms: due to neuroma formation, which causes ectopic stimuli leading to central sensitization, or because of Wallerian degeneration—a process that induces functional and structural changes in adjacent intact nerve fibers, leading to hyperalgesia.

The most common ultrasonographic finding in peripheral nerve injury is a fascicular enlargement, reflecting intraneural edema. This typically manifests as a hypoechoic, thickened segment of the nerve extending over several centimeters, and may be observed already in the early stages of peripheral nerve lesion. Strain-induced nerve lesions—such as sciatic nerve injury following hip arthroplasty- exemplify this pattern.

In cases of neuroma-in-continuity, ultrasound demonstrates a localized, spindle-shaped, hypoechoic nerve enlargement lacking internal fascicular structure but with preservation of the epineurium [141].

Certain nerves are particularly susceptible to injury with limited potential for spontaneous recovery. These include the C5 nerve root, the ulnar nerve and the peroneal nerve.

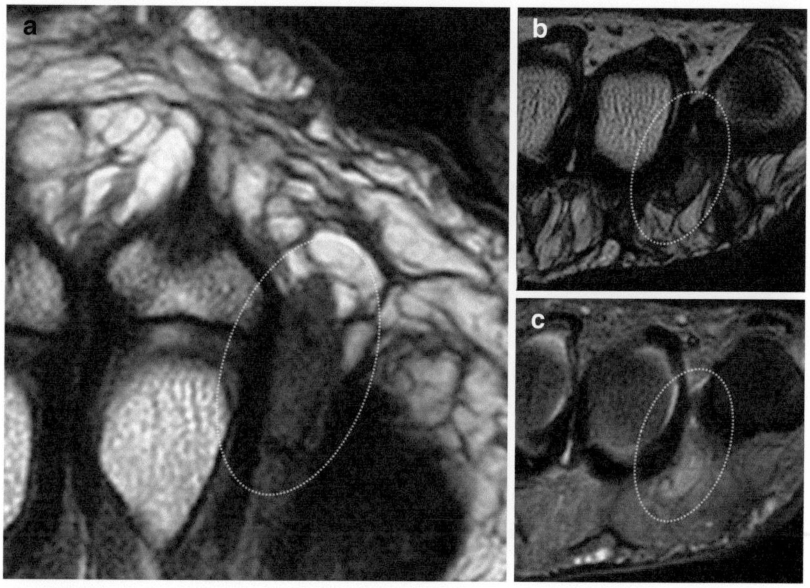

Fig. 7.22 Morton's neuroma: Axial T1 (**a**) at the level of the metatarsal heads shows a fusiform, isointense enlargement of the plantar digital nerve (arrows) within the third intermetatarsal space. Coronal T2 (**b**) and coronal STIR (**c**) demonstrate the neuroma (dotted circle) as a predominantly low-signal-intensity lesion

Peripheral nerve injuries can result in the development of painful neuromas. A neuroma represents a non-neoplastic proliferation of disorganized nerve fibers and connective tissue, typically appearing within 1–12 months following injury. It constitutes the undirected attempt of disrupted fascicles during reinnervation. Concomitant injury to adjacent connective tissue promotes scarring and fibrosis, further impairing axonal and directing aberrant growth [148].

Pain manifests in form of neuropathic pain, arising both from central sensitization and from Wallerian degeneration. The latter occurs as adjacent, otherwise intact nerve fibers undergo maladaptive changes in response to the injury environment, thereby contributing to increased nociceptive signaling.

Possible cause represent traumatic nerve injury, unsuccessful surgical repair, iatrogenic lesion, or chronic mechanical irritation such as traction or repetitive stress (e.g., Morton neuroma).

Terminal (stump) neuromas classically form following complete nerve transection (Sunderland grade V), occurring either unintentionally or as a sequela of surgical amputation.

A neuroma-in-continuity (associated with Sunderland grade III or IV) represents an initially fusiform enlargement at the site of injury. Progressive deposition of scar tissue ensues, which may involve either the entire nerve or only a portion of it [149] (Figs. 7.23 and 7.24).

Pain—typically burning or stabbing in quality—constitutes the typical clinical manifestation of a neuroma. It is usually well localized to the side of the lesion and may be provoked even by light tactile stimulation (allodynia).

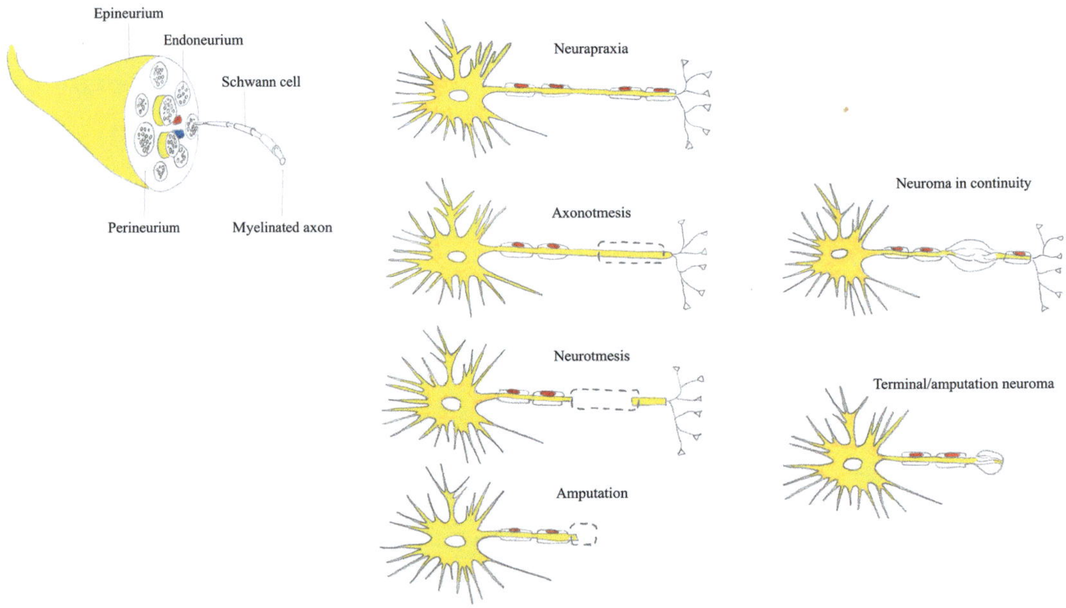

Fig. 7.23 Diagram illustrating nerve anatomy and types of nerve injuries. The left side shows a cross-section of a nerve, the right side depicts the stages of nerve injuries and illustrates neuroma formation

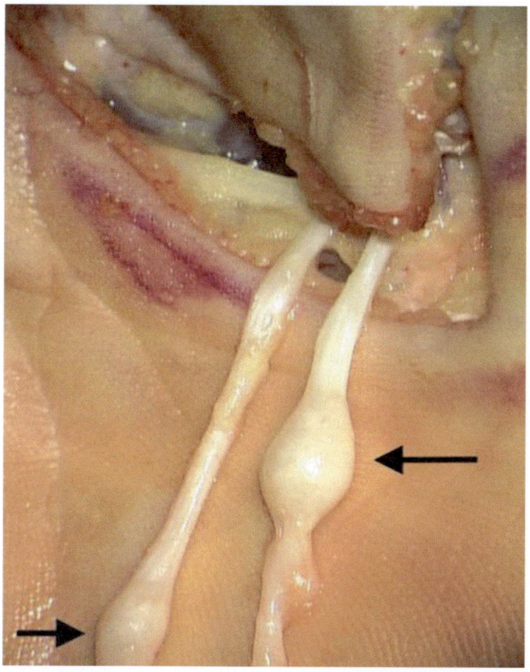

Fig. 7.24 An anatomical diagram showing neuroma formation (arrow) of two palmar digital nerves of the hand after trauma

Subcutaneous neuromas are typically more painful than subfascial neuromas. This difference is attributed to the distinct characteristics of the surrounding tissue; the subcutaneous location is more exposed to inflammatory mediators, which amplify nociceptive stimuli and thereby contribute to heightened pain perception.

Accurate diagnosis of neuromas relies heavily on thorough medical history, which may provide insight into the mechanism of nerve injury. Electrophysiological studies may depict a nerve conduction block at the site of the lesion.

On ultrasound, neuromas appear as hypoechoic bulbous or fusiform enlargements of the nerve, with disruption and loss of the normal fascicular "honeycomb" architecture.

On MRI, a neuroma can be identified as an inhomogeneous hyperintensity in T2 -weighted sequence, often accompanied by contrast enhancement.

Patients are initially treated conservatively including anticonvulsants (e.g., gabapentin, Ppregabalin), antidepressants (e.g., duloxetin, amitriptylin), and opioids. Local injections of anesthetics or corticosteroids can be considered for symptomatic relief. Minimally invasive procedures such as radiofrequency ablation and cryotherapy have also been described in literature.

However, these measures often provide only temporary benefit, and surgical intervention is frequently required.

Surgical techniques range from external neurolysis—to release scar tissue-, surgical transection for terminal neuromas, to excision of the neuroma and subsequent coaptation of the proximal and distal nerve ends. Split repair presents an option when only part of the nerve is affected, and involves the selective excision of the neuroma-affected fascicles while preserving the intact fascicles. The resulting defect is bridged with a nerve graft.

The removement of adjacent fibrotic tissue and coverage of the nerve with vascularized soft tissue, improves the local microenvironment and supports regeneration [147, 149, 151].

The application of synthetic nerve conduits following neuroma resection has been discussed in literature but has not yet been widely adopted in clinical practice.

Isolated resection of a neuroma may provide initial pain relief; however, recurrence of pain is common over time. Wrapping or covering the residual nerve stump with soft tissue has been shown to reduce the reoccurrence of pain.

Additional therapeutic options for refractory neuropathic pain include neuromodulation techniques—such as spinal cord stimulation, peripheral nerve stimulation and intrathecal drug delivery—as well as ablative surgical procedures including neurectomy, dorsal rhizotomy, and dorsal root entry zone lesioning (DREZ).

7.2.1 Facial Nerve Palsy

In principle, every cranial nerve is susceptible to injury; however, the facial nerve is the most commonly affected and therefore warrants particular attention and should be mentioned (Fig. 7.25).

The causes for facial nerve injury are various and include the following:

Idiopathic facial nerve palsy (Bell palsy) represents the most frequent cause, accounting for approximately 70% of cases, and is a diagnosis of exclusion [152].

It is thought to be associated with preceding viral infections. Recovery may take up to one year, and a small proportion of patients do not achieve complete recovery.

Bell's palsy most commonly affects individuals between the age of 15–45 years of age.

Infection—Bacterial infections such as acute otitis media or viral infections such as herpes zoster

Iatrogenic—Surgical interventions of the cerebellopontine angle (e.g., vestibular schwannoma resection)

Traumatic—Temporal bone fractures

Neoplastic—Tumors affecting the nerve, including facial and acoustic neuromas, meningiomas, or arachnoid cysts

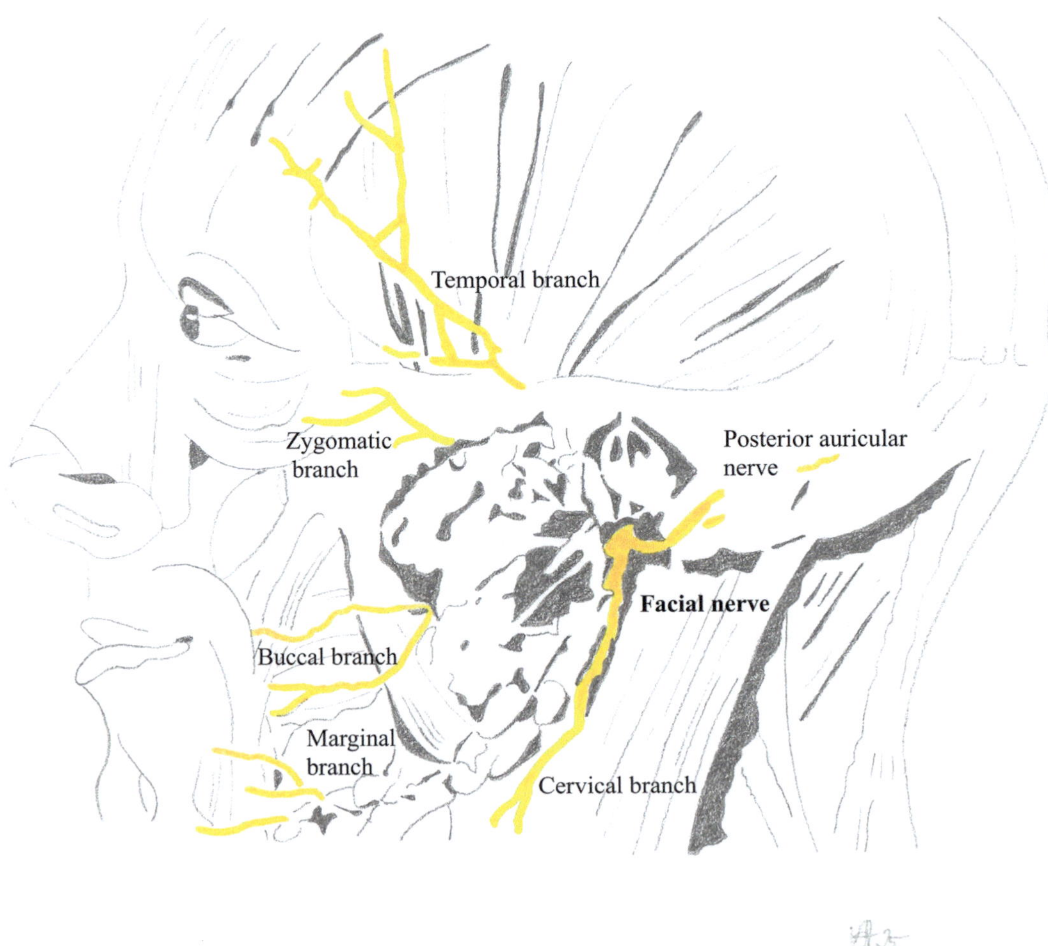

Fig. 7.25 Anatomical drawing showing a lateral view of the face to demonstrate the facial nerve and its terminal branches

Facial nerve palsies are usually unilateral. Bilateral involvement is rare and may indicate an underlying systemic condition, such as Lyme disease, multiple sclerosis, or Guillain-Barré syndrome.

Anatomically, the facial nerve traverses a narrow canal within the temporal bone, particularly in the labyrinthine segment, making it susceptible to ischemic injury from compression.

Regarding the clinical examination, the *House-Brackmann score* is used to evaluate the degree of paresis [153] (Table 7.2).

Imaging studies, including magnetic resonance imaging (MRI) and computed tomography (CT) may help to identify the underlying causes. Electrophysiological assessment is recommended to evaluate the functional status of the facial nerve and guide prognosis and management.

In terms of treatment, conservative therapy should focus on eyecare (artificial tears, watch glass bandage) to prevent corneal injury and facial muscles exercises to maintain tone and prevent atrophy[155].

Idiopathic facial palsy is usually treated with corticosteroids and analgesics over approximately 10 days.

Antibiotics are indicated if the palsy is secondary to bacterial infection, such as acute otitis media.

Table 7.2 House-Brackmann score evaluating the severity of facial nerve palsy

House-Brackmann score	
Grade	Description
I	Normal function
II	Mild dysfunction; slight asymmetry of the mouth
III	Visible weakness of the affected side, eyebrow lifting may not be possible, complete eye closure with maximal effort, obvious asymmetry of the mouth
IV	Severe synkinesis, eyebrow lifting is not possible, incomplete eye closure, asymmetry of the mouth
V	Severe dysfunction with barely perceptible motion
VI	No movement, no synkinesis, loss of muscle tone

Reconstructive surgery in facial nerve is technically demanding, and optimal approaches remain debated [156].

The primary goal of surgery is dynamic facial reanimation, when feasible.

Regarding reconstruction, various surgical techniques are available including:

Nerve transfers: Hypoglossal-to-facial-nerve transfer, direct masseteric-to-facial nerve transposition (MNT), and cross-facial nerve grafting (CFNG).

Muscle-based procedures: Free functional muscle transfers (e.g., gracilis or latissimus dorsi), temporalis-lengthening myoplasty (involving coronoid osteotomy and harvesting the fascia lata **Combinations** of nerve transfers and muscle procedures tailored to the individual case and combinations of all of the above-mentioned procedures [157].

Previously, incomplete facial nerve palsy (better than House-Brackmann grade IV) was considered a relative contraindication for nerve transfer surgery; current practice no longer considers this a limitation.

Cross facial nerve grafting for unilateral facial palsy involves connecting branches of the healthy facial nerve to the paralyzed side using a sural nerve graft [158]. Frequently taken donor branches are those from the zygomaticofacial trunk. Surgical techniques vary in terms of graft coaptation sites and whether a one or two-stage procedure is employed [161].

Some authors prefer to perform a two-stage surgical approach in cases of incomplete facial nerve palsy to asure axonal sprouting towards the desired direction, often using the tinel sign to monitor nerve sprouting. In such cases, there is an inherent risk of misdirected axonal sprouting from the paretic nerve toward the healthy side, which may compromise functional recovery.

Facial nerve reconstructive procedures are typically performed within 6–12 months of paralysis onset to optimize functional recovery.

CFGN is a widely utilized technique because it allows the restoration of spontaneous, emotionally mediated facial movements. However, outcomes are sometimes unpredictable. Limitations are related to the facial nerve providing a relatively limited number of motor axons, which may affect the degree of muscle reinnervation. Another disadvantage represents the fact that sacrificing donor branches on the healthy side, can potentially compromise facial function and may cause sensory deficits.

The *direct masseteric-to-facial-nerve transfer* is a gladly taken donor nerve for reinnervating the lower face, due to its high motor axon count, its proximity to the facial nerve, and the ability to perform direct coaptation without a graft. This avoids the power loss associated with multiple coaptation sites in grafted transfers.

Unlike CFGN, the MNT does not provide spontaneous or dissociated facial movements, which constitutes the main drawback of this technique.

Interestingly, some reports describe cases of spontaneous smiling after MNT [162].

Combining CFNG with MNT for reinnervation of the facial nerve has been reported to produce favorable funcional outcomes. However, older patients or those with greater preoperative resting asymmetry may achieve less satisfactory results [159, 160].

The *hypoglossal-to-facial nerve transfer* was first described by Korte in 1901 and involves transposition of the hypoglossal nerve to the paralyzed facial nerve either via direct coaptation or with an interposed nerve graft.

One of the earliest nerve transfer procedures for facial nerve palsy was the spinal accessory to facial nerve transfer, described in 1879.

Due to limited restoration of facial movement following surgery, coupled with concomitant swallowing and speech difficulties arising from hemiparesis of the tongue, this technique did not achieve widespread adoption. Subsequent modifications were introduced, using only fascicles of the hypoglossal nerve as a donor, rather than sacrificing the entire nerve, to perform a "supercharge" nerve transfer, thereby augmenting the residual muscle strength [163].

Muscle transpositions and free functional muscle transfers remain viable options for patients with long standing facial nerve palsy and extensive denervated musculature.

Selection of the most appropriate surgical intervention depends on the severity and duration of facial nerve palsy, the availability of suitable donor nerves, the patient's overall clinical status and age and, ultimately, the surgeon's expertise.

7.2.2 Obstetric Brachial Plexus Palsy

Obstetric brachial plexus palsy (OBPP), first described by Duchenne and Erb in 1872 and 1874, and later by Klumpke in 1885, refers to a lesion of the brachial plexus occurring during birth.

The incidence of OBPP is estimated to range from 0.1 to 6.3 cases per 1,000 live births [165]. The condition is more prevalent in developing countries compared to industrialized nations.

Maternal risk factors include overweight, diabetes mellitus, and multiparity. Neonates with a high birth weight (>4,000 g) or head circumference greater than 52 cm are at increased risk. Additional contributing factors include inexperience of the obstetrician, use of operative delivery instruments such as forceps or vacuum extractors, prolonged labor, uterine anomalies, and abnormal fetal position [168, 171].

The pathophysiologic mechanism involves traction of the fetal head while the shoulder remains impacted in the birth canal, resulting in stretching of the brachial plexus.

The severity of paresis is variable, ranging from transient stretch injury to complete nerve root avulsion.

The upper brachial plexus is more often affected due to the traction mechanism, predominantly involving nerve roots C5 and C6, with occasional involvement of C7, resulting in Erb's palsy.

Spontaneous recovery occurs in more than 50% of affected infants, with reports ranging up to 92% [169]. Nevertheless, although shoulder abduction and elbow flexion often recover well, hand function frequently remains impaired.

The **Narakas Classification** stratifies lesions into four groups—upper Erb's lesion, extended Erb's lesion, total palsy, and total palsy with Horner syndrome (Table 7.3). Due to the mechanism of OBPP, isolated lesions of the lower brachial plexus (C8-T1, Klumpke's palsy) are classically uncommon [170].

The occurrence of a Horner syndrome, which indicates sympathetic neural involvement, suggests a more severe brachial plexus injury with spinal root avulsion. This may also be associated with phrenic nerve injury, representing an increased risk of respiratory complications in neonates [173].

Another important issue facing the medical team in OBPP is the resulting muscular imbalance of the shoulder girdle. Involvement of the upper spinal roots leads to weakness of the supraspinatus, infraspinatus, and rhomboid muscles due to lesions of the suprascapular and dorsal scapular nerves, respectively. Consequently, this results in diminished external rotation and abduction of the arm, producing an internally rotated, flail-like arm.

In total plexus injuries, additional weakness of the deltoid, subscapularis and pectoralis muscles is observed. While this also produces a flail arm, internal rotation is generally less pronounced.

Diagnosis can be straightforward in cases of distinct paresis or avulsion.

However, minor stretch injuries pose significant diagnostic challenges, particularly in infants who are not able to follow verbal instructions.

Various assessment tools are available with the active movement scale (AMS) being both reliable and easy to implement. This scale quantifies upper limb movement in infants during play, using an eight-point grading system. Additional useful evaluations include the Towel test and the Cookie test.

Accurate clinical assessment requires repeated examinations. Differential diagnosis such as clavicular or humeral fractures, and septic arthritis, must be excluded.

Eventually, surgical exploration remains the most definitive diagnostic approach in OBPP, allowing intraoperative nerve stimulation, neurolysis, and, when indicated, primary nerve reconstruction.

Table 7.3 Narakas classification to categorize the type of brachial plexus lesion

Narakas classification			
Name	Involved roots	Paresis	Likely outcome
Narakas 1—Upper Erb's	C5, C6	Abduction/external rotation of the shoulder, elbow flexion, normal wrist, and hand function	Spontaneous recovery in ~80% possible
Narakas 2—Extended Erb's	C5, C6, C7	Abduction/external rotation of the shoulder, elbow flexion, wrist drop	Spontaneous recovery in ~60% possible
Narakas 3—Total palsy	C5, C6, C7, C8, T1	Complete flaccid palsy	Spontaneous recovery in ~30–50% possible especially shoulder and elbow recovery (worse for hand)
Narakas 4—Total palsy with Horner syndrome[a]	C5, C6, C7, C8, T1	Complete flaccid palsy with Horner Syndrome[a]	Surgery necessary

[a]Horner syndrome = miosis, ptosis, enophathlmus

The optimal timing for surgical intervention varies in literature ranging from 3 and 7 months.

For C5-C6 lesions, the waiting period is typically 3–4 months, whereas C7–Th1 lesions may warrant up to 7 months, reflecting difference in axonal regrowth distance.

Recovery of biceps muscle function by 3 months is generally considered a favorable prognostic indicator for spontaneous recovery.

Surgical management depends on lesion severity and may include shoulder reduction and rebalancing procedures, neurolysis, nerve grafting, or nerve transfers. Physiotherapy represents an essential part in the therapy of OBPP to prevent contractions and shoulder dysplasia.

Shoulder arthrodesis may be considered as a salvage therapy in patients with total brachial plexus palsy who experience pain associated with a flail arm. This intervention is typically reserved for later stages of management.

Isolated upper plexus injuries (Narakas 1 and 2) are classically post-ganglionic lesions and are amenable to reconstructive surgery via nerve grafting. In contrast, total plexus injuries (Narakas 3 and 4) are more likely preganglionic, often requiring nerve transfer surgeries due to the potential presence of nerve root avulsion.

7.2.3 Traumatic Brachial Plexus Injury (BPI)

The brachial plexus is formed by the ventral spinal nerve roots C5–Th1 and is particularly vulnerable to traumatic injury. Trauma resulting from motorcycle or car accidents, accounts for approximately 80–90% of all **traumatic brachial plexus injuries** [176, 177, 208]. Other etiologies include sports-related injuries, as well as penetrating trauma such as stab and gunshot wounds, particularly in developing countries. Non-traumatic causes of brachial plexus injury include neoplasms, iatrogenic injury, or inflammatory processes.

Brachial plexus injury (BPI) most commonly affect male patients between 15 and 25 years of age [179].

Several classification systems exist for BPI, with the most commonly utilized outlined below:

Location of injury [178]:

- Upper BPI ➔ Erb-Duchenne, C5–C6 spinal nerve roots
- Extended upper BPI ➔ C5–C7 spinal nerve roots
- Lower BPI ➔ Dejerine-Klumpke, C8–Th1 spinal nerve roots
- Complete lesion

Form of injury:

- Traction without macroscopic injury of nerve fibers (neurapraxia)
- Post-ganglionic injury (rupture) ➔ Involves the spinal nerve, trunks or divisions
- Pre-ganglionic injury between the spinal ganglion and the spinal cord ➔ Involves the proximal axons of the primary afferent and efferent nerves (Fig. 7.26)

Unfavorable prognostic factors for recovery following brachial plexus injury include lesions of the inferior trunk, which require axonal regeneration over a longer distance, prolonged pain exceeding six months (with intensity and duration potentially correlating with lesion severity), and the presence of Horner syndrome, indicating involvement of spinal nerve roots C8–Th2 [180].

In cases of nerve discontinuity, neuroma formation at the proximal nerve stump is frequently observed.

The clinical presentation varies widely depending on the extent of injury, ranging from sensory-motor deficits in specific nerve distributions to complete paralysis of the upper extremity. Chronic BPI's commonly manifest with muscle atrophy and vegetative disturbances

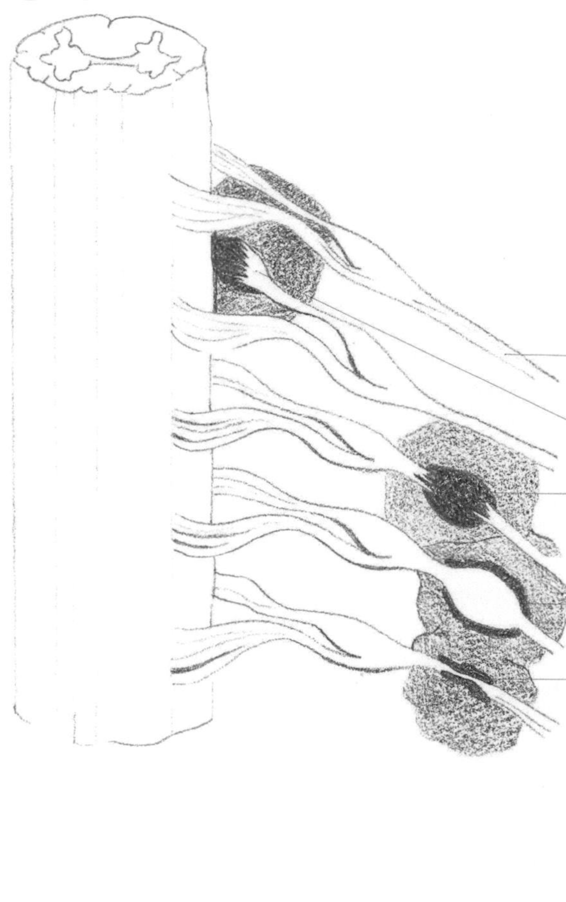

Fig. 7.26 Drawing demonstrating different types of brachial plexus injury

including alterations in blood flow, temperature regulation, and perspiration.

As many patients present as polytrauma patients, they often require intensive care treatment for concomitant injuries. Consequently, brachial plexus injury may initially be overlooked.

Diagnostic evaluation includes MR-neurography, ultrasound and myelo-CT scans. Electrophysiological studies are also critical, contributing both to initial diagnosis and postoperative follow-up [181].

Patients should undergo clinical and electrophysical reassessment every four weeks following trauma. Surgical intervention is indicated if no signs of spontaneous recovery are observed after approximately four months, with the maximum waiting period generally considered to be 9–10 months.

While literature reports vary regarding the optimal timing till surgery, the consensus emphasizes that surgical management should ideally occur within one year of injury. The principle "**time is nerve**" underscores the importance of timely intervention.

Surgical treatment options include neurolysis, nerve reconstruction, and nerve transfer procedures.

7.2.3.1 Nerve Root Avulsion or Brachial Plexus Avulsion (BPA)

Brachial plexus avulsion (**BPA**) is a preganglionic form of brachial plexus injury, most commonly resulting from traction forces.

It was first described in 1872 by Duchenne, who observed such injuries in neonates (OBPP).

Clinically, BPA typically presents with complete paralysis, anesthesia, and hyperhidrosis in the affected region. The Hoffman-Tinel sign is absent, and neuroma formation is not observed at the infraganglionic level.

Avulsion of nerve roots C8–Th2 may result in Horner syndrome [187].

Approximately 80% of patients with root avulsion injury eventually develop neuropathic (deafferentation) pain [188–190]. Pathophysiologically, injury to the Lissauer tract and the dorsal horn of the spinal cord leads to an initially reduced activity in the superficial neurons and the substantia gelatinosa, followed by abnormal activity in the deeper laminae (particularly lamina V). This aberrant neuronal activity culminates in central sensitization. The resulting pain is classically continuous, burning in quality and interrupted by episodic pain exacerbations [140, 191].

Magnetic resonance imaging and CT myelography are key diagnostic tools in BPA. Radiological indicators include pseudomeningoceles, characterized by cerebrospinal fluid collections within the dural pouches of the affected segments, reflecting perineural tear. Additional findings may include hemorrhage, edema, and displacement of the spinal cord [195].

In l chronic cases, fatty infiltration of the paraspinal muscles secondary to atrophy can be visualized in the T2-weighted MRI sequences.

Electrophysiological testing demonstrates absent motor nerve conduction, while sensory nerve action potentials remain intact due to preservation of the dorsal root ganglion.

Electromyography typically reveals denervation potentials, such as fibrillation potentials and positive sharp waves, approximately 14 days after injury [196].

Spontaneous regeneration does not occur in root avulsion injuries and surgical intervention is required.

Nevertheless, conservative management should not be neglected, both preoperatively and postoperatively. This includes physiotherapy and passive mobilization to prevent joint stiffness, electrotherapy to preserve muscle fibers, and use of supportive splints to stabilize the shoulder.

Management of deafferentation pain begins with pharmacological therapy. Anticonvulsants (e.g., pregabalin, gabapentin, carbamazepine), antidepressants (e.g., duloxetine) and opioids are commonly employed.

However, the overall success rate of conservative treatment is low, and many patients will ultimately require neurosurgical interventions such as dorsal root entry zone lesioning (DREZ) or spinal cord stimulation (SCS).

DREZ lesion involves the targeted generation of small lesions via thermocoagulation in the Lissauer tract and the dorsal horn (Lamina I-V), called tractotomy, disrupting hyperexcitable neuronal circuits and thereby reducing pain [198, 199] (Fig. 7.27).

Spinal cord stimulation BPA-related pain was first described in 1974 by Sweet and Wepsic. This minimally invasive, reversible procedure is based on the gate-control-theory, wherein electrical stimulation inhibits nociceptive transmission by modulating A∂ & C-fibers.

7.2.4 Lumbar Plexus Injury

Lumbar plexus injury (**LPI**) may result from direct trauma (e.g., fractures or hip dislocations), iatrogenic causes (e.g., hip arthroplasty), gynecological factors (e.g., pregnancy, pelvic tumors), inflammatory or metabolic diseases (e.g., type II diabetes mellitus, sarcoidosis, osteomyelitis), or as a sequala of radiation therapy [200, 201].

Although less common than brachial plexus injury, lumbar plexus injury is more frequently observed in women, reflecting its association with gynecological etiologies.

The hallmark clinical manifestation is lower back pain, which may occur with or without radiation to the lower extremity.

Additional features may include sensory disturbances, autonomic dysfunction such as lsphincter impairment, and muscle atrophy in chronic cases.

Differential diagnosis should carefully exclude spinal cord pathologies (e.g., spinal ste-

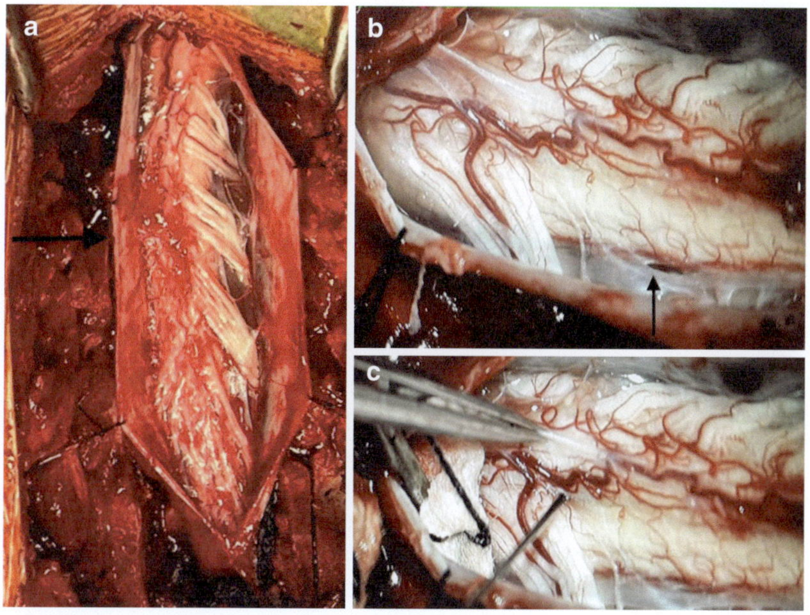

Fig. 7.27 Intraoperative pictures of the cervical spinal cord. Picture **a** demonstrates nerve root avulsion C5–C8 on the right side (arrow) after opening the dura to visualize the spinal cord. Note, that the unaffected left side provides visualization of the spinal nerve roots. Pictures **b** and **c** show the spinal root avulsion viewed under the microscope (arrow), and the technique of thermocoagulation (**c**)

nosis, intervertebral disc herniation, neoplasms, cauda equina syndrome) and mononeuropathies.

The underlying pathophysiological mechanisms vary by etiology and include traction injury, fibrosis or scar formation, direct compression, or neoplastic infiltration.

MRI and electrodiagnostic studies are essential to confirm the diagnosis. In cases where neoplastic involvement is suspected, positron emission tomography scan (PET-CT) is recommended.

Treatment strategies range from conservative management—comprising analgesia and physiotherapy—to surgical interventions such as tumor resection, neurolysis, nerve grafting, or nerve transfer.

Due to the anatomical location of the lumbar plexus within the bony pelvis, surgical approaches are technically more challenging compared with those for the brachial plexus.

7.3 Iatrogenic Nerve Injuries

Iatrogenic nerve injuries represent a distinct pathological subgroup and are more common than often assumed.

These lesions may occur through a variety of mechanisms, including direct trauma, traction, compression, ischemia, exposure to neurotoxic agents (e.g., local anesthetics), or thermal damage. In contrast to other forms of peripheral nerve injury, iatrogenic lesions are classically isolated, and are not commonly associated with concomitant injuries.

Patients frequently do not recognize these injuries, and referral to a specialist is often delayed [202, 203].

Non-surgical causes include needle-induced trauma following injections or nerve blocks, compression by hematoma, tourniquet- or cast-related injury, and delayed complications of radiation therapy.

Direct surgical mechanisms of nerve damage implicate transection, compression, contusion, excision, or coagulation.

An additional emerging cause is the use of foreign materials in aesthetic procedures. These may elicit an immune-mediated response with or without secondary compressive neuropathy. Importantly, current evidence does not support a role of direct neurotoxicity in these cases. Treatment generally involves surgical nerve decompression with or without neurolysis and—when necessary— extensive excision of the foreign material.

Commonly affected nerves are summarized in Table 7.4:

Table 7.4 Common iatrogenic nerve lesions

Affected nerve	Cause
Accessory nerve	Lymph node biopsy/resection
Median nerve	Carpal tunnel surgery
Sciatic nerve, femoral nerve	Hip arthroplasty surgery, trauma surgery, endoscopic procedures, varicose vein surgery
Radial nerve	Trauma surgery
Inguinal nerve	Hernia surgery
Facial nerve	Maxillofacial/otologic surgery

Therapy of iatrogenic nerve lesions is highly dependent on the underlying mechanism of injury. Complete transection of a nerve classically requires surgical intervention, whereas injuries resulting from exposure to neurotoxic agents may be appropriately managed with a conservative "watchful waiting" approach.

7.4 Ballistic Nerve Injuries

Although uncommon in most European countries, ballistic trauma represents an important mechanism of peripheral nerve injury in other regions of the world, and warrants discussion. Gunshot wounds are associated with complex pathophysiological mechanisms, and approximately 30–60% of cases ultimately require meticulous surgical repair [204].

Ballistic injuries caused by bullets result in direct tissue penetration, high-energy impacts with secondary damages to surrounding structures, and additional thermal injury.

By contrast, shrapnel injuries typically produce multiple small wounds of varying depth across different tissues and organs. Over time, retained fragments may provoke chronic foreign body inflammatory reactions, which can contribute to neuropathic pain.

High-resolution ultrasonography is considered to be the preferred imaging modality as it provides rapid diagnostic information, thus enabling early surgical intervention.

Two main surgical strategies have been described in the literature, depending on the extent of damage. In cases of small shrapnel-induced injuries, the associated inflammatory response often results in neuroma and scar formation, for which interfascicular neurolysis may be an appropriate option. The thermal component of gunshot wounds, however, can lead to pronounced intraneural fibrosis, making surgical intervention more challenging.

In severe cases characterized by intractable neuropathic pain, nerve grafting has been reported to provide more effective symptom relief than neurolysis.

> Nonetheless, grafting cannot be considered universally superior. In cases involving extensive neuromas in continuity with dense fibrosis, grafting seems to be the better surgical approach though.

Comprehensive internal neurolysis may be sufficient to restore a satisfactory motor function.

Regardless of the reconstructive strategy, extensive and precise debridement of the surrounding connective tissue is essential to optimize the neural environment thereby preventing further scarring [205].

7.5 Peripheral Nerve Tumors

7.5.1 Schwannoma (Neurinoma)

Schwannomas are well-circumscribed, round, solid tumors that typically demonstrate a hyperechoic margin on ultrasonographic examination. They are eccentric in relation to the long axis of the affected nerve, and may occasionally contain cystic degeneration, necrosis, or calcifications—a variant referred to as *ancient schwannoma*.

Histopathologically, schwannomas are composed of alternating Antoni A and Antoni B regions, exhibit high cellularity, and frequently contain hyalinized blood vessels [206].

They originate from a single nerve fascicle and are characterized by a displacing rather than an infiltrative growth pattern.

Schwannomas account for approximately 5% of all benign soft-tissue neoplasms [209].

The most frequently affected nerves are located in the upper extremities, with the ulnar, median and radial nerve being the most common site of origin. Less frequently, with a prevalence of 1–10%, schwannomas can be found in the lower extremities [207].

Management depends on clinical presentation. Small, asymptomatic tumors can be observed with regular follow-up. Surgical resection is indicated in cases of progressive tumor growth or the development of neurological symptoms.

Due to their non-infiltrative, eccentric growth pattern, tumor resection can usually be performed without damage to the fascicle (Fig. 7.28).

For patients who are not suitable candidates for surgery, such as those unable to tolerate general anesthesia, radiosurgery may serve as an alternative treatment option.

7.5.2 Neurofibroma

Neurofibromas represent the most common type of peripheral nerve sheath tumor. Approximately 90% occur sporadically, while the remaining 10% are associated with **Neurofibromatosis (NF)** [213].

They may present as isolated or localized lesions (cutaneous or intraneural), diffuse forms—often related to Neurofibromatosis-, or as extensive soft tissue masses. Both sexes are affected equally.

Solitary neurofibromas are classically manifest as isolated lesions presenting as slow-growing, non-invasive, well-circumscribed masses.

On ultrasonography, the generally demonstrate central localization along the nerve axis and may appear as a hyperechoic center surrounded by a hypoechoic rim. Compared with schwannomas, neurofibromas are more frequently heterogenous, demonstrate lower vascularity and present a greater propensity for intraneural infiltration.

Histologically, neurofibromas consist of a mixture of schwann cells, perineural cells and fibroblasts. They may arise from multiple non-functional fascicles.

On MRI, characteristic findings may include the "target sign"—which describes a hyperechoic central area surrounded by a hypoechoic peripheral rim—and the "split fat sign" [214, 215].

Whole-body imaging is recommended in patients with neurofibromas, gven their association with syndromic conditions such as Neurofibromatosis.

Plexiform neurofibromas are large, diffuse tumors characterized by extensive involvement along one or more nerves of the trunk or extremi-

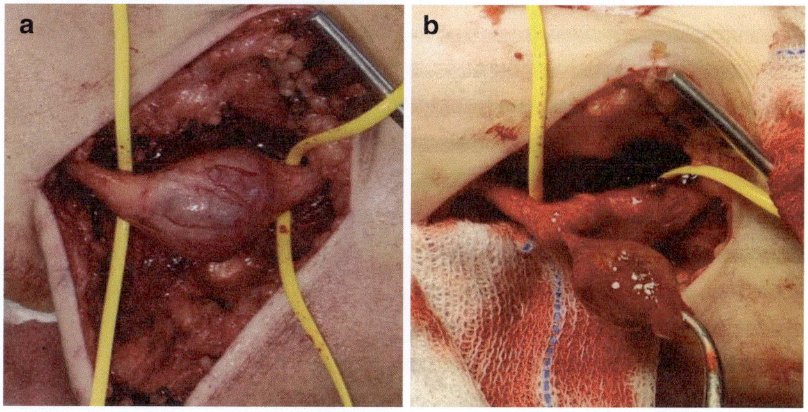

Fig. 7.28 Two-panel image showing a schwannoma of the median nerve prior to (**a**) and during surgical excision (**b**)

ties [219]. They are dysmorphic with a heterogenic echogenicity and ill-defined margins disrupting the normal nerve architecture. They may infiltrate adjacent tissues and are strongly associated with Neurofibromatosis type 1 (NF1) [216].

Diffuse neurofibromas are superficially located mass lesions involving the epidermis and the subcutaneous tissue, most commonly in the head and neck region. They exhibit a plaque-like, infiltrative growth pattern [218].

Occasionally, neurofibromas may mimic schwannomas, with a single fascicle entering and exiting the lesion; however, histopathological evaluation confirms the diagnosis of neurofibroma.

Sonographic differential diagnosis include cellulitis, hemangioma, or angiolipoma, as those lesions may infiltrate subcutaneous fat and occasionally demonstrate fatty proliferation [220].

Clinically, neurofibromas may remain asymptomatic or produce neurological deficits and pain depending on the extent of neural infiltration.

Plexiform variants are typically presenting with pain and carry an increased risk of malignant transformation, thus biopsy may be indicated.

Management principles largely resemble those for schwannomas. Surgical interventions typically reserved for symptomatic relief—particularly pain—with the objective of preserving neurological function and and mitigating the risk of malignant transformation (Fig. 7.29).

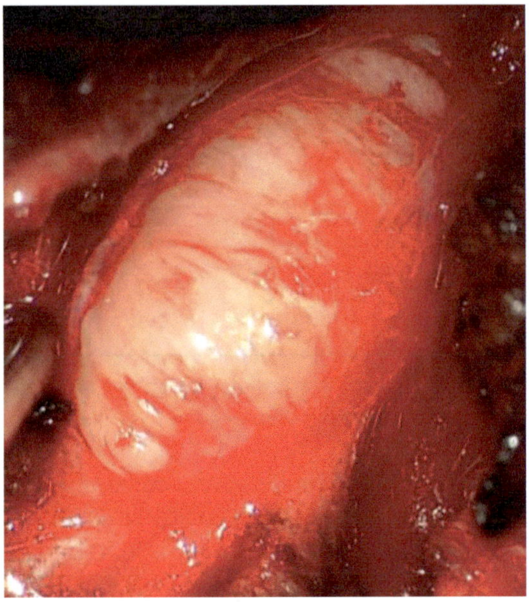

Fig. 7.29 Anatomical image representing a neurofibroma of the ulnar nerve

In clinical practice, Schwannomas and Neurofibromas are undistinguishable on the basis of clinical presentation and imaging alone; definite diagnosis requires histopathological examination.

7.5.3 Perineurioma

Perineurioma represents a rare entity of benign, slow-growing nerve sheath tumors usually affecting adolescents and young adults. The precise pathophysiology remains unclear, however, a genetic basis is presumed.

Clinically, it is characterized by slowly progressive, painless motor deficits with concomitant atrophy of the corresponding musculature. Sensory deficits are not seen [223].

On ultrasonography, perineuriomas appear as hypoechoic thickening of the affected nerve with variable vascularity. The MRI typically demonstrates fusiform nerve enlargement with increase signal intensity and may show the characteristic “onion-bulb appearance”, with occasional contrast enhancement (Fig. 7.30).

Electromyography often reveals features of long-standing chronic lesion, reflecting the fact that motor deficits are frequently recognized rather late by patients.

The differential diagnosis includes schwannomas, neurofibromas, chronic inflammatory demyelinating polyneuropathy (CIPD), or Charcot-Marie-Tooth disease [224].

When located at anatomical bottleneck sites, perineuriomas may be electrophysiologically indistinguishable from entrapment neuropathies.

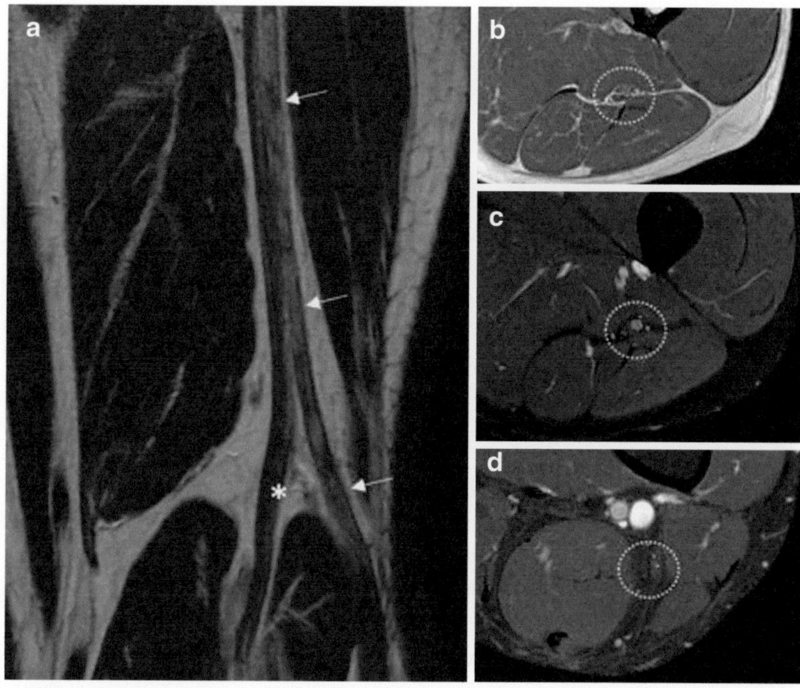

Fig. 7.30 Perineurioma of the sciatic nerve: (**a**) coronal T2-TSE image reveals long-segment enlargement of the sciatic nerve, predominantly affecting its peroneal division (arrows). The tibial division (asterix) shows normal anatomy and signal intensity. (**b**) (PD), (**c**) (PD-SPAIR), and (**d**) (T1-SPAIR) demonstrate preserved fascicular architecture with increased fascicular signal intensity and mild contrast enhancement (arrowhead). TSE Turbo spin echo, PD Proton density, PD-SPAIR Proton density spectral adiabatic inversion recovery

Histopathological confirmation is recommended and can be achieved through biopsy of a non-functional fascicle.

Perineuriomas exhibit very slow growth and malignant transformation has not been reported.

Total resection should not be aimed due to high risk of functional deficits. Decompression of hypertrophic fascicle via epineurotomy may be considered. In more severe cases, nerve reconstruction procedures and tendon transfers are indicated.

> Nerve grafting is generally not feasible, as these lesions tend to be located proximally, often requiring grafts of prohibitive length. In perineuriomas of the sciatic nerve, the tibial and the peroneal components remain confined to separated nerve sheaths, allowing for nerve transfer strategies to be effective in selected cases.

7.5.4 Nerve Sheath Ganglion

Nerve sheath ganglia account for approximately 18% of non-traumatic peroneal nerve lesions [225].

These lesions are well-organized cystic structures located within the epineurium of peripheral nerves. They vary considerably in size and and may reach dimensions of up to 10 cm. The precise etiopathogenesis remains unclear, however, the most widely accepted hypothesis involves articular origin, as these cysts are often communicating with the adjacent synovial joint via an articular nerve branch [226] (Fig. 7.31).

The common peroneal nerve at the fibular head is the most frequently affected site, with rare involvement of the tibial nerve [227].

In the upper extremity, the ulnar nerve at the cubital tunnel is the most common location.

Sonographically, a polycystic anechoic tumor, lacking vascularization, can be identified. They appear as a nodule aligned along the nerve resem-

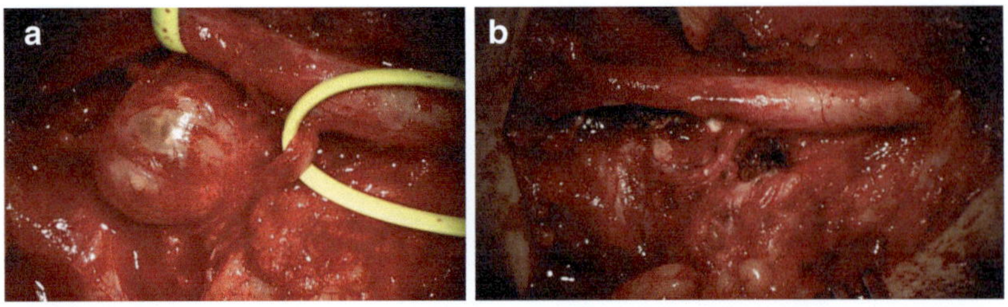

Fig. 7.31 Anatomical illustration presenting a nerve sheath ganglion of the ulnar nerve. Picture **a** demonstrates a branch of the ulnar nerve (yellow loop) encircling the ganglion. **b** demonstrates the postoperative view following resection of the ganglion

bling a "string of pearls", with fascicles displaced toward the periphery.

Clinically, nerve sheath ganglia are usually asymptomatic unless compressing the nerve or an adjacent vessel. When symptomatic, patients commonly present with localized pain and numbness in the distribution of the affected nerve. Muscle weakness occurs less frequently.

7.5.5 Neurofibromatosis (NF)

Neurofibromatosis (NF) describes a rare hereditary disorder classified among the phacomatoses. It is characterized by the development of predominantly benign tumors of the peripheral nerves and skin, though central nervous system manifestations may also occur. Neurological symptoms are variable; notably up to one-third of affected individuals remain asymptomatic.

Patients with NF may develop a spectrum of peripheral nerve sheath tumors including neurofibromas, plexiform neurofibromas, and schwannomas.

Based on genetic alterations and clinical phenotype, neurofibromatosis is divided into two major subtypes [232, 234]:

Neurofibromatosis Type 1 = (NF1, Recklinghausen Disease)

- Approximately 96% of all neurofibromatoses
- 1:3000 of all birth (50% sporadic, 50% hereditary)
- No prevalence regarding race or sex
- Autosomal dominant, mutation of the neurofibrim 1 (NF I) gene (= TumorSuppressor gene) on chromosome 17q11.2
- Manifestation in early childhood
- NF1-patients present with at least two of the following clinical signs (Fig. 7.32):
  - Six or more café-au-lait-spots
  - Two or more neurofibromas
  - Axillary or inguinal freckling
  - Optic glioma
  - At least two hamartomas of the iris ("Lisch-nodules"—no visual impairment)
  - Typical bone changes (dysplasia of the sphenoid bone, thinning of the long bones)
  - First-degree relative with NF1

A distinction should be made between neurofibromatosis type 1 (NF1) and **NF1-like syndromes**. In contrast to NF 1, NF1-like syndromes are not associated with pathogenic genetic mutations and are characterized by the absence of neurofibromas and lisch nodules.

Life expectancy in patients with NF1 is reduced by approximately 15 years compared with the general population [236].

Comprehensive assessment should include genetic testing as well as neuropsychological evaluation to identify cognitive or psychological impairments associated with this disorder.

Regarding the therapeutic management, regular follow-up using MRI and PET-CT imaging is recommended for early detection of complications (Fig. 7.33).

Surgical resection is indicated in symptomatic neurofibromas, although recurrence rates remain high.

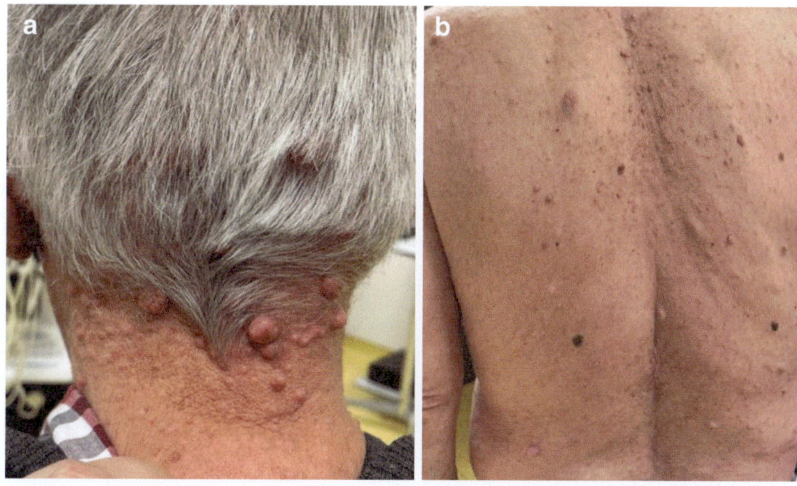

Fig. 7.32 Clinical presentation of a NF1 patient: Cutaneous neurofibromas (**a**, **b**) and café-au-lait-spots

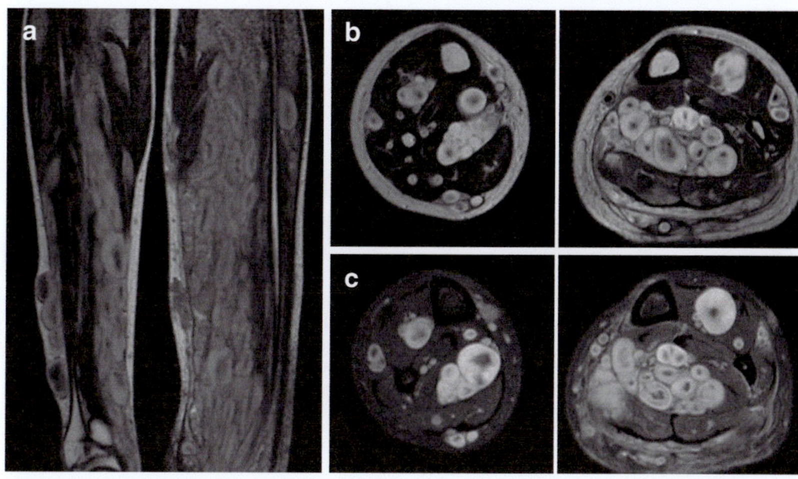

Fig. 7.33 Benign PNST: Plexiform neurofibromas in NF1: The images demonstrate innumerable neurofibromas, including plexiform neurofibromas involving the sciatic nerves (**a**—coronal T2) and their branches (**b**—axial T2-TSE and **c**—PD-SPAIR). TSE Turbo spin echo, PD-SPAIR Proton density spectral adiabatic inversion recovery

Approximately 4.6% of plexiform neurofibromas undergo malignant transformation, often headed by the onset of pain or progressive neurological deficits [237]. In such cases, wide surgical resection is recommended.

The use of MEK-inhibitors (e.g., selumetinib) has demonstrated efficacy in reducing tumor volume and improving tumor-related pain, muscle strength, and overall quality of life [238]. Additional MEK-inhibitors as well as tyrosine kinase inhibitors are currently under clinical investigation.

In optic gliomas, chemotherapy represents the first-line therapy.

Neurofibromatosis Type 2 = (NF2, Bilateral Acoustic or Central Neurofibroma)

- Approximately 3% of all neurofibromatoses
- Between 1:33,000 and 1:87,410 births
- Autosomal dominant, mutation of the NF2 gene merlin (cell wall protein, tumor suppression) on chromosome 22q12
- Manifestation in childhood or early adulthood
- Clinical signs: (frequently) bilateral schwannomas—most commonly vestibular schwannomas, meningeomas, ependymomas

In patients suspected with **neurofibromatosis type 2 (NF 2)**, an MRI of the entire neuroaxis is recommended to identify or exclude additional tumor sites.

NF2 patients should undergo regular audiological assessments in conjunction with serial MRI examinations to monitor for tumor progression and associated complications.

Surgical resection is considered first-line treatment in symptomatic tumors. However, recurrence rates are high—representing approximately 44%—and surgery carries significant risks, most notably hearing loss and facial nerve palsy [239, 240].

Radiation therapy may be considered as an alternative in selected cases, though it is associated with an increased risk for malignant transformation. The VEGF- Inhibitor bevacizumab has shown efficacy in reducing tumor volume and in improving hearing outcomes in some patients.

Schwannomatosis

Schwannotmatosis is a distinct clinical entity, separated from NF 2, yet very similar to it regarding genetics and clinical presentation, which can complicate accurate diagnosis.

The defining criterion for schwannomatosis is the presence of multiple schwannomas in the absence of vestibular schwannomas (i.e. without involvement of cranial nerve VIII) [241].

Peripheral nerves are most commonly affected, followed by the spine, with 89% and 74% respectively [242] (Fig. 7.34). Cranial nerve schwannomas are rare; when present, the trigeminal nerve is the most commonly affected.

The predominant symptom is chronic pain, which can be severe and debilitating. The risk for malignant transformation is considered low.

The primary therapeutic objective is symptomatic relief and preservation of neurological function via surgical resection. Chemotherapy or immunotherapy have no established role in schwannomatosis. In selected cases, e.g., patients who are not eligible for surgery, radiotherapy can be considered.

- Rare condition (<1%)
- Many common clinical manifestations with NF2
- Unclear genetic origin but frequently mutation of SMARCB or LZTR1 gene
- Incidence 1:40,000 (85% spontaneous, 15% hereditary)
- Patients are classically ≥30 years of age
- Diagnosis: ≥2 Schwannomas without vestibular tumor and without NF2 mutation
  1 schwannoma + first degree relative with schwannomatosis

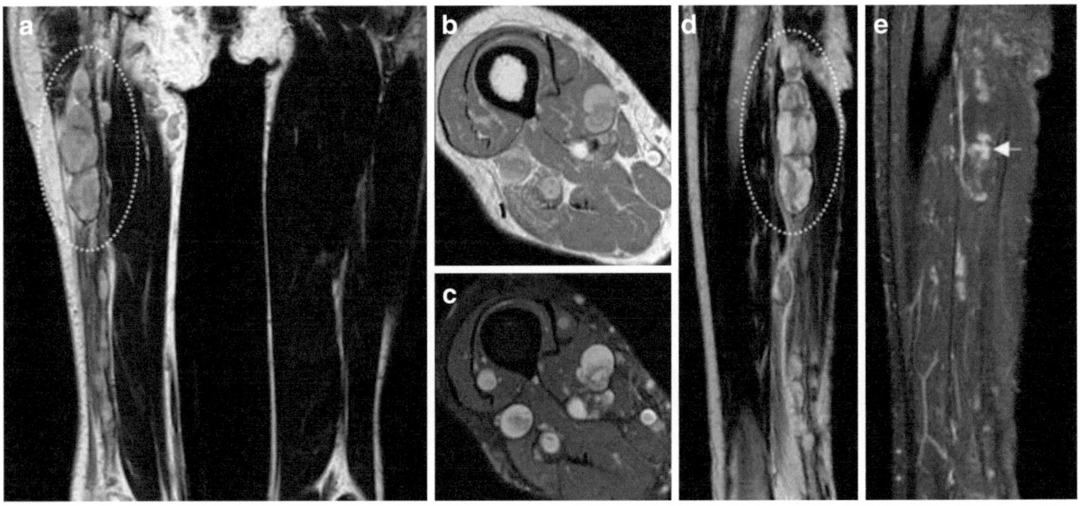

Fig. 7.34 Schwannomatosis: (**a**) (coronal T2-TSE), (**b**) (axial PD), (**c**) (axial PD-SPAIR) and (**d**) (sagittal T2-TSE) demonstrate multiple schwannomas in the thigh. The dotted circle indicates the sciatic nerve. (**e**) (Sagittal T1-SPIR) shows heterogeneous contrast enhancement (arrow). TSE Turbo spin echo

Genetic testing needs to be performed to differentiate schwannomatosis from NF2

- Clinical signs: pain, hypesthesia/paresthesia, rarely motor weakness

7.5.6 Malignant Peripheral Nerve Tumors (MPNSTs)

Malignant peripheral nerve tumors are rare soft tissue sarcomas with an incidence of 1 per 100,000 individuals, affecting both sexes equally. Between 10–20% of cases occur in the pediatric population [244].

50% of MPNSTs arise in patients with neurofibromatosis type 1 (NF1), who have a life-time risk of approximately 10%.

Around 10% of MPNST patients have a prior history of radiation exposure.

They may develop de novo from a peripheral nerve or through malignant transformation of a pre-existing benign nerve sheath tumor.

MPNSTs are classified with the group of soft tissue sarcomas.

They demonstrate a marked tendency for local invasion and metastatic spread, most commonly to regional lymph nodes and the lungs.

Five-year overall survival rate ranges between 30–60% with a median survival rate of ~6 years [248].

They are usually located in the proximal limbs and the trunk (mediastinum, retroperitoneum).

Clinically, a rapidly growing mass with early symptoms of pain, sensory deficits (hypesthesia), and motor deficits may raise the suspicion for malignancy [245].

Pain at rest or **nocturnal pain** is a strong indicator of malignancy!

Regarding imaging studies, MRI is the modality of choice typically revealing a large tumor mass of more than 5 cm in size having an irregular shape with infiltrative margins, a heterogenic appearance and peritumoral edema. Hemorrhage and necrosis, as well as increased angiogenesis is observed [249] (Fig. 7.35).

As MPNSTs demonstrate a higher metabolic activity compared with benign tumors, 18F-FDG PET/CT imaging may aid in establishing diagnosis.

Nevertheless, histopathological confirmation is essential in terms of diagnosis. Needle biopsies are discouraged as nearly half of the patients may develop new deficits or pain following biopsy. Open biopsy may be performed in cases with diagnostic uncertainty prior to definite treatment.

PET-CT guided biopsy is an emerging technique that may help guide surgical strategy [250].

Surgical resection with negative margins remain the cornerstone of therapy and is the strongest prognostic factor [251].

Nerve reconstruction following tumor resection rarely restores function but may reduce pain.

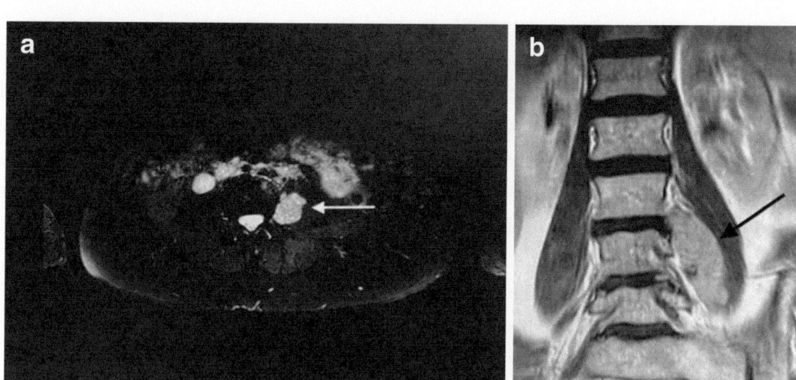

Fig. 7.35 MPNST: (**a**) (axial T2-SPAIR) and (**b**) (coronal T1) demonstrate a MPNST reaching from the left lumbar spinal nerves L3 to L5

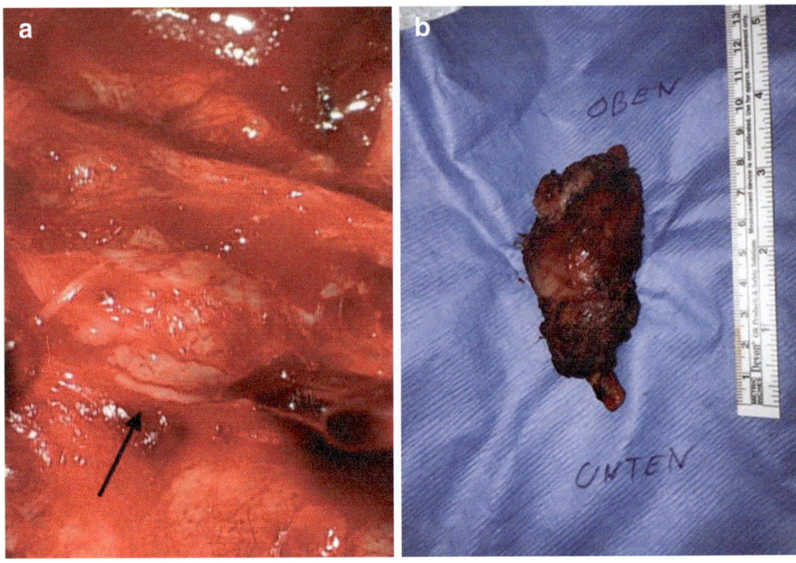

Fig. 7.36 Two-panel image showing surgical and specimen details: MPNST from lumbar spinal nerves L3–L5 paravertebral left (**a**). (**b**) Shows the resected tumor

Despite high perioperative morbidity and recurrence rates, aggressive surgical management offers the best outcomes (Fig. 7.36).

Chemotherapy (e.g., ifosfamid, doxorubicin) has shown limited efficacy [253].

Radiotherapy lacks strong evidence but may provide local control, especially in tumors >5 cm, reducing the risk for recurrence.

Outcomes are generally worse in NF1-associated MPNSTs compared with sporadic cases.

Tumors located more distally within the body are associated with improved outcomes.

The *Triton tumor* represents a rare histological variant of MPNST—accounting for approximately 5% of all cases. It is most frequently encountered in patients with NF1 [254].

Histopathologically, these tumors arise from Schwann cells as a rhabdomyoblastic differentiation with immunohistochemical positivity for S-100 protein. Clinically, they typically present as enlarging firm masses originating from medium- to large-sized peripheral nerves.

Given their highly aggressive biological behavior, the standard treatment consists of radical surgical resection combined with adjuvant chemoradiotherapy. Despite these interventions, the overall prognosis remains poor.

Metastases affecting the peripheral nerves, including the plexuses, may occurs either through direct infiltration by solid tumors or as remote metastases of cancerous diseases like lymphoma or leukemia.

Routes of dissemination include endoneural spread, lymphatic invasion, or hematogenous metastases. Locally invasive tumors—particularly those of the head and neck region (squamous cell carcinoma, breast carcinoma, or lung carcinoma)—tend to infiltrate the brachial plexus. These lesions should be carefully distinguished from "true" metastatic deposits.

Tumor-associated neuropathic pain is common in patients with MPNST or peripheral nerve metastases, necessitating comprehensive pain management strategies. Clinical presentation usually becomes apparent with the onset of neurological deficits or pain and must be differentiated from treatment-related neuropathies secondary to chemotherapy or radiation. The typical clinical picture is that of a mononeuropathy with focal sensory and motor impairments in the distribution of the affected nerve.

Diagnosis is established through detailed clinical history, complemented by electrophysiological studies and magnetic resonance imaging (Fig. 7.37). Where feasible, surgical resection remains the treatment of choice.

Owing to the high recurrence and progressive rates, patients require close surveillance with MRI examnations performed at three-months intervals.

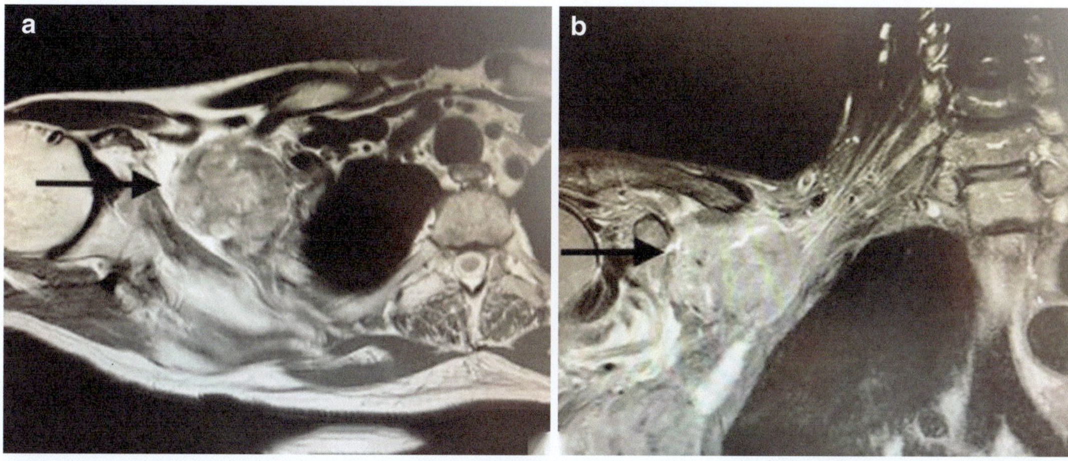

Fig. 7.37 Metastasis of a melanoma located at the right brachial plexus reaching from retro- to infraclavicular is shown in (**a**) (T2) and (**b**) (STIR)

7.5.7 Rare Tumors

Desmoid Tumor

Desmoid tumors are fibroblastic soft-tissue neoplasms characterized by locally aggressive and infiltrative growth, but without metastatic potential. They exhibit a high propensity for local recurrence following treatment [257]. A notable predilection for female patients compared with males has been observed.

The tumors typically originate from the muscle fascia or aponeurosis, with the abdominal wall fascia representing the most frequent site of involvement [258]. Other commonly affected locations include the neck, shoulder girdle, extremities, or pelvis (Fig. 7.38).

Clinically, their infiltrative nature leads to pain and weakness of the involved musculature or adjacent nerves. On examination, patients often describe a firm, scar-like mass that is readily palpable and may elicit pain upon compression.

Different treatment options are available including surgical resection—with or without adjuvant radiation—chemotherapy or isolated limb perfusion (ILP) [259] (Fig. 7.39).

However, surgical intervention carries a substantial risk of functional impairment and is associated with high recurrence rates.

Given these challenges, some experts advocate for conservative strategy of active surveillance, as none of the currently available treatment options consistently achieve satisfactory long-term outcomes.

Neurolymphomatosis

Neurolymphomatosis represents a condition characterized by the direct infiltration of peripheral nerves—including cranial nerves—by B-cell Non-Hodgkin lymphomas, and less frequently T-cell Lymphomas. It demonstrates rapid progression, with pain being the predominant clinical presentation. However, the full clinical spectrum of polyneuropathy or mononeuropathy may also be observed [260].

Diagnosis is challenging, as MRI demonstrates limited sensitivity of approximately 40%.

More reliable diagnostic modalities include PET-CT or nerve biopsy, the latter achieving a sensitivity exceeding 80% [261] (Fig. 7.40).

The first-line treatment consists of chemotherapy, following therapeutic protocols similar to those employed in central nervous system lymphomas, with reported response rates of approximately 82% [262]. Combination therapy with adjunctive radiotherapy may also be considered.

Surgical intervention is not regarded as a therapeutic option. Nevertheless, in selected cases—

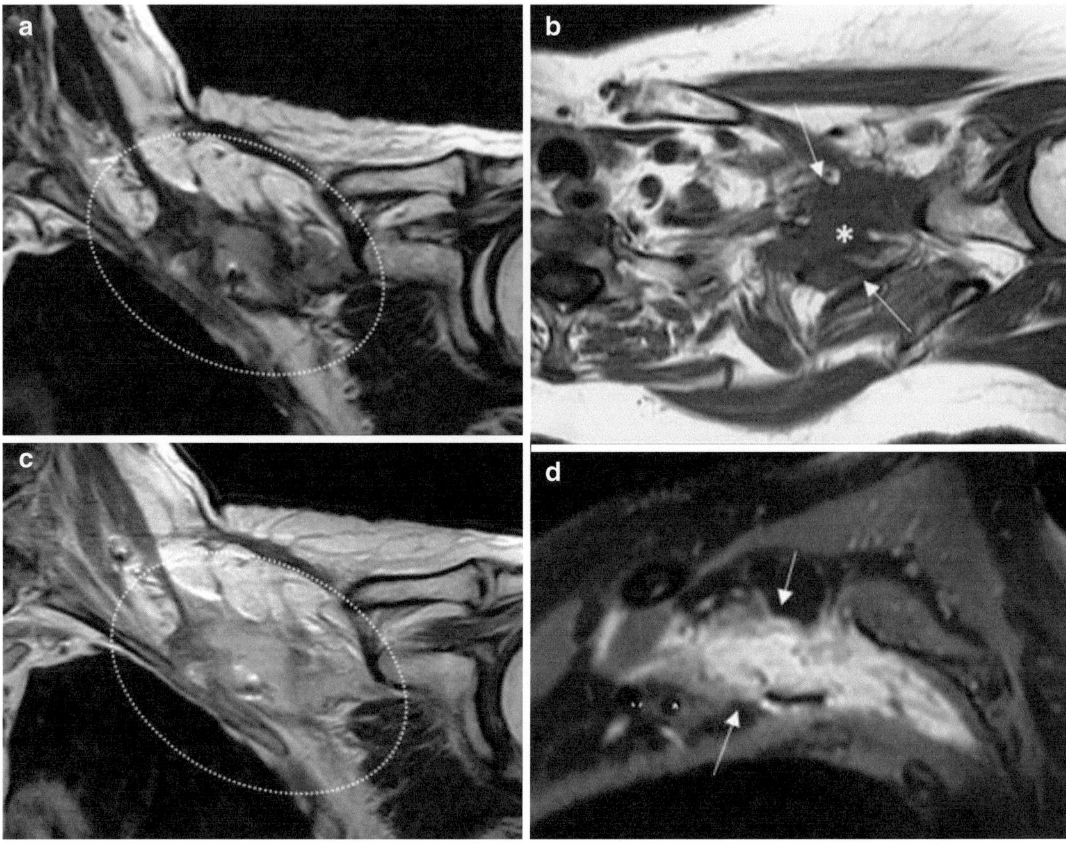

Fig. 7.38 Retro- and infraclavicular desmoid tumor: Large mass with a heterogenous, predominantly T2-hyperintense signal and T1-isointense appearance (**a**—coronal T2-TSE, **b**—axial T1-TSE), extending along the brachial plexus down to the level of the trunk divisions, cords and terminal branches (dotted circle, asterix and arrow). (**c**) (Coronal T1-TSE) and (**d**) (sagittal T1-SPIR) demonstrate intense contrast enhancement (dotted circle and arrows). TSE Turbo spin echo, SPIR Spectral presaturation with inversion recovery

such as those with severe intractable pain or large compressive lesions—surgical resection may be performed for symptomatic relief.

Despite these measures, prognosis remains poor, with a mean life expectancy of approximately 10 months.

Lipomatosis of the Nerve/Fibrolipomatous Hamartoma of the Nerve/Neural Fibrolipoma

Lipomatosis of the nerve, also referred to fibrolipomatous hamartoma or neural fibrolipoma, is a rare benign entity characterized by abnormal proliferation of fibroadipose tissue within the epineurium, resulting in separation and distortion of nerve fascicles. The disorder most commonly affects nerves of the distal extremities, with the median nerve being the predominant site of involvement [263].

An association with macrodactyly is well recognized, occurring in approximately 30% of cases [264].

Neural fibrolipomas are more frequently observed in children compared adults and are distinguished by their slow growth and abundant intraneural adipose tissue.

Clinically, symptomatic patients present with pain, paresthesia, or motor weakness in the distribution of the affected nerve.

From a diagnostic perspective, ultrasound is often sufficient to establish diagnosis. MRI pro-

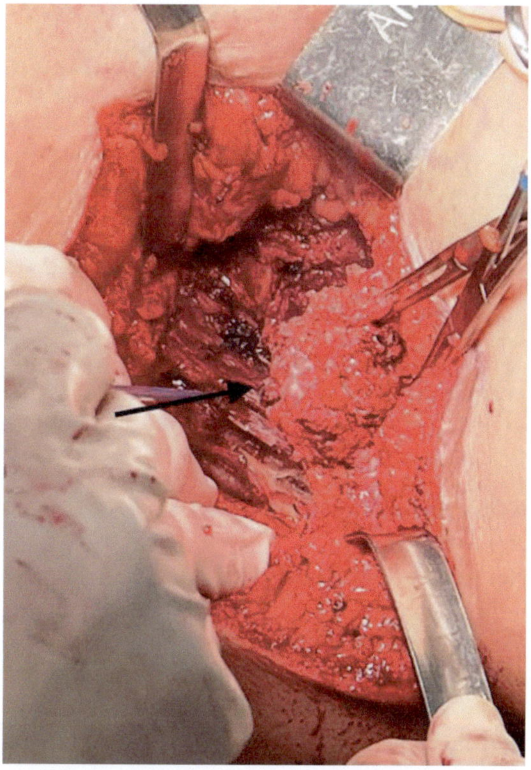

Fig. 7.39 Intraoperative image showing a desmoid tumor (arrow) of the proximal sciatic nerve. It represents as a firm mass

vides complementary evaluation, allowing more detailed assessment of the extent of nerve involvement (Fig. 7.41).

Management is typically focused on surgical decompression with the aim to preserve neurological function. Radical excision is generally avoided due to the high risk of significant neurological deficit.

Intraneural Hemangioma

Intraneural hemangiomas are exceedingly rare benign vascular tumors with a predilection for female patients. The median nerve is the most frequently affected nerve [266].

Patients typically present with a sudden onset of pain, attributed to mechanical compression of the involved nerve. Unlike many other intraneural lesions, sensory or motor disturbances are generally absent.

Diagnostic evaluation relies on ultrasound, MRI, and angiography which together facilitate assessment of both intraneural involvement and vascular supply.

Preoperative embolization is often recommended to reduce the risk of intraoperative bleeding. Partial resection of the tumor may suffice for

Fig. 7.40 Neurolymphoma: (**a**) FDG-PET/CT demonstrates linear abnormal uptake along the right brachial plexus, which shows normal signal intensity on sagittal STIR (**b**). (**c**) Sagittal STIR image reveals denervation changes (asterix) affecting the subscapularis, supraspinatus and infraspinatus muscles. FDG PET/CT Positron emission tomography/computed tomography scan

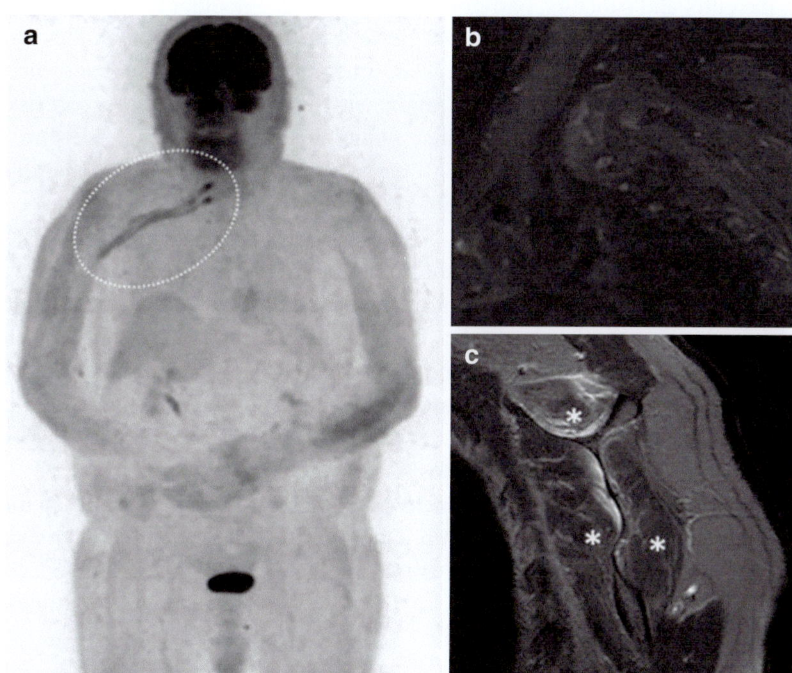

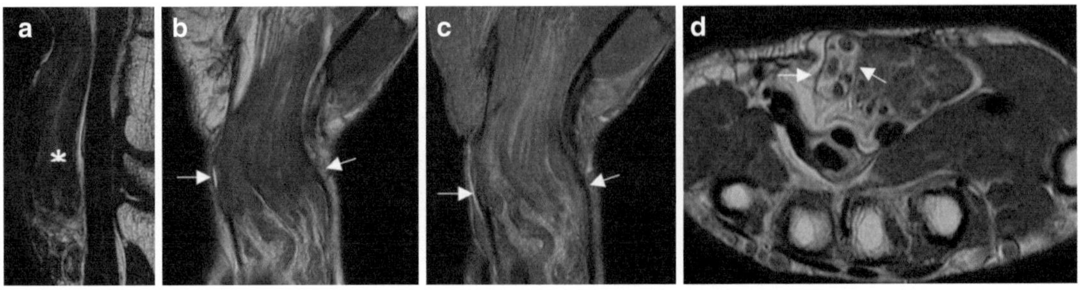

Fig. 7.41 Fibrolipoma of the median nerve: Sagittal TS-TSE (**a**), coronal T1-TSE (**b**), and PD-SPIR (**c**) MRI of the wrist at the level of the carpal tunnel demonstrate a mass-like expansion of the median nerve (asterix and arrows) with multiple enlarged neural fascicles, extending from the forearm to the hand. Axial T1-TSE (**d**) demonstrates enlarged neural fascicles containing macroscopic fat (arrows). TSE Turbo spin echo, PD-SPIR Proton density spectral presaturation with inversion recovery

symptomatic relief; however, reoccurrence has been reported. Total resection can prevent reccurrence but usually necessitates excision of the affected nerve, leading to permanent neurological deficits [267].

Postoperative radiotherapy, with or without preoperative embolization, has been described as an adjective treatment option [268].

Granular Cell Tumor (Abrikossoff Tumor)

Granular cell tumors are benign neoplasms of Schwann cell origin. They most frequently arise in the cutis and subcutis, particularly in the head and neck region—most notably in the oral cavity—and less commonly in the gastrointestinal tract of middle-aged adults. The tumor was first described in 1926 by the Russian pathologist Abrikossoff [269].

Involvement of small to medium-sized nerves is typical.

Malignant transformation is rare, occurring in approximately 1-2% of cases, and is associated with infiltration of adjacent tissues [270].

Clinically, granular cell tumors are often asymptomatic, slow-growing, painless nodules discovered incidentally.

Biopsy will establish the diagnosis.

Surgical excision is the treatment of choice, followed by close clinical follow-up. The roles of chemotherapy and radiotherapy are limited in this context.

Nerve Sheath Myxoma (NSM) and Neurothekeoma

Nerve sheath myxoma (NSM) and **neurothekeoma** are rare benign schwann cell-derived tumors most commonly arising in the cutis and subcutis of the upper and lower extremities in children and young adults. Histologically, NSM is characterized by hypocellular, spindle-shaped cells with elongated processes, whereas neurothekeoma demonstrates a more cellular appearance composed of spindle and epitheloid cells.

Clinically, these lesions present as painless nodular formatios, although pain may rarely occur. Imaging modalities such as ultrasound and MRI typically lack specificity, as these tumors closely resemble other soft tissue neoplasms [271].

Surgical excision remains the therapy of choice and is generally curative.

Paraganglioma

Paragangliomas are rare neuroendocrine tumors most commonly located in the head and neck region, typically arising in close proximity to the lower cranial nerves or the carotid artery.

While the majority are sporadic, approximately 10% are associated with familial syndromes [273].

Histologically, paragangliomas are composed of neural cells derived from the sympathetic and parasympathetic nervous system and often function as catecholamine-secreting tumors.

Diagnosis is established through biochemical testing—most commonly 24-hours urinary measurement of catecholamines and metanephrins—combined with imaging modalities such as MRI [274].

Surgical resection is the treatment of choice in solitary tumors. Particularly attention must be given to perioperative hemodynamic management, as tumor manipulation may precipitate significant blood pressure fluctuations.

Approximately 10% of paragangliomas exhibit malignant transformation with metastatic potential. In such cases, treatment options include tumor mass resection to decrease catecholamine load within the body, embolization, cryoablation, or radiofrequency ablation [275]. Conventional chemotherapy and radiotherapy are generally ineffective; however, both may be considered in a palliative setting for advanced disease [276].

Malignant Melanotic Nerve Sheath Tumor (MMNST)

Malignant melanotic nerve sheath tumors (MMNSTs) are pigmented tumors originating from the schwann cells, representing less than 1% of all nerve sheath tumors [277]. The spinal nerves constitute their most frequent site of occurrence [278].

The initial clinical manifestation often include pain and dysesthesia followed by motor weakness.

Magnetic resonance imaging typically demonstrates a well-circumscribed mass, that appears hypointense on T2-weighted sequence with homogeneous contrast enhancement after gadolinium administration, resembling the imaging characteristics of schwannomas or neurofibromas.

Despite the benign radiological appearance, MMNSTs frequently display aggressive biological behavior with a high risk of recurrence and metastatic dissemniation.

Gross total surgical resection remains the mainstay of therapy. Adjuvant radiotherapy may be considered, particularly in cases of incomplete resection or high risk features (Fig. 7.42).

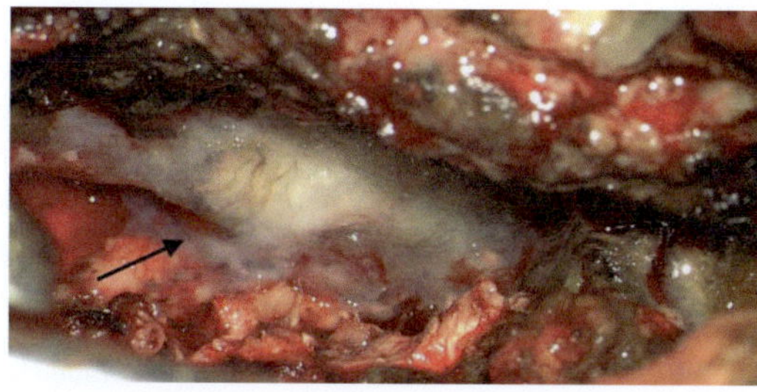

Fig. 7.42 *MMNST* of the spinal nerve S1

Further Reading

1. Trescot AM, editor. Peripheral nerve entrapments: clinical diagnosis and management. Springer; 2016. https://doi.org/10.1007/978-3-319-27482-5.
2. Yu M, Wang SM. Anatomy, head and neck, occipital nerves. In: StatPearls. StatPearls Publishing; 2022.
3. Hock G, Johnson A, Barber P, Papa C. Current clinical concepts: rehabilitation of thoracic outlet syndrome. J Athl Train. 2024;59(7):683–95. https://doi.org/10.4085/1062-6050-0138.22.
4. Maślanka K, Zielinska N, Karauda P, Balcerzak A, Georgiev G, Borowski A, Drobniewski M, Olewnik Ł. Congenital, acquired, and trauma-related risk factors for thoracic outlet syndrome-review of the literature. J Clin Med. 2023;12(21):6811. https://doi.org/10.3390/jcm12216811.
5. Masocatto NO, Da-Matta T, Prozzo TG, Couto WJ, Porfirio G. Thoracic outlet syndrome: a narrative review. Síndrome do desfiladeiro torácico: uma revisão narrativa. Rev Col Bras Cir. 2019;46(5):e20192243. https://doi.org/10.1590/0100-6991e-20192243.
6. Maru S, Dosluoglu H, Dryjski M, Cherr G, Curl GR, Harris LM. Thoracic outlet syndrome in children and young adults. Eur J Vasc Endovasc Surg. 2009;38(5):560–4. https://doi.org/10.1016/j.ejvs.2009.06.015.
7. Panther EJ, Reintgen CD, Cueto RJ, Hao KA, Chim H, King JJ. Thoracic outlet syndrome: a review. J Shoulder Elb Surg. 2022;31(11):e545–61. https://doi.org/10.1016/j.jse.2022.06.026.
8. Jones MR, Prabhakar A, Viswanath O, Urits I, Green JB, Kendrick JB, Brunk AJ, Eng MR, Orhurhu V, Cornett EM, Kaye AD. Thoracic outlet syndrome: a comprehensive review of pathophysiology, diagnosis, and treatment. Pain Ther. 2019;8(1):5–18. https://doi.org/10.1007/s40122-019-0124-2. Epub 2019 Apr 29. PMID: 31037504; PMCID: PMC6514035.
9. Jones SJ, Miller JMM. Spurling test. [Updated 2023 Aug 8]. In: StatPearls [Internet]. Treasure Island: StatPearls Publishing; 2025. Available from: https://www.ncbi.nlm.nih.gov/books/NBK493152/.

10. Leider JD, Derise OC, Bourdreaux KA, Dierks GJ, Lee C, Varrassi G, Sherman WF, Kaye AD. Treatment of suprascapular nerve entrapment syndrome. Orthop Rev. 2021;13(2):25554. https://doi.org/10.52965/001c.25554.
11. Knipe H, Vadera S, Feger J, et al. Suprascapular neuropathy. Radiopaedia.org. 2024. https://doi.org/10.53347/rID-37641.
12. Katzer A, Niedermauntel WP, Rump J. Das parsonage-turner-syndrom [Parsonage-Turner Syndrome – case report]. Z Orthop Unfall. 2017;155(6):705–7. https://doi.org/10.1055/s-0043-114416.
13. England JD, Sumner AJ. Neuralgic amyotrophy: an increasingly diverse entity. Muscle Nerve. 1987;10(1):60–8. https://doi.org/10.1002/mus.880100112.
14. Cignetti NE, Cox RS, Baute V, McGhee MB, van Alfen N, Strakowski JA, Boon AJ, Norbury JW, Cartwright MS. A standardized ultrasound approach in neuralgic amyotrophy. Muscle Nerve. 2023;67(1):3–11. https://doi.org/10.1002/mus.27705.
15. Holle JF, Limmroth V, Windisch W, Zimmerman M. Neuralgic amyotrophy. Dtsch Arztebl Int. 2024;121(15):483–9. https://doi.org/10.3238/arztebl.m2024.0077.
16. Winter J, Karir A, Clark TA, Giuffre JL. Surgical treatment of parsonage turner syndrome with primary nerve transfers: a case series and cadaver dissection. Ann Plast Surg. 2022;89(3):301–5. https://doi.org/10.1097/SAP.0000000000003265. PMID: 35993685.
17. Kim DH, Sung DH, Chang MC. Diagnosis of hourglass-like constriction neuropathy of the radial nerve using high-resolution magnetic resonance neurography: a report of two cases. Diagnostics (Basel, Switzerland). 2020;10(4):232. https://doi.org/10.3390/diagnostics10040232.
18. Van Eijk JJ, Groothuis JT, Van Alfen N. Neuralgic amyotrophy: an update on diagnosis, pathophysiology, and treatment. Muscle Nerve. 2016;53(3):337–50. https://doi.org/10.1002/mus.25008.
19. Hashizume H, Inoue H, Nagashima K, Hamaya K. Posterior interosseous nerve paralysis related to focal radial nerve constriction secondary to vasculitis. J Hand Surg (Edinburgh, Scotland). 1993;18(6):757–60. https://doi.org/10.1016/0266-7681(93)90239-c.
20. Yongwei P, Guanglei T, Jianing W, Shuhuan W, Qingtai L, Wen T. Nontraumatic paralysis of the radial nerve with multiple constrictions. J Hand Surg Am. 2003;28(2):199–205. https://doi.org/10.1053/jhsu.2003.50007.
21. Wang Y, Liu T, Song L, Zhang Z, Zhang Y, Ni J, Lu L. Spontaneous peripheral nerve palsy with hourglass-like fascicular constriction in the upper extremity. J Neurosurg. 2019;131(6):1876–86. https://doi.org/10.3171/2018.8.JNS18419.
22. He R, Yu JL, Jin HL, Ng L, Wang JC, Li X, Gai TT, Zhou Y, Li DP. Hourglass-like constriction of the anterior interosseous nerve in the left forearm: a case report. World J Clin Cases. 2023;11(17):4194–201. https://doi.org/10.12998/wjcc.v11.i17.4194. PMID: 37388800; PMCID: PMC10303608.
23. Pan YW, Wang S, Tian G, Li C, Tian W, Tian M. Typical brachial neuritis (Parsonage-Turner Syndrome) with hourglass-like constrictions in the affected nerves. J Hand Surg Am. 2011;36(7):1197–203. https://doi.org/10.1016/j.jhsa.2011.03.041.
24. Granata G, Tomasello F, Sciarrone MA, Stifano V, Lauretti L, Luigetti M. Neuralgic amyotrophy and hourglass nerve constriction/nerve torsion: two sides of the same coin? A clinical review. Brain Sci. 2024;14(1):67. https://doi.org/10.3390/brainsci14010067.
25. Hangge PT, Breen I, Albadawi H, Knuttinen MG, Naidu SG, Oklu R. Quadrilateral space syndrome: diagnosis and clinical management. J Clin Med. 2018;7(4):86. https://doi.org/10.3390/jcm7040086.
26. Khan IA, Launico MV, Varacallo MA. Anatomy, shoulder and upper limb, arm quadrangular space. In: StatPearls. StatPearls Publishing; 2025.
27. Ekholm R, Ponzer S, Törnkvist H, Adami J, Tidermark J. The Holstein-Lewis humeral shaft fracture: aspects of radial nerve injury, primary treatment, and outcome. J Orthop Trauma. 2008;22(10):693–7. https://doi.org/10.1097/BOT.0b013e31818915bf.
28. Chang G, Ilyas AM. Radial nerve palsy after humeral shaft fractures: the case for early exploration and a new classification to guide treatment and prognosis. Hand Clin. 2018;34(1):105–12. https://doi.org/10.1016/j.hcl.2017.09.011.
29. O'Gorman CM, Kassardjian C, Sorenson EJ. Musculocutaneous neuropathy. Muscle Nerve. 2018;58(5):726–9. https://doi.org/10.1002/mus.26186.
30. Kissel JA, Leonardelli C. Isolated musculocutaneous neuropathy: a case report. J Can Chiropr Assoc. 2019;63(3):162–70.
31. Aldossari RM, Galecio Castillo MC, Hameed S. Benediction sign. In: StatPearls. StatPearls Publishing; 2024. https://www.ncbi.nlm.nih.gov/books/NBK554458/.
32. Dydyk AM, Negrete G, Sarwan G, Cascella M. Median nerve injury. In: StatPearls. StatPearls Publishing; 2023.
33. Suranyi L. Median nerve compression by Struthers ligament. J Neurol Neurosurg Psychiatry. 1983;46(11):1047–9. https://doi.org/10.1136/jnnp.46.11.1047.
34. Tosin D, Antoniadis G, Wirtz CR, Pedro MT. Seltenes Kompressionssyndrom des N. medianus durch den Processus supracondylaris und das Struthers-Ligament [Rare compression syndrome of the median nerve due to a supracondylar humeral process and a ligament of Struthers]. Handchir Mikrochir Plast Chir. 2024;56(1):101–5. https://doi.org/10.1055/a-2234-4636.

35. Caetano EB, Sabongi Neto JJ, Vieira LA, Caetano MF, de Bona JE, Simonatto TM. Struthers' ligament and supracondylar humeral process: an anatomical study and clinical implications. Acta Ortop Bras. 2017;25(4):137–42. https://doi.org/10.1590/1413-785220172504168330.
36. Struthers J. On a peculiarity of the humerus and humeral artery. J. Hand Surg Eur Vol. 2007;32(1):54–6. https://doi.org/10.1016/j.jhsb.2006.09.001.
37. Bilge T, Yalaman O, Bilge S, Cokneşeli B, Barut S. Entrapment neuropathy of the median nerve at the level of the ligament of Struthers. Neurosurgery. 1990;27(5):787–9. https://doi.org/10.1097/00006123-199011000-00017.
38. Aydinlioglu A, Cirak B, Akpinar F, Tosun N, Dogan A. Bilateral median nerve compression at the level of Struthers' ligament. Case report. J Neurosurg. 2000;92(4):693–6. https://doi.org/10.3171/jns.2000.92.4.0693.
39. Shah Mardan QNM, Al-Khayarin A, Bouri F, Muneer M. Lacertus fibrosus release in proximal median nerve entrapment: a systematic review. Int Orthop. 2025;49(5):1167–74. https://doi.org/10.1007/s00264-025-06493-5.
40. Apard T, Martinel V, Batby G, Draznieks G, Descamps J. Lacertus syndrome: recent advances. Hand Surg Rehabil. 2024;43(4):101738. https://doi.org/10.1016/j.hansur.2024.101738.
41. Bassett FH 3rd, Spinner RJ, Schroeter TA. Brachial artery compression by the lacertus fibrosus. Clin Orthop Relat Res. 1994;307:110–6.
42. Dang AC, Rodner CM. Unusual compression neuropathies of the forearm, part II: median nerve. J Hand Surg Am. 2009;34(10):1915–20. https://doi.org/10.1016/j.jhsa.2009.10.017.
43. Tang JB. Median nerve compression: lacertus syndrome versus superficialis-pronator syndrome. J Hand Surg Eur Vol. 2021;46(9):1017–22. https://doi.org/10.1177/17531934211024092.
44. Hagert E, Jedeskog U, Hagert CG, Marín Fermín T. Lacertus syndrome: a ten year analysis of two hundred and seventy five minimally invasive surgical decompressions of median nerve entrapment at the elbow. Int Orthop. 2023;47(4):1005–11. https://doi.org/10.1007/s00264-023-05709-w.
45. Akhondi H, Varacallo MA. Anterior interosseous syndrome. In: StatPearls. StatPearls Publishing; 2023.
46. Li N, Russo K, Rando L, Gulotta-Parrish L, Sherman W, Kaye AD. Anterior interosseous nerve syndrome. Orthop Rev. 2022;14(4):38678. https://doi.org/10.52965/001c.38678.
47. Schantz K, Riegels-Nielsen P. The anterior interosseous nerve syndrome. J Hand Surg (Edinburgh, Scotland). 1992;17(5):510–2. https://doi.org/10.1016/s0266-7681(0.
48. Krishnan KR, Sneag DB, Feinberg JH, Wolfe SW. Anterior interosseous nerve syndrome reconsidered: a critical analysis review. JBJS Rev. 2020;8(9):e2000011. https://doi.org/10.2106/JBJS.RVW.20.00011.
49. Hartz CR, Linscheid RL, Gramse RR, Daube JR. The pronator teres syndrome: compressive neuropathy of the median nerve. J Bone Joint Surg Am Vol. 1981;63(6):885–90.
50. Dididze M, Tafti D, Sherman AL. Pronator teres syndrome. In: StatPearls. StatPearls Publishing; 2023.
51. Fuss FK, Wurzl GH. Median nerve entrapment. Pronator teres syndrome. Surgical anatomy and correlation with symptom patterns. Surg Radiol Anat: SRA. 1990;12(4):267–71. https://doi.org/10.1007/BF01623702.
52. Adler JA, Wolf JM. Proximal median nerve compression: pronator syndrome. J Hand Surg Am. 2020;45(12):1157–65. https://doi.org/10.1016/j.jhsa.2020.07.006.
53. Balcerzak AA, Ruzik K, Tubbs RS, Konschake M, Podgórski M, Borowski A, Drobniewski M, Olewnik Ł. How to differentiate pronator syndrome from carpal tunnel syndrome: a comprehensive clinical comparison. Diagnostics (Basel, Switzerland). 2022;12(10):2433. https://doi.org/10.3390/diagnostics12102433.
54. Osiak K, Elnazir P, Walocha JA, Pasternak A. Carpal tunnel syndrome: state-of-the-art review. Folia Morphol. 2022;81(4):851–62. https://doi.org/10.5603/FM.a2021.0121.
55. Chen CH, Wu T, Sun JS, Lin WH, Chen CY. Unusual causes of carpal tunnel syndrome: space occupying lesions. J Hand Surg Eur Vol. 2012;37(1):14–9. https://doi.org/10.1177/1753193411414352.
56. Sharrak S, Das JM. Hand nerve compression syndromes. In: StatPearls. StatPearls Publishing; 2023.
57. Joshi A, Patel K, Mohamed A, Oak S, Zhang MH, Hsiung H, Zhang A, Patel UK. Carpal tunnel syndrome: pathophysiology and comprehensive guidelines for clinical evaluation and treatment. Cureus. 2022;14(7):e27053. https://doi.org/10.7759/cureus.27053.
58. Genova A, Dix O, Saefan A, Thakur M, Hassan A. Carpal tunnel syndrome: a review of literature. Cureus. 2020;12(3):e7333. https://doi.org/10.7759/cureus.7333.
59. Davis DD, Kane SM. Median nerve palsy. In: StatPearls. StatPearls Publishing; 2023. https://www.ncbi.nlm.nih.gov/books/NBK557890/.
60. Becker RE, Manna B. Anatomy, shoulder and upper limb, ulnar nerve. In: StatPearls. StatPearls Publishing; 2023.
61. Ferre-Martinez A, Miguel-Pérez M, Möller I, Ortiz-Miguel S, Pérez-Bellmunt A, Ruiz N, Sanjuan X, Agullo J, Ortiz-Sagristà J, Martinoli C. Possible points of ulnar nerve entrapment in the arm and forearm: an ultrasound, anatomical, and histological study. Diagnostics (Basel, Switzerland). 2023;13(7):1332.
62. Cloete D, Lahri S. Ulnar nerve injury and Froment's test: a case report. Cureus. 2019;11(12):e6335. https://doi.org/10.7759/cureus.6335.

63. Bains S, Rocha Cabrero F. Electrodiagnostic evaluation of ulnar neuropathy. In: StatPearls. StatPearls Publishing; 2022.
64. Caetano EB, Sabongi Neto JJ, Vieira LA, Caetano MF. The arcade of Struthers: an anatomical study and clinical implications. Rev Bras Ortop. 2017;52(3):331–6. https://doi.org/10.1016/j.rboe.2016.07.006.
65. Sivak WN, Hagerty SE, Huyhn L, Jordan AC, Munin MC, Spiess AM. Diagnosis of ulnar nerve entrapment at the arcade of Struthers with electromyography and ultrasound. Plast Reconstr Surg Glob Open. 2016;4(3):e648. https://doi.org/10.1097/GOX.0000000000000628.
66. Granger A, Sardi JP, Iwanaga J, Wilson TJ, Yang L, Loukas M, Oskouian RJ, Tubbs RS. Osborne's ligament: a review of its history, anatomy, and surgical importance. Cureus. 2017;9(3):e1080. https://doi.org/10.7759/cureus.1080.
67. Floranda EE, Jacobs BC. Evaluation and treatment of upper extremity nerve entrapment syndromes. Prim Care. 2013;40(4):925, ix. https://doi.org/10.1016/j.pop.2013.08.009.
68. Chen SH, Tsai TM. Ulnar tunnel syndrome. J Hand Surg Am. 2014;39(3):571–9. https://doi.org/10.1016/j.jhsa.2013.08.102.
69. Chauhan M, Anand P, Das JM. Cubital tunnel syndrome. In: StatPearls. StatPearls Publishing; 2023.
70. Anderson D, Woods B, Abubakar T, Koontz C, Li N, Hasoon J, Viswanath O, Kaye AD, Urits I. A comprehensive review of cubital tunnel syndrome. Orthop Rev. 2022;14(3):38239. https://doi.org/10.52965/001c.38239.
71. Qing C, Zhang J, Wu S, Ling Z, Wang S, Li H, Li H. Clinical classification and treatment of cubital tunnel syndrome. Exp Ther Med. 2014;8(5):1365–70. https://doi.org/10.3892/etm.2014.1983.
72. Bordes SJ Jr, Jenkins S, Bang K, Turgut M, Iwanaga J, Loukas M, Spinner RJ, Dumont AS, Tubbs RS. Ulnar nerve subluxation and dislocation: a review of the literature. Neurosurg Rev. 2021;44(2):793–8. https://doi.org/10.1007/s10143-020-01286-3.
73. Mirza A, Mirza JB, Thomas TL Jr. Classification and treatment of ulnar nerve subluxation following endoscopic cubital tunnel release. J Hand Surg Glob Online. 2020;2(4):232–9. https://doi.org/10.1016/j.jhsg.2020.05.001.
74. Catalano LW 3rd, Barron OA. Anterior subcutaneous transposition of the ulnar nerve. Hand Clin. 2007;23(3):339, vi. https://doi.org/10.1016/j.hcl.2007.06.005.
75. Lleva JMC, Munakomi S, Chang KV. Ulnar neuropathy. In: StatPearls. StatPearls Publishing; 2023. https://www.ncbi.nlm.nih.gov/books/NBK534226/.
76. Campbell WW, Pridgeon RM, Sahni SK. Entrapment neuropathy of the ulnar nerve at its point of exit from the flexor carpi ulnaris muscle. Muscle Nerve. 1988;11(5):467–70. https://doi.org/10.1002/mus.880110509.
77. Agarwal A, Chandra A, Jaipal U, et al. Imaging in the diagnosis of ulnar nerve pathologies—a neoteric approach. Insights Imaging. 2019;10:37. https://doi.org/10.1186/s13244-019-0714-x.
78. Moneim MS. Ulnar nerve compression at the wrist. Ulnar tunnel syndrome. Hand Clin. 1992;8(2):337–44.
79. Earp BE, Floyd WE, Louie D, Koris M, Protomastro P. Ulnar nerve entrapment at the wrist. J Am Acad Orthop Surg. 2014;22(11):699–706. https://doi.org/10.5435/JAAOS-22-11-699.
80. Aleksenko D, Varacallo MA. Guyon canal syndrome. In: StatPearls. StatPearls Publishing; 2023.
81. Maroukis BL, Ogawa T, Rehim SA, Chung KC. Guyon canal: the evolution of clinical anatomy. J Hand Surg Am. 2015;40(3):560–5. https://doi.org/10.1016/j.jhsa.2014.09.026.
82. Inaparthy PK, Anwar F, Botchu R, Jähnich H, Katchburian MV. Compression of the deep branch of the ulnar nerve in Guyon's canal by a ganglion: two cases. Arch Orthop Trauma Surg. 2008;128(7):641–3. https://doi.org/10.1007/s00402-008-0636-4.
83. Depukat P, Mizia E, Klosinski M, Dzikowska M, Klimek-Piotrowska W, Mazur M, Kuniewicz M, Bonczar T. Anatomy of Guyon's canal – a systematic review. Folia Med Cracov. 2014;54(2):81–6.
84. Ramage JL, Varacallo MA. Anatomy, shoulder and upper limb, hand Guyon canal. In: StatPearls [Internet]. Treasure Island: StatPearls Publishing; 2025. Retrieved from https://www.ncbi.nlm.nih.gov/books/NBK534814/.
85. Fadel ZT, Samargandi OA, Tang DT. Variations in the anatomical structures of the Guyon canal. Plast Surg (Oakville, ON). 2017;25(2):84–92. https://doi.org/10.1177/2292550317694851.
86. Węgiel A, Karauda P, Zielinska N, Tubbs RS, Olewnik Ł. Radial nerve compression: anatomical perspective and clinical consequences. Neurosurg Rev. 2023;46(1):53. https://doi.org/10.1007/s10143-023-01944-2.
87. Spinner RJ, Poliakoff MB, Tiel RL. The origin of "Saturday night palsy"? Neurosurgery. 2002;51(3):737–41. https://doi.org/10.1097/00006123-200209000-00023.
88. Glover NM, Black AC, Murphy PB. Anatomy, shoulder and upper limb, radial nerve. In: StatPearls [Internet]. Treasure Island: StatPearls Publishing; 2025. Retrieved from https://www.ncbi.nlm.nih.gov/books/NBK534840/.
89. Gragossian A, Varacallo MA. Radial nerve injury. In: StatPearls. StatPearls Publishing; 2023.
90. Ansari FH, Juergens AL. Compressive radial mononeuropathy. In: StatPearls. StatPearls Publishing; 2023.
91. Latef TJ, Bilal M, Vetter M, Iwanaga J, Oskouian RJ, Tubbs RS. Injury of the radial nerve in the arm: a review. Cureus. 2018;10(2):e2199. https://doi.org/10.7759/cureus.2199.

92. Lubahn JD, Cermak MB. Uncommon nerve compression syndromes of the upper extremity. J Am Acad Orthop Surg. 1998;6(6):378–86. https://doi.org/10.5435/00124635-199811000-00006.
93. Bowman J, Curnutte B, Andrews K, Stirton J, Ebraheim N, Mustapha AA. Lateral intermuscular septum as cause of radial nerve compression: case report and review of the literature. J Surg Case Rep. 2018;2018(8):rjy226. https://doi.org/10.1093/jscr/rjy226.
94. Streib E. Upper arm radial nerve palsy after muscular effort: report of three cases. Neurology. 1992;42(8):1632–4. https://doi.org/10.1212/wnl.42.8.1632.
95. Laumonerie P, Dufournier B, Vari N, Manchec O, Tibbo ME, Cintas P, Mansat P, Faruch-Bifeld M. Atraumatic proximal radial nerve entrapment. Illustrative cases and systematic review of literature. Eur J Orthop Surg Traumatol: Orthop Traumatol. 2022;32(5):811–20. https://doi.org/10.1007/s00590-021-.
96. Prasartritha T, Liupolvanish P, Rojanakit A. A study of the posterior interosseous nerve (PIN) and the radial tunnel in 30 Thai cadavers. J Hand Surg Am. 1993;18(1):107–12. https://doi.org/10.1016/0363-5023(93)90253-Y.
97. Hazani R, Engineer NJ, Mowlavi A, Neumeister M, Lee WP, Wilhelmi BJ. Anatomic landmarks for the radial tunnel. Eplasty. 2008;8:e37.
98. Henry AK. Extensile exposure. 2nd ed. Edinburgh: Churchill Livingstone; 1973. p. 91–100. [Google Scholar].
99. Mohana-Borges AVR, Silva LTSD, Mohana-Borges RS, Statum S, Jerban S, Wu Y, Barrère V, Souza SAL, Chung CB. Neurovascular crossing patterns between leash of Henry and deep branch of radial nerve: implications for neurointervention and diagnostic imaging. Skeletal Radiol. 2025;54(3):493.
100. Wheeler R, DeCastro A. Posterior interosseous nerve syndrome. In: StatPearls. StatPearls Publishing; 2023.
101. Carr D, Davis P. Distal posterior interosseous nerve syndrome. J Hand Surg Am. 1985;10(6 Pt 1):873–8. https://doi.org/10.1016/s0363-5023(85)80165-9.
102. Patterson JMM, Medina MA, Yang A, Mackinnon SE. Posterior interosseous nerve compression in the forearm, AKA radial tunnel syndrome: a clinical diagnosis. Hand (New York, NY). 2024;19(2):228–35. https://doi.org/10.1177/15589447221122822.
103. Saratsiotis J, Myriokefalitakis E. Diagnosis and treatment of posterior interosseous nerve syndrome using soft tissue manipulation therapy: a case study. J Bodyw Mov Ther. 2010;14(4):397–402. https://doi.org/10.1016/j.jbmt.2009.11.002.
104. Portilla Molina AE, Bour C, Oberlin C, Nzeusseu A, Vanwijck R. The posterior interosseous nerve and the radial tunnel syndrome: an anatomical study. Int Orthop. 1998;22(2):102–6. https://doi.org/10.1007/s002640050218.
105. Cha J, York B, Tawfik J. Posterior interosseous nerve compression. Eplasty. 2014;14:ic4.
106. Massey EW, Pleet AB. Handcuffs and cheiralgia paresthetica. Neurology. 1978;28(12):1312–3. https://doi.org/10.1212/wnl.28.12.1312.
107. Anthony JH, Hadeed A, Hoffler CE. Cheiralgia paresthetica. In: StatPearls [Internet]. Treasure Island: StatPearls Publishing; 2025. Retrieved from https://www.ncbi.nlm.nih.gov/books/NBK545200/.
108. Tosun N, Tuncay I, Akpinar F. Entrapment of the sensory branch of the radial nerve (Wartenberg's syndrome): an unusual cause. Tohoku J Exp Med. 2001;193(3):251–4. https://doi.org/10.1620/tjem.193.251.
109. Marco C, Miguel-Pérez M, Pérez-Bellmunt A, Ortiz-Sagristà JC, Martinoli C, Möller I, Ortiz Miguel S, Agulló P. Anatomical causes of compression of the sciatic nerve in the pelvis. Piriform syndrome. Causas anatómicas de compresión del nervio ciático en la pelvis. Síndrome piriforme. Rev Esp Cir Ortop Traumatol (Engl Ed). 2019;63(6):424–30. https://doi.org/10.1016/j.recot.2019.06.002.
110. Davis D, Taqi M, Vasudevan A. Sciatica. In: StatPearls. StatPearls Publishing; 2024.
111. Hicks BL, Lam JC, Varacallo MA. Piriformis syndrome. In: StatPearls. StatPearls Publishing; 2023.
112. Probst D, Stout A, Hunt D. Piriformis syndrome: a narrative review of the anatomy, diagnosis, and treatment. PM R: J Inj Funct Rehabil. 2019;11(Suppl 1):S54–63. https://doi.org/10.1002/pmrj.12189.
113. Kirschner JS, Foye PM, Cole JL. Piriformis syndrome, diagnosis and treatment. Muscle Nerve. 2009;40(1):10–8. https://doi.org/10.1002/mus.21318.
114. Brochado JF, Pereira J. Behind the pain: understanding and treating piriformis syndrome. Cureus. 2024;16(10):e70750. https://doi.org/10.7759/cureus.70750.
115. Stafford GH, Villar RN. Ischiofemoral impingement. J Bone Joint Surg Br Vol. 2011;93(10):1300–2. https://doi.org/10.1302/0301-620X.93B10.26714.
116. Lee S, Kim I, Lee SM, Lee J. Ischiofemoral impingement syndrome. Ann Rehabil Med. 2013;37(1):143–6. https://doi.org/10.5535/arm.2013.37.1.143.
117. Wu WT, Chang KV, Mezian K, Naňka O, Ricci V, Chang HC, Wang B, Hung CY, Özçakar L. Ischiofemoral impingement syndrome: clinical and imaging/guidance issues with special focus on ultrasonography. Diagnostics (Basel). 2022;13(1):139. https://doi.org/10.3390/diagnostics13010139. PMID: 36611431; PMCID: PMC9818255.
118. Bradshaw C, McCrory P, Bell S, Brukner P. Obturator nerve entrapment. A cause of groin pain in athletes. Am J Sports Med. 1997;25(3):402–8. https://doi.org/10.1177/036354659702500322.
119. Tipton JS. Obturator neuropathy. Curr Rev Musculoskelet Med. 2008;1(3–4):234–7. https://doi.org/10.1007/s12178-008-9030-7.

120. Grossman MG, Ducey SA, Nadler SS, Levy AS. Meralgia paresthetica: diagnosis and treatment. J Am Acad Orthop Surg. 2001;9(5):336–44. https://doi.org/10.5435/00124635-200109000-00007.
121. Scholz C, Hohenhaus M, Pedro MT, Uerschels AK, Dengler NF. Meralgia paresthetica: relevance, diagnosis, and treatment. Dtsch Arztebl Int. 2023;120(39):655–61. https://doi.org/10.3238/arztebl.m2023.0170.
122. Jokela T, Löppönen P. Saphenous nerve compression in the differential diagnosis of knee pain. Case study and a review of the literature. Trauma Case Rep. 2025;57:101183. https://doi.org/10.1016/j.tcr.2025.101183.
123. Porr J, Chrobak K, Muir B. Entrapment of the saphenous nerve at the adductor canal affecting the infrapatellar branch – a report on two cases. J Can Chiropr Assoc. 2013;57(4):341–9.
124. Beltran LS, Bencardino J, Ghazikhanian V, Beltran J. Entrapment neuropathies III: lower limb. Semin Musculoskelet Radiol. 2010;14(5):501–11. https://doi.org/10.1055/s-0030-1268070.
125. Feger J. Saphenous neuropathy. Reference article. Radiopaedia.org. 2025. https://doi.org/10.53347/rID-92705.
126. Chang KV, Mezian K, Naňka O, Wu WT, Lou YM, Wang JC, Martinoli C, Özçakar L. Ultrasound imaging for the cutaneous nerves of the extremities and relevant entrapment syndromes: from anatomy to clinical implications. J Clin Med. 2018;7(11):457. https://doi.org/10.3390/jcm7110457.
127. Poage C, Roth C, Scott B. Peroneal nerve palsy: evaluation and management. J Am Acad Orthop Surg. 2016;24(1):1–10. https://doi.org/10.5435/JAAOS-D-14-00420.
128. Lezak B, Massel DH, Varacallo MA. Peroneal nerve injury. In: StatPearls. StatPearls Publishing; 2024.
129. Fortier LM, Markel M, Thomas BG, Sherman WF, Thomas BH, Kaye AD. An update on peroneal nerve entrapment and neuropathy. Orthop Rev. 2021;13(2):24937. https://doi.org/10.52965/001c.24937.
130. Anselmi SJ. Common peroneal nerve compression. J Am Podiatr Med Assoc. 2006;96(5):413–7. https://doi.org/10.7547/0960413.
131. Liu Z, Zhou J, Zhao L. Anterior tarsal tunnel syndrome. J Bone Joint Surg Br Vol. 1991;73(3):470–3. https://doi.org/10.1302/0301-620X.73B3.1670452.
132. Kanbe K, Kubota H, Shirakura K, Hasegawa A, Udagawa E. Entrapment neuropathy of the deep peroneal nerve associated with the extensor hallucis brevis. J Foot Ankle Surg. 1995;34(6):560–2. https://doi.org/10.1016/S1067-2516(09)80078-1.
133. Ferkel E, Davis WH, Ellington JK. Entrapment neuropathies of the foot and ankle. Clin Sports Med. 2015;34(4):791–801. https://doi.org/10.1016/j.csm.2015.06.002.
134. Brown CL, Worts P, Borom A. Superficial peroneal nerve entrapment: diagnosis and surgical management. A retrospective study of 46 patients. Foot Ankle Orthop. 2019;4(4):2473011419S00120. https://doi.org/10.1177/2473011419S00120.
135. Tzika M, Paraskevas G, Natsis K. Entrapment of the superficial peroneal nerve: an anatomical insight. J Am Podiatr Med Assoc. 2015;105(2):150–9. https://doi.org/10.7547/0003-0538-105.2.150.
136. Ghosh SK, Raheja S, Tuli A. Potential sites of compression of tibial nerve branches in foot: a cadaveric and imaging study. Clin Anat (New York, NY). 2013;26(6):768–79. https://doi.org/10.1002/ca.22203.
137. Nelson SC. Tarsal tunnel syndrome. Clin Podiatr Med Surg. 2021;38(2):131–41. https://doi.org/10.1016/j.cpm.2020.12.001.
138. Jain S, Mannan K. The diagnosis and management of Morton's neuroma: a literature review. Foot Ankle Spec. 2013;6(4):307–17. https://doi.org/10.1177/1938640013493464.
139. Bhatia M, Thomson L. Morton's neuroma – current concepts review. J Clin Orthop Trauma. 2020;11(3):406–9. https://doi.org/10.1016/j.jcot.2020.03.024.
140. Lovaglio AC, Socolovsky M, Di Masi G, Bonilla G. Treatment of neuropathic pain after peripheral nerve and brachial plexus traumatic injury. Neurol India. 2019;67(Suppl 1):S32–7. https://doi.org/10.4103/0028-3886.250699.
141. Graesser EA, Parsons MS, Olafsen NP, Dy CJ, Brogan DM. Advances in imaging of traumatic nerve injuries. J Am Acad Orthop Surg. 2024. https://doi.org/10.5435/JAAOS-D-24-00889. Advance online publication.
142. Dahlin LB, Wiberg M. Nerve injuries of the upper extremity and hand. EFORT Open Rev. 2017;2(5):158–70. https://doi.org/10.1302/2058-5241.2.160071.
143. Robinson LR. Traumatic injury to peripheral nerves. Muscle Nerve. 2000;23(6):863–73. https://doi.org/10.1002/(sici)1097-4598(200006)23:6<863::aid-mus4>3.0.co;2-0.
144. Bhandari PS. Management of peripheral nerve injury. J Clin Orthopa Trauma. 2019;10(5):862–6. https://doi.org/10.1016/j.jcot.2019.08.003.
145. Zimmermann KS, Aman M, Harhaus L, Boecker AH. Improving outcomes in traumatic peripheral nerve injuries to the upper extremity. Eur J Orthop Surg Traumatol: Orthop Traumatol. 2024;34(7):3687–97. https://doi.org/10.1007/s00590-023-03751-3.
146. Minarelli J, Davis EL, Dickerson A, Moore WC, Mejia JA, Gugala Z, Olmsted-Davis EA, Davis AR. Characterization of neuromas in peripheral nerves and their effects on heterotopic bone formation. Mol Pain. 2019;15:1744806919838191. https://doi.org/10.1177/1744806919838191.
147. Krishnan KG, Pinzer T, Schackert G. Coverage of painful peripheral nerve neuromas with vascularized soft tissue: method and results. Neurosurgery. 2005;56(2 Suppl):369–78. https://doi.org/10.1227/01.neu.0000156881.10388.d8.

148. Neumeister MW, Winters JN. Neuroma. Clin Plast Surg. 2020;47(2):279–83. https://doi.org/10.1016/j.cps.2019.12.008.
149. Yang H, Dong Y, Wang Z, Lai J, Yao C, Zhou H, Alhaskawi A, Hasan Abdullah Ezzi S, Kota VG, Hasan Abdulla Hasan Abdulla M, Lu H. Traumatic neuromas of peripheral nerves: diagnosis, management and future perspectives. Front Neurol. 2023;13:1039529. https://doi.org/10.3389/fneur.2022.1039529.
150. Burchiel KJ, Johans TJ, Ochoa J. The surgical treatment of painful traumatic neuromas. J Neurosurg. 1993;78(5):714–9. https://doi.org/10.3171/jns.1993.78.5.0714.
151. Poppler LH, Parikh RP, Bichanich MJ, Rebehn K, Bettlach CR, Mackinnon SE, Moore AM. Surgical interventions for the treatment of painful neuroma: a comparative meta-analysis. Pain. 2018;159(2):214–23. https://doi.org/10.1097/j.pain.0000000000001101.
152. Walker NR, Mistry RK, Mazzoni T. Facial nerve palsy. In: StatPearls. StatPearls Publishing; 2023.
153. House JW, Brackmann DE. Facial nerve grading system. Otolaryngol Head Neck Surg. 1985;93(2):146–7. https://doi.org/10.1177/019459988509300202.
154. Spencer CR, Irving RM. Causes and management of facial nerve palsy. Br J Hosp Med (London, England : 2005). 2016;77(12):686–91. https://doi.org/10.12968/hmed.2016.77.12.686.
155. Owusu JA, Stewart CM, Boahene K. Facial nerve paralysis. Med Clin North Am. 2018;102(6):1135–43. https://doi.org/10.1016/j.mcna.2018.06.011.
156. Hazin R, Azizzadeh B, Bhatti MT. Medical and surgical management of facial nerve palsy. Curr Opin Ophthalmol. 2009;20(6):440–50. https://doi.org/10.1097/ICU.0b013e3283313cbf.
157. Peng GL, Azizzadeh B. Cross-facial nerve grafting for facial reanimation. Facial Plast Surg: FPS. 2015;31(2):128–33. https://doi.org/10.1055/s-0035-1549046.
158. Harb JL, Ein LJ. The role of the cross face nerve graft in facial reanimation and endoscopic harvest of the sural nerve. Atlas Oral Maxillofac Surg Clin North Am. 2023;31(1):25–31. https://doi.org/10.1016/j.cxom.2022.09.003.
159. Hontanilla B, Olivas J, Cabello Á, Marré D. Cross-face nerve grafting versus masseteric-to-facial nerve transposition for reanimation of incomplete facial paralysis: a comparative study using the FACIAL CLIMA evaluating system. Plast Reconstr Surg. 2018;142(2):179e–91e. https://doi.org/10.1097/PRS.0000000000004612.
160. Kollar B, Weiss JBW, Kiefer J, Eisenhardt SU. Functional outcome of dual reinnervation with cross-facial nerve graft and masseteric nerve transfer for facial paralysis. Plast Reconstr Surg. 2024;153(6):1178e–90e. https://doi.org/10.1097/PRS.0000000000010888.
161. Collar R, Boahene KDO. Cross-facial nerve grafting (CFNG), procedure. In: Kountakis SE, editor. Encyclopedia of otolaryngology, head and neck surgery. Springer; 2013. https://doi.org/10.1007/978-3-642-23499-6_361.
162. Kleijwegt MC, Wever C, Hensen EF, Jansen JC, Koot RW, Malessy MJA. Reestablishment of the smile after hypoglossal-facial nerve transfer: what can we learn? J Neurol Surg Part B Skull Base. 2023;85(5):546–52. https://doi.org/10.1055/a-2128-5191.
163. Flores LP. Surgical results of the hypoglossal-facial nerve jump graft technique. Acta Neurochir. 2007;149(12):1205–10. https://doi.org/10.1007/s00701-007-1412-x.
164. Volk GF, Geitner M, Geißler K, Thielker J, Raslan A, Mothes O, Dobel C, Guntinas-Lichius O. Functional outcome and quality of life after hypoglossal-facial jump nerve suture. Front Surg. 2020;7:11. https://doi.org/10.3389/fsurg.2020.00011.
165. Vaquero G, Ramos A, Martinez JC, Valero P, Nunez-Enamorado N, Simon-De Las Heras R, Camacho-Salas A. Paralisis braquial obstetrica: incidencia, seguimiento evolutivo y factores pronosticos [Obstetric brachial plexus palsy: incidence, monitoring of progress and prognostic factors]. Rev Neurol. 2017;65(1):19–25.
166. Louden E, Marcotte M, Mehlman C, Lippert W, Huang B, Paulson A. Risk factors for brachial plexus birth injury. Children (Basel, Switzerland). 2018;5(4):46. https://doi.org/10.3390/children5040046.
167. Shenaq SM, Armenta AH, Roth FS, Lee RT, Laurent JP. Current management of obstetrical brachial plexus injuries at Texas Children's Hospital Brachial Plexus Center and Baylor College of Medicine. Semin Plast Surg. 2005;19(1):42–55. https://doi.org/10.1055/s-2005-867107.
168. Gosk J, Rutowski R. Analiza czynników ryzyka okołoporodowych uszkodzen splotu ramiennego [Analysis of risk factors for perinatal brachial plexus palsy]. Ginekol Pol. 2005;76(4):270–6.
169. O'Berry P, Brown M, Phillips L, Evans SH. Obstetrical brachial plexus palsy. Curr Probl Pediatr Adolesc Health Care. 2017;47(7):151–5. https://doi.org/10.1016/j.cppeds.2017.06.003.
170. Al-Qattan MM, El-Sayed AA, Al-Zahrani AY, Al-Mutairi SA, Al-Harbi MS, Al-Mutairi AM, Al-Kahtani FS. Narakas classification of obstetric brachial plexus palsy revisited. J Hand Surg Eur Vol. 2009;34(6):788–91. https://doi.org/10.1177/1753193409348185.
171. Bahm J, Ocampo-Pavez C, Disselhorst-Klug C, Sellhaus B, Weis J. Obstetric brachial plexus palsy: treatment strategy, long-term results, and prognosis. Dtsch Arztebl Int. 2009;106(6):83–90. https://doi.org/10.3238/arztebl.2009.0083. Epub 2009 Feb 6. PMID: 19562016; PMCID: PMC2695299.
172. van Ouwerkerk WJR. Preoperative investigations in obstetric brachial plexus palsy. Semin

Plast Surg. 2005;19(1):17–23. https://doi.org/10.1055/s-2005-867113.
173. Sawires M, Berek K. Horner-Syndrom: Neuroanatomie, pathophysiologische Grundlagen und diagnostische Verfahren. J Neurol Neurochir Psychiatr. 2011;12(1):12–8. Retrieved from https://www.kup.at/journals/summary/10834.
174. Socolovsky M, Costales JR, Paez MD, Nizzo G, Valbuena S, Varone E. Obstetric brachial plexus palsy: reviewing the literature comparing the results of primary versus secondary surgery. Child's Nerv Syst: ChNS. 2016;32(3):415–25. https://doi.org/10.1007/s00381-015-2971-4.
175. Pejkova S, Filipce V, Peev I, Nikolovska B, Jovanoski T, Georgieva G, Srbov B. Brachial plexus injuries – review of the anatomy and the treatment options. Prilozi (Makedonska akademija na naukite i umetnostite. Oddelenie za medicinski nauki). 2021;42(1):91–103. https://doi.org/10.2478/prilozi-2021-0008.
176. Coene LN. Mechanisms of brachial plexus lesions. Clin Neurol Neurosurg. 1993;95 Suppl:S24–9. https://doi.org/10.1016/0303-8467(93)90030-k.
177. Li GY, Xue MQ, Wang JW, Zeng XY, Qin J, Sha K. Traumatic brachial plexus injury: a study of 510 surgical cases from multicenter services in Guangxi, China. Acta neurochir. 2019;161(5):899–906. https://doi.org/10.1007/s00701-019-03871-y.
178. Thatte MR, Babhulkar S, Hiremath A. Brachial plexus injury in adults: diagnosis and surgical treatment strategies. Ann Indian Acad Neurol. 2013;16(1):26–33. https://doi.org/10.4103/0972-2327.107686.
179. Shin AY, Spinner RJ, Steinmann SP, Bishop AT. Adult traumatic brachial plexus injuries. J Am Acad Orthop Surg. 2005;13(6):382–96. https://doi.org/10.5435/00124635-200510000-00003.
180. Rorabeck CH, Harris WR. Factors affecting the prognosis of brachial plexus injuries. J Bone Joint Surg Br Vol. 1981;63-B(3):404–7. https://doi.org/10.1302/0301-620X.63B3.7263755.
181. Doi K, Otsuka K, Okamoto Y, Fujii H, Hattori Y, Baliarsing AS. Cervical nerve root avulsion in brachial plexus injuries: magnetic resonance imaging classification and comparison with myelography and computerized tomography myelography. J Neurosurg. 2002;96(3 Suppl):277–84. https://doi.org/10.3171/spi.2002.96.3.0277.
182. Kaiser R, Waldauf P, Haninec P. Types and severity of operated supraclavicular brachial plexus injuries caused by traffic accidents. Acta Neurochir. 2012;154(7):1293–7. https://doi.org/10.1007/s00701-012-1291-7.
183. Wu KY, Spinner RJ, Shin AY. Traumatic brachial plexus injury: diagnosis and treatment. Curr Opin Neurol. 2022;35(6):708–17. https://doi.org/10.1097/WCO.0000000000001124.
184. Lurje A. Concerning surgical treatment of traumatic injury of the upper division of the brachial plexus (Erb's-type). Ann Surg. 1948;127(2):317–26.
185. Bertelli JA, Ghizoni MF. Nerve root grafting and distal nerve transfers for C5–C6 brachial plexus injuries. J Hand Surg Am. 2010;35(5):769–75. https://doi.org/10.1016/j.jhsa.2010.01.004.
186. Bertelli JA, Ghizoni MF. Brachial plexus avulsion injury repairs with nerve transfers and nerve grafts directly implanted into the spinal cord yield partial recovery of shoulder and elbow movements. Neurosurgery. 2003;52(6):1385–90. https://doi.org/10.1227/01.neu.0000065134.21334.d7.
187. Bertelli JA, Ghizoni MF. Use of clinical signs and computed tomography myelography findings in detecting and excluding nerve root avulsion in complete brachial plexus palsy. J Neurosurg. 2006;105(6):835–42. https://doi.org/10.3171/jns.2006.105.6.835.
188. Hruby LA. Deafferentation pain following brachial plexus avulsion injuries. In: Aszmann OC, Farina D, editors. Bionic limb reconstruction. Springer; 2021. pp. 171–6. https://doi.org/10.1007/978-3-030-60746-3_16.
189. Samii M, Bear-Henney S, Lüdemann W, Tatagiba M, Blömer U. Treatment of refractory pain after brachial plexus avulsion with dorsal root entry zone lesions. Neurosurgery. 2001;48(6):1269–77.
190. Bertelli JA, Ghizoni MF. Pain after avulsion injuries and complete palsy of the brachial plexus: the possible role of nonavulsed roots in pain generation. Neurosurgery. 2008;62(5):1104–14. https://doi.org/10.1227/01.neu.0000325872.37258.12.
191. Hanakawa T. Neural mechanisms underlying deafferentation pain: a hypothesis from a neuroimaging perspective. J Orthop Sci. 2012;17(3):331–5. https://doi.org/10.1007/s00776-012-0209-9.
192. Bourne S, Bhaskar A, Thakur M. Basic anatomy and physiology of pain pathways. Neurosurg Clin N Am. 2014;25(4):629–38. https://doi.org/10.1016/j.nec.2014.06.001.
193. Teixeira MJ, da Paz MG, Bina MT, Santos SN, Raicher I, Galhardoni R, Fernandes DT, Yeng LT, Baptista AF, de Andrade DC. Neuropathic pain after brachial plexus avulsion–central and peripheral mechanisms. BMC Neurol. 2015;15:73. https://doi.org/10.1186/s12883-015-0329-x.
194. Marchand S. Physiopathology of pain. In: Saba L, editor. Neuroimaging of pain. Springer; 2017. https://doi.org/10.1007/978-3-319-48046-6_4.
195. Carvalho GA, Nikkhah G, Matthies C, Penkert G, Samii M. Diagnosis of root avulsions in traumatic brachial plexus injuries: value of computerized tomography myelography and magnetic resonance imaging. J Neurosurg. 1997;86(1):69–76. https://doi.org/10.3171/jns.1997.86.1.0069.
196. Terzis JK, Novikov ML. Radiological and electrophysiological detection of nerve roots avulsion in patients with birth-related brachial plexus paralysis. Semin Plast Surg. 2005;19(1):24–41. https://doi.org/10.1055/s-2005-867112.

197. Leechavengvongs S, Witoonchart K, Uerpairojkit C, Thuvasethakul P, Malungpaishrope K. Combined nerve transfers for C5 and C6 brachial plexus avulsion injury. J Hand Surg Am. 2006;31(2):183–9. https://doi.org/10.1016/j.jhsa.2005.09.019.
198. Chalil A, Wang Q, Abbass M, Santyr BG, MacDougall KW, Staudt MD. Dorsal root entry zone lesioning for brachial plexus avulsion injuries: case series and literature review. Front Pain Res (Lausanne, Switzerland). 2021;2:749801. https://doi.org/10.3389/fpain.2021.749801.
199. Gebreyohanes AMH, Ahmed AI, Choi D. Dorsal root entry zone lesioning for brachial plexus avulsion: a comprehensive literature review. Oper Neurosurg (Hagerstown, MD). 2021;20(4):324–33. https://doi.org/10.1093/ons/opaa447.
200. Dydyk AM, Hameed S. Lumbosacral plexopathy. In: StatPearls. StatPearls Publishing; 2023. https://www.ncbi.nlm.nih.gov/books/NBK556030/.
201. Grunert P, Drazin D, Iwanaga J, Schmidt C, Alonso F, Moisi M, Chapman JR, Oskouian RJ, Tubbs RS. Injury to the lumbar plexus and its branches after lateral fusion procedures: a cadaver study. World Neurosurg. 2017;105:519–25. https://doi.org/10.1016/j.wneu.2017.06.027.
202. Kretschmer T, Antoniadis G, Braun V, Rath SA, Richter HP. Evaluation of iatrogenic lesions in 722 surgically treated cases of peripheral nerve trauma. J Neurosurg. 2001;94(6):905–12. https://doi.org/10.3171/jns.2001.94.6.0905.
203. Hara T, Tatebe M, Kurahashi T, Hirata H. Iatrogenic peripheral nerve injuries – common causes and treatment: a retrospective single-center cohort study. J Orthop Sci. 2021;26(6):1119–23. https://doi.org/10.1016/j.jos.2020.09.009.
204. Stepan JG. Ballistic nerve injuries: state of the evidence and approach to the patient based on experience. J Hand Surg Glob Online. 2024;6(5):743–8. https://doi.org/10.1016/j.jhsg.2024.01.021.
205. Meade A, Hembd A, Cho MJ, Zhang AY. Surgical treatment of upper extremity gunshot injures: an updated review. Ann Plast Surg. 2021;86(3S Suppl 2):S312–8. https://doi.org/10.1097/SAP.0000000000002634.
206. Hilton DA, Hanemann CO. Schwannomas and their pathogenesis. Brain Pathol (Zurich, Switzerland). 2014;24(3):205–20. https://doi.org/10.1111/bpa.12125.
207. Albert P, Patel J, Badawy K, Weissinger W, Brenner M, Bourhill I, Parnell J. Peripheral nerve schwannoma: a review of varying clinical presentations and imaging findings. J Foot Ankle Surg. 2017;56(3):632–7.
208. Li X, Zhong G, Xu X, Wang K, Zhu Y, Qi X, Lv J, Wang Y, Shao S. Surgical strategies for peripheral nerve schwannoma based on the intraoperative neurophysiological monitoring panel. Laparosc Endosc Robot Surg. 2019;2(3):65–9. https://doi.org/10.1016/j.lers.2019.06.001.
209. Khamlichi H, Mailleux P. The "tail sign" in intramuscular schwannoma. J Belg Soc Radiol. 2020;104(1):43. https://doi.org/10.5334/jbsr.2157.
210. Gosk J, Gutkowska O, Urban M, Wnukiewicz W, Reichert P, Ziółkowski P. Results of surgical treatment of schwannomas arising from extremities. Biomed Res Int. 2015;2015:547926. https://doi.org/10.1155/2015/547926.
211. Guedes F, et al., editors. Diagnostic assessment and treatment of peripheral nerve tumors. Springer International Publishing; 2021.
212. Messersmith L, Krauland K. Neurofibroma. In: StatPearls. StatPearls Publishing; 2023. https://www.ncbi.nlm.nih.gov/books/NBK539707/.
213. Skovronsky DM, Oberholtzer JC. Pathologic classification of peripheral nerve tumors. Neurosurg Clin N Am. 2004;15(2):157–66. https://doi.org/10.1016/j.nec.2004.02.005.
214. Lin J, Martel W. Cross-sectional imaging of peripheral nerve sheath tumors: characteristic signs on CT, MR imaging, and sonography. AJR Am J Roentgenol. 2001;176(1):75–82. https://doi.org/10.2214/ajr.176.1.1760075.
215. Deka JB, Shah R, Jiménez M, Bhatnagar N, Bravo-Sánchez A, Piñas-Bonilla I, Abián-Vicén J, Jiménez F. A retrospective analysis of high resolution ultrasound evaluation of the "split fat sign" in peripheral nerve sheath tumors. Healthcare (Basel, Switzerland). 2023;11(24):3147. https://doi.org/10.3390/healthcare11243147.
216. Abbas O, Bhawan J. Cutaneous plexiform lesions. J Cutan Pathol. 2010;37(6):613–23. https://doi.org/10.1111/j.1600-0560.2010.01529.x.
217. St-Amant M, Weerakkody Y, Sharma R, et al. Plexiform neurofibroma. Radiopaedia.org. n.d. https://doi.org/10.53347/rID-19088. Accessed 30 May 2024.
218. Hassell DS, Bancroft LW, Kransdorf MJ, Peterson JJ, Berquist TH, Murphey MD, Fanburg-Smith JC. Imaging appearance of diffuse neurofibroma. AJR Am J Roentgenol. 2008;190(3):582–8. https://doi.org/10.2214/AJR.07.2589.
219. Kumar BS, Gopal M, Talwar A, Ramesh M. Diffuse neurofibroma of the scalp presenting as circumscribed alopecic patch. Int J Trichology. 2010;2(1):60–2. https://doi.org/10.4103/0974-7753.66919.
220. Ravi AK, Ram R, Lindberg MR, Pandey T. Diffuse infiltrative neurofibroma: a clinical, radiological, and histological conundrum. Skeletal Radiol. 2014;43(12):1773–8. https://doi.org/10.1007/s00256-014-1965-8.
221. Chen W, Jia JW, Wang JR. Soft tissue diffuse neurofibromas: sonographic findings. J Ultrasound Med. 2007;26(4):513–8. https://doi.org/10.7863/jum.2007.26.4.513.
222. Zhou HY, Jiang S, Ma FX, Lu H. Peripheral nerve tumors of the hand: clinical features, diagnosis, and treatment. World J Clin Cases. 2020;8(21):5086–98. https://doi.org/10.12998/wjcc.v8.i21.5086.

223. Brand C, Pedro MT, Pala A, Heinen C, Scheuerle A, Braun M, Antoniadis G. Perineurioma: a rare entity of peripheral nerve sheath tumors. J Neurol Surg A Cent Eur Neurosurg. 2022;83(1):1–5. https://doi.org/10.1055/s-0041-1726110.
224. Wang LM, Zhong YF, Zheng DF, Sun AP, Zhang YS, Dong RF, Pan Y. Intraneural perineurioma affecting multiple nerves: a case report and literature review. Int J Clin Exp Pathol. 2014;7(6):3347–54.
225. Visser LH. High-resolution sonography of the common peroneal nerve: detection of intraneural ganglia. Neurology. 2006;67(8):1473–5. https://doi.org/10.1212/01.wnl.0000240070.98910.bc.
226. Lu H, Chen L, Jiang S, Shen H. A rapidly progressive foot drop caused by the posttraumatic intraneural ganglion cyst of the deep peroneal nerve. BMC Musculoskelet Disord. 2018;19(1):298. https://doi.org/10.1186/s12891-018-2229-x.
227. Tseng KF, Hsu HC, Wang FC, Fong YC. Nerve sheath ganglion of the tibial nerve presenting as a Baker's cyst: a case report. Knee Surg Sports Traumatol Arthrosc. 2006;14(9):880–4. https://doi.org/10.1007/s00167-006-0062-5.
228. Gillies RM, Burrows C. Nerve sheath ganglion of the superficial radial nerve. J Hand Surg (Edinburgh, Scotland). 1991;16(1):94–5. https://doi.org/10.1016/0266-7681(91)90139-f.
229. Panwar J, Mathew A, Thomas BP. Cystic lesions of peripheral nerves: are we missing the diagnosis of the intraneural ganglion cyst? World J Radiol. 2017;9(5):230–44. https://doi.org/10.4329/wjr.v9.i5.230.
230. Solomon J, Warren K, Dombi E, Patronas N, Widemann B. Automated detection and volume measurement of plexiform neurofibromas in neurofibromatosis 1 using magnetic resonance imaging. Comput Med Imaging Graph. 2004;28(5):257–65. https://doi.org/10.1016/j.compmedimag.2004.03.002.
231. Borofsky S, Levy LM. Neurofibromatosis: types 1 and 2. AJNR Am J Neuroradiol. 2013;34(12):2250–1. https://doi.org/10.3174/ajnr.A3534.
232. Ferner RE. Neurofibromatosis 1 and neurofibromatosis 2: a twenty first century perspective. Lancet Neurol. 2007;6(4):340–51. https://doi.org/10.1016/S1474-4422(07)70075-3.
233. Tamura R. Current understanding of neurofibromatosis type 1, 2, and schwannomatosis. Int J Mol Sci. 2021;22(11):5850. https://doi.org/10.3390/ijms22115850.
234. von Deimling A, Krone W, Menon AG. Neurofibromatosis type 1: pathology, clinical features and molecular genetics. Brain Pathol (Zurich, Switzerland). 1995;5(2):153–62. https://doi.org/10.1111/j.1750-3639.1995.tb00589.x.
235. Kim TK, Park YS, Nakagawa I. Clinical and genetic overview of neurofibromatosis type 2 (NF2). J Korean Neurosurg Soc. 2025;68(3):272–7. https://doi.org/10.3340/jkns.2025.0048.
236. Rasmussen SA, Yang Q, Friedman JM. Mortality in neurofibromatosis 1: an analysis using U.S. death certificates. Am J Hum Genet. 2001;68(5):1110–8. https://doi.org/10.1086/320121.
237. Ducatman BS, Scheithauer BW, Piepgras DG, Reiman HM, Ilstrup DM. Malignant peripheral nerve sheath tumors. A clinicopathologic study of 120 cases. Cancer. 1986;57(10):2006–21. https://doi.org/10.1002/1097-0142(19860515)57:10<2006::aid-cncr2820571022>3.0.co;2-6.
238. Armstrong AE, Belzberg AJ, Crawford JR, Hirbe AC, Wang ZJ. Treatment decisions and the use of MEK inhibitors for children with neurofibromatosis type 1-related plexiform neurofibromas. BMC Cancer. 2023;23(1):553. https://doi.org/10.1186/s12885-023-10996-y.
239. Evans DG. Neurofibromatosis type 2 (NF2): a clinical and molecular review. Orphanet J Rare Dis. 2009;4:16. https://doi.org/10.1186/1750-1172-4-16.
240. Maniakas A, Saliba I. Neurofibromatosis type 2 vestibular schwannoma treatment: a review of the literature, trends, and outcomes. Otol Neurotol. 2014;35(5):889–94. https://doi.org/10.1097/MAO.0000000000000272.
241. Radek M, Tomasik B, Wojdyn M, Snopkowska-Wiaderna D, Błaszczyk M, Radek A. Neurofibromatosis type 2 (NF 2) or schwannomatosis?–case report study and diagnostic criteria. Neurol Neurochir Pol. 2016;50(3):219–25. https://doi.org/10.1016/j.pjnns.2016.02.005.
242. Schraepen C, Donkersloot P, Duyvendak W, Plazier M, Put E, Roosen G, Vanvolsem S, Wissels M, Bamps S. What to know about schwannomatosis: a literature review. Br J Neurosurg. 2022;36(2):171–4. https://doi.org/10.1080/02688697.2020.1836323.
243. MacCollin M, Chiocca EA, Evans DG, Friedman JM, Horvitz R, Jaramillo D, Lev M, Mautner VF, Niimura M, Plotkin SR, Sang CN, Stemmer-Rachamimov A, Roach ES. Diagnostic criteria for schwannomatosis. Neurology. 2005;64(11):1838–45. https://doi.org/10.1212/01.WNL.0000163982.78900.AD.
244. Amirian ES, Goodman JC, New P, Scheurer ME. Pediatric and adult malignant peripheral nerve sheath tumors: an analysis of data from the surveillance, epidemiology, and end results program. J Neuro-Oncol. 2014;116(3):609–16. https://doi.org/10.1007/s11060-013-1345-6.
245. Knight SWE, Knight TE, Santiago T, Murphy AJ, Abdelhafeez AH. Malignant peripheral nerve sheath tumors-a comprehensive review of pathophysiology, diagnosis, and multidisciplinary management. Children (Basel, Switzerland). 2022;9(1):38. https://doi.org/10.3390/children9010038.
246. Yao C, Zhou H, Dong Y, Alhaskawi A, Hasan Abdullah Ezzi S, Wang Z, Lai J, Goutham Kota V, Hasan Abdulla Hasan Abdulla M, Lu H. Malignant peripheral nerve sheath tumors: latest concepts in

disease pathogenesis and clinical management. Cancers. 2023;15(4):1077. https://doi.org/10.3390/cancers15041077.

247. Somatilaka BN, Sadek A, McKay RM, Le LQ. Malignant peripheral nerve sheath tumor: models, biology, and translation. Oncogene. 2022;41(17):2405–21. https://doi.org/10.1038/s41388-022-02290-1.

248. Imura Y, Outani H, Takenaka S, Yasuda N, Nakai S, Nakai T, Wakamatsu T, Tamiya H, Hamada K, Kakunaga S. Clinical outcomes and prognostic factors for patients with malignant peripheral nerve sheath tumour. Sarcoma. 2021;2021:8335290. https://doi.org/10.1155/2021/8335290.

249. Chhabra A, Soldatos T, Durand DJ, Carrino JA, McCarthy EF, Belzberg AJ. The role of magnetic resonance imaging in the diagnostic evaluation of malignant peripheral nerve sheath tumors. Indian J Cancer. 2011;48(3):328–34. https://doi.org/10.4103/0019-509x.84945.

250. Brahmi M, Thiesse P, Ranchere D, Mognetti T, Pinson S, Renard C, Decouvelaere AV, Blay JY, Combemale P. Diagnostic accuracy of PET/CT-guided percutaneous biopsies for malignant peripheral nerve sheath tumors in neurofibromatosis type 1 patients. PLoS One. 2015;10(10):e0138386.

251. Dunn GP, Spiliopoulos K, Plotkin SR, Hornicek FJ, Harmon DC, Delaney TF, Williams Z. Role of resection of malignant peripheral nerve sheath tumors in patients with neurofibromatosis type 1. J Neurosurg. 2013;118(1):142–8. https://doi.org/10.3171/2012.9.JNS101610.

252. Prudner BC, Ball T, Rathore R, Hirbe AC. Diagnosis and management of malignant peripheral nerve sheath tumors: current practice and future perspectives. Neurooncol Adv. 2019;2(Suppl 1):i40–9. https://doi.org/10.1093/noajnl/vdz047.

253. Sobczuk P, Teterycz P, Czarnecka AM, Świtaj T, Koseła-Paterczyk H, Kozak K, Falkowski S, Rutkowski P. Systemic treatment for advanced and metastatic malignant peripheral nerve sheath tumors-a sarcoma reference center experience. J Clin Med. 2020;9(10):3157. https://doi.org/10.3390/jcm9103157.

254. Brooks JS, Freeman M, Enterline HT. Malignant "Triton" tumors. Natural history and immunohistochemistry of nine new cases with literature review. Cancer. 1985;55(11):2543–9. https://doi.org/10.1002/1097-0142(19850601)55:11<2543::aid-cncr2820551105>3.0.co;2-4.

255. Ram R, Gardner J, Alapati S, Jambhekar K, Pandey T, Montgomery C, Nicholas R. Malignant triton tumor (malignant peripheral nerve sheath tumor with rhabdomyoblastic differentiation) occurring in a vascularized free flap reconstruction graft. Int J Surg Pathol. 2017;25(5):462–7.

256. Kretschmer T, editor. Nervenchirurgie: trauma, tumor. Springer: Kompression; 2014.

257. Bektas M, Bell T, Khan S, Tumminello B, Fernandez MM, Heyes C, Oton AB. Desmoid tumors: a comprehensive review. Adv Ther. 2023;40(9):3697–722. https://doi.org/10.1007/s12325-023-02592-0.

258. Kasper B, Ströbel P, Hohenberger P. Desmoid tumors: clinical features and treatment options for advanced disease. Oncologist. 2011;16(5):682–93. https://doi.org/10.1634/theoncologist.2010-0281.

259. Al-Jazrawe M, Au M, Alman B. Optimal therapy for desmoid tumors: current options and challenges for the future. Expert Rev Anticancer Ther. 2015;15(12):1443–58. https://doi.org/10.1586/14737140.2015.1096203.

260. Baehring JM, Batchelor TT. Diagnosis and management of neurolymphomatosis. Cancer J (Sudbury, Mass). 2012;18(5):463–8. https://doi.org/10.1097/PPO.0b013e31826c5ad5.

261. Choi YJ, Shin JA, Kim YH, Cha SJ, Cho JY, Kang SH, Yi SY, Lee HR. Neurolymphomatosis of brachial plexus in patients with non-Hodgkin's lymphoma. Case Rep Oncol Med. 2013;2013:492329. https://doi.org/10.1155/2013/492329.

262. Gan HK, Azad A, Cher L, Mitchell PL. Neurolymphomatosis: diagnosis, management, and outcomes in patients treated with rituximab. Neuro Oncol. 2010;12(2):212–5. https://doi.org/10.1093/neuonc/nop021.

263. Silverman TA, Enzinger FM. Fibrolipomatous hamartoma of nerve. A clinicopathologic analysis of 26 cases. Am J Surg Pathol. 1985;9(1):7–14. https://doi.org/10.1097/00000478-198501000-00004.

264. Agarwal S, Haase SC. Lipofibromatous hamartoma of the median nerve. J Hand Surg Am. 2013;38(2):392–7. https://doi.org/10.1016/j.jhsa.2012.10.042.

265. Siqueira MG, Martins RS, Foroni L, de Oliveira AJM, Lordelo G, Heise CO. Fibrolipomatous hamartoma of the median nerve: an unusual cause of carpal tunnel syndrome. Clin Case Reports. 2023;11(3):e7022. https://doi.org/10.1002/ccr3.7022.

266. Doğramaci Y, Kalaci A, Sevinç TT, Yanat AN. Intraneural hemangioma of the median nerve: a case report. J Brachial Plex Peripher Nerve Inj. 2008;3:5. https://doi.org/10.1186/1749-7221-3-5.

267. Patel CB, Tsai TM, Kleinert HE. Hemangioma of the median nerve: a report of two cases. J Hand Surg Am. 1986;11(1):76–9. https://doi.org/10.1016/s0363-5023(86)80108-3.

268. Châtillon CE, Guiot MC, Jacques L. Lipomatous, vascular, and chondromatous benign tumors of the peripheral nerves: representative cases and review of the literature. Neurosurg Focus. 2007;22(6):E18. https://doi.org/10.3171/foc.2007.22.6.19.

269. Neelon D, Lannan F, Childs J. Granular cell tumor. In: StatPearls. StatPearls Publishing; 2023.

270. Rose B, Tamvakopoulos GS, Yeung E, Pollock R, Skinner J, Briggs T, Cannon S. Granular cell tumours: a rare entity in the musculoskeletal system. Sarcoma. 2009;2009:765927. https://doi.org/10.1155/2009/765927.

271. Khashaba H, Hafez E, Burezq H. Nerve sheath myxoma: a rare tumor, a case report and literature review. Int J Surg Case Rep. 2020;73:183–6. https://doi.org/10.1016/j.ijscr.2020.07.030. Epub 2020 Jul 15. PMID: 32693231; PMCID: PMC7533628.
272. Kao EY, Kernig ML. Neurothekeoma. In: StatPearls. StatPearls Publishing; 2022.
273. Bravo EL, Gifford RW Jr. Current concepts. Pheochromocytoma: diagnosis, localization and management. N Engl J Med. 1984;311(20):1298–303. https://doi.org/10.1056/NEJM198411153112007.
274. Joynt KE, Moslehi JJ, Baughman KL. Paragangliomas: etiology, presentation, and management. Cardiol Rev. 2009;17(4):159–64. https://doi.org/10.1097/CRD.0b013e3181a6de40.
275. Pacak K, Fojo T, Goldstein DS, Eisenhofer G, Walther MM, Linehan WM, Bachenheimer L, Abraham J, Wood BJ. Radiofrequency ablation: a novel approach for treatment of metastatic pheochromocytoma. J Natl Cancer Inst. 2001;93(8):648–9. https://doi.org/10.1093/jnci/93.8.648.
276. Huang H, Abraham J, Hung E, Averbuch S, Merino M, Steinberg SM, Pacak K, Fojo T. Treatment of malignant pheochromocytoma/paraganglioma with cyclophosphamide, vincristine, and dacarbazine: recommendation from a 22-year follow-up of 18 patients. Cancer. 2008;113(8):2020–8.
277. Benson JC, Marais MD, Flanigan PM, Bydon M, Giannini C, Spinner RJ, Folpe AL. Malignant melanotic nerve sheath tumor. AJNR Am J Neuroradiol. 2022;43(12):1696–9. https://doi.org/10.3174/ajnr.A7691.
278. Meyer A, Billings SD. What's new in nerve sheath tumors. Virchows Archiv: Int J Pathol. 2020;476(1):65–80. https://doi.org/10.1007/s00428-019-02671-0.

Good to Know: Based on Examples

8

<u>Overall rule regarding nerve transfers:</u>
Incomplete lesions ➔ Intraplexal donor
Complete lesions ➔ Extraplexal donor

The *spinal accessory nerve* represents an exception as it is frequently taken as a donor in nerve transfer procedures, including cases of incomplete brachial plexus lesions. Its clinical utility derives from its consistent functional reliability and its close anatomical relationship to the brachial plexus, which facilitates surgical accessibility and effective axonal nerve transfer.

8.1 Nerve Compression

Median Nerve—Carpal Tunnel Syndrome
Outcomes following median nerve decompression are generally favorable, whereas recovery after ulnar nerve surgery tends to be less predictable, with comparatively low functional improvement.
Anatomical landmarks for the carpal tunnel (Fig. 8.1):

Proximal ulnar side ➔ Pisiforme bone
Middle square ➔ Safe square
Proximal median side ➔ Palmar cutaneous branch of the median nerve
Distal ➔ Arcus palmaris and recurrent motor branch of the median nerve

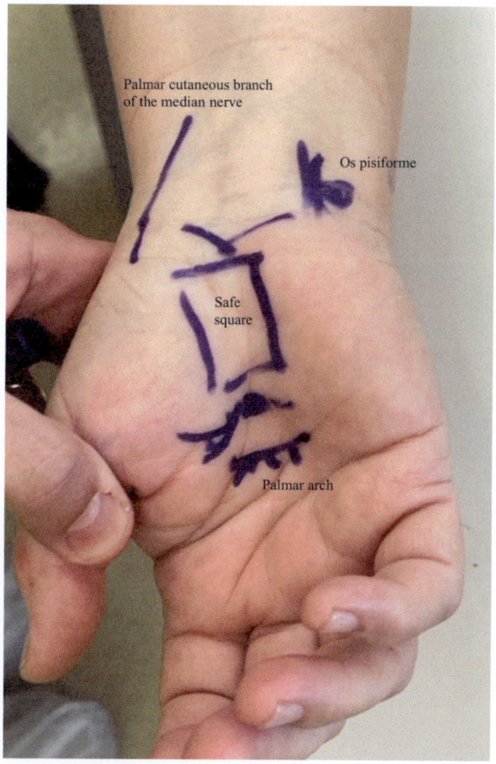

Fig. 8.1 Schematic anatomy of the carpal tunnel with its anatomical borders

> Position the third digital nerve toward the thenar eminence, noting that the **recurrent branch** typically terminates near the fingertip

K. Hobitsch, *Peripheral Nerve Surgery - A Compendium*,
https://doi.org/10.1007/978-3-032-03409-0_8

Ulnar Nerve—Cubital Tunnel Syndrome

To delineate the course of the ulnar nerve distal to the cubital tunnel, identify the midpoint between the medial and the lateral epicondyle and locate the pisiform bone. An imaginary line connecting these landmarks can be used to approximate the distal path of the nerve.

Early surgical intervention is critical, as the ulnar nerve demonstrate limited regenerative capacity, and delayed treatment may compromise functional recovery.

The role of **anterior transposition of the ulnar nerve** during cubital tunnel surgery remains controversial. Even in cases of recurrent cubital tunnel syndrome or subluxation of the ulnar nerve, the indication for transposition of the ulnar nerve is debated.

Studies have shown that there is no significant difference in the outcome between simple ulnar nerve decompression and decompression combined with anterior transposition of the ulnar nerve. In fact, anterior transposition of the ulnar nerve may be associated with a higher incidence of complications [1–3].

Anterior transposition requires extensive exposure of the nerve and circumferential mobilization, which may compromise its vascular supply, increase susceptibility to external pressure, and potentially hinder regeneration.

Effective decompression of the ulnar nerve at the cubital tunnel necessitates division of the proximal muscular aponeurosis (arcade of Struthers) as well as the distal muscular fascia of the flexor carpi ulnaris (Fig. 8.2).

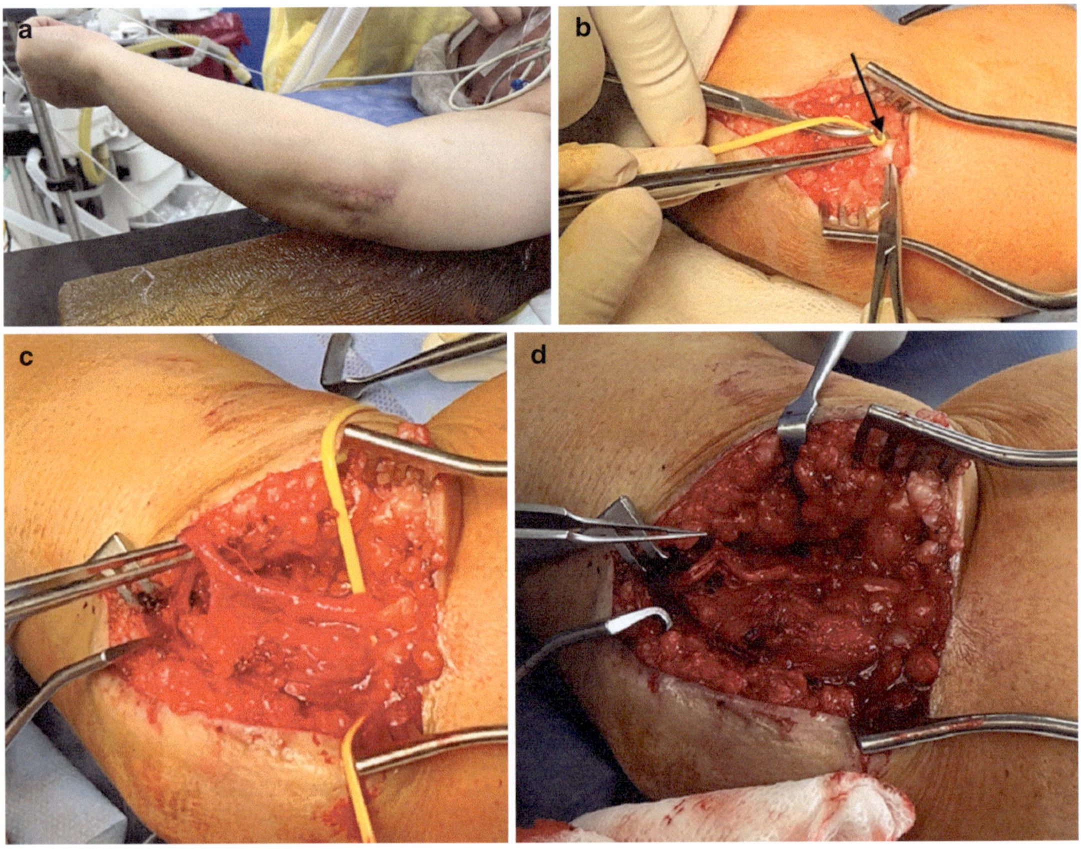

Fig. 8.2 Intraoperative images demonstrating anterior transposition of the ulnar nerve in a patient with recurrent cubital tunnel syndrome: (**a**) represents the typical positioning of the patient's arm. The ulnar nerve is detected (**b**, arrow) and dissected (**c**) to be then positioned more anteriorly in the subcutaneous tissue of the arm (**d**)

Care should be taken to preserve the medial antebrachial cutaneous branch of the ulnar nerve, as inadvertent injury can predispose the patient to neuroma formation.

Thoracic Outlet Syndrome

During thoracic outlet syndrome (TOS) surgery, the inferior trunk of the brachial plexus should be identified first, as it is particularly susceptible to traction or overdistension.

Case Presentation:

Female patient, 48 years

History:

The patient underwent combined neurogenic and vascular TOS surgery 1.5 years ago via a supra- and infraclavicular approach together with the vascular surgeon. At that time, resection of the anterior scalene muscle and partial resection of the cervical rib were performed.

The patient remained symptom-free for approximately 2 months postoperatively, after which pain recurred. The pain was described as continuous and electrifying, localized primarily to the distal ulnar region with antegrade radiation to the upper arm. Symptoms were aggravated by certain body positions. Paresthesia was also present, including hypersensitivity to temperature changes with fingertips turning blue upon cold exposure.

Clinical Presentation:

On physical examination, atrophy of the thenar and hypothenar muscles was visible and slight weakness of the interossei muscles could be objectified.

Magnetic resonance imaging revealed the brachial plexus in close contact with transverse process of thoracic vertebrae 7 (Th7).

Surgical Plan:

The operative plan involved removal of the fibrotic tissue and, if necessary, resection of the transverse process via a supraclavicular approach.

Intraoperative Findings:

Upon identification of the brachial plexus trunks, the transverse process of Th7 was palpated directly beneath the plexus, compressing the inferior trunk.

Initial dissection between the inferior trunk and the subclavian artery was planned; however, extensive fibrotic tissue necessitated a more inferior approach. The compressive bony structure was successfully resected, alleviating the mechanical compression of the inferior trunk (Fig. 8.3).

Considerations during surgery: During dissection, the brachial plexus trunks are continuously subjected to traction. It is essential to frequently adjust both the patient's limb position and the retractors to minimize the risk of iatrogenic nerve injury. All three trunks of the brachial plexus should be clearly identified. Additionally, the phrenic nerve must be visualized and protected throughout the procedure to prevent inadvertent transection.

Pudendal Nerve

If pudendal nerve compression syndrome is suspected, a diagnostic pudendal nerve block should be performed prior to considering surgical intervention.

Surgery can be performed via either a dorsal transgluteal approach, which provides exposure of the entire nerve, or a ventral perineal apporach.

Common compressive structures include the sacrotuberal ligament (the most frequent cause), scarring, varicose veins, or an additional fascia.

The pudendal nerve arises from S2, S3, and S4, giving rise to the inferior rectal, perineal, and dorsal nerve of the penisor clitoris. Functionally, approximately 50% of fibers are sensory, 20% motor, and 30% autonomic [4]. Nerve compression predominantly affects the sensitive fibers causing pain in the perineal or in the clitoral/penile area that worsens when sitting. Severe long-standing conditions may involve urinary and fecal disturbances as well as sexual dysfunction.

Females are more often affected than males.

Both the pathophysiology and surgical management remain controversial, with debate regarding existence of the syndrome, outcomes, and possible placebo effects.

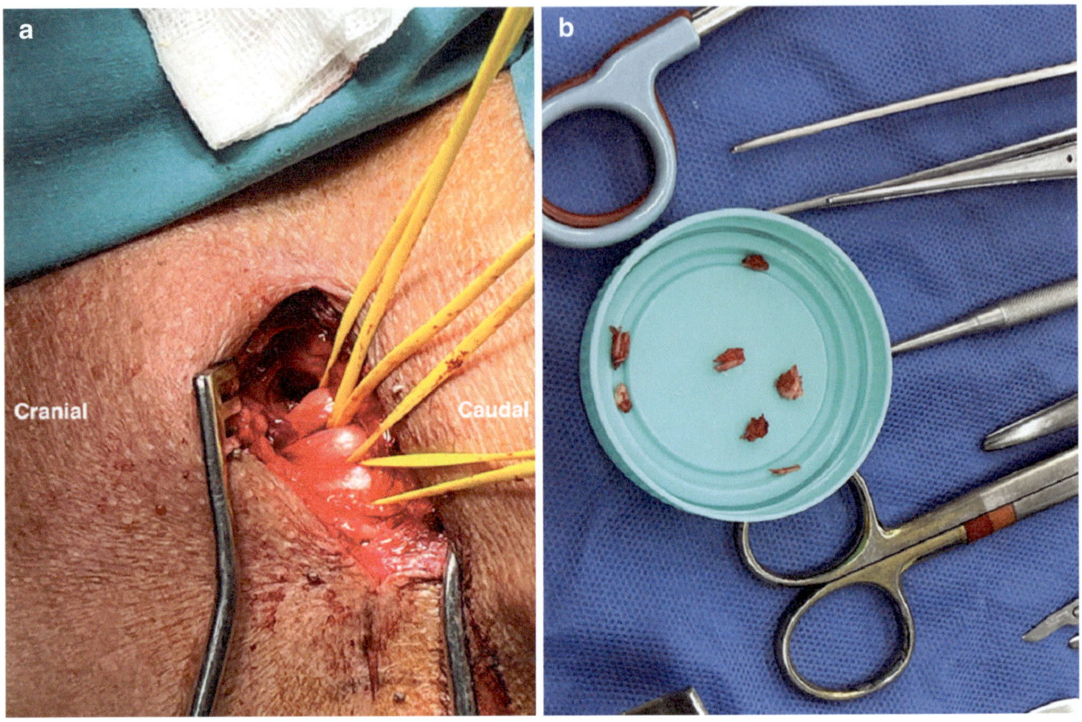

Fig. 8.3 TOS surgery: Supraclavicular approach revealing the trunks (**a**). (**b**) shows part of the resected transverse process of Th7

Conservative treatment should be attempted first, including analgesics, antidepressants, and physiotherapy. Positive response to at least three diagnostic nerve blocks are generally required before surgical intervention is indicated.

Surgical decompression can be performed via transgluteal, transperineal, or transvaginal approaches. The pudendal nerve is classically decompressed within the Alcock's canal and at sites between the sacrospinous and sacrotuberous ligaments. In cases of surgical failure, neuromodulation may be considered as a final therapeutic option.

Lateral Femoral Cutaneous Nerve

Surgical intervention may be considered in patients with **meralgia paresthetica** who fail conservative management. The following approaches are commonly employed:

The lateral femoral cutaneous nerve may be transected and the proximal nerve stump placed deep within the surrounding tissue. The transection should be performed as proximally as possible, allowing the nerve to retract into the pelvis where it is no longer subjected to compressive forces. This technique effectively reliefs pain but carries the risk of permanent sensory loss in the lateral thigh.

The second option would be decompression of the nerve at the inguinal canal, typically by incising the inguinal ligament (Fig. 8.4). While this approach preserves sensory function, it has a higher risk of symptom recurrence compared with nerve resection.

A longitudinal incision medial to the anterior superior iliac spine provides direct access to the inguinal canal and the lateral femoral cutaneous nerve.

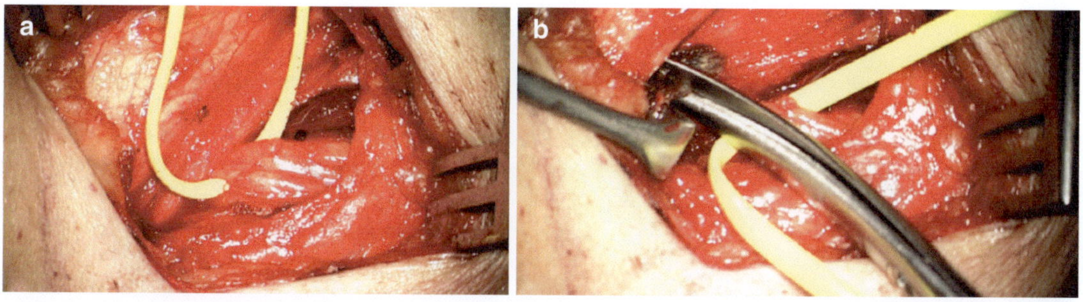

Fig. 8.4 Intraoperative images of lateral femoral cutaneous nerve (**a**, yellow loop, which is decompressed by incision of the inguinal ligament (**b**)

8.2 Tumor

Median Nerve
Case Presentation:

Female patient, 67 years,

Clinical Presentation:

A patient presented with paresthesia and pain in the hand for six months. At the same time, she could palpate a nodule on the inner aspect of the upper arm.

The MRI demonstrated a well-circumscribed mass along the course of the median nerve suggestive of a schwannoma.

Intraoperative Findings:

Intraoperatively, the lesion did not exhibit the typical characteristics of a schwannoma, as no fascicle could be clearly observed entering or exiting the tumor (Fig. 8.5). Nevertheless, histopathological examination confirmed diagnosis of a median nerve schwannoma.

Sciatic Nerve
Case Presentation:

Female patient 22 years

Clinical Presentation:

She presented at the hospital with continuous pain for four months, predominantly affecting the tibial nerve innervated dermatome of the lower extremity. Physical examination revealed no motor deficits in the lower extremities.

The MRI identified a mass arising from the sciatic nerve.

Surgical Plan:

Tumor resection via transgluteal approach was planned.

Intraoperative Findings:

Intraoperatively, the tumor was found to be closely adherent to the tibial component of sciatic nerve, correlating with the patient's tibial-distributed pain (Fig. 8.6).

Sciatic Nerve Lesion

- Anatomical landmarks: The sciatic nerve is located between the lateral aspect of the greater trochanter and medial ischial tuberosity. Knowledge of these bony landmarks facilitates save identification of the nerve during surgery.
- The **transgluteal approach** is indicated for stab wounds, tumor resection, sciatic nerve compression at the sciatic notch, and iatrogenic nerve injury following hip surgery.
- Other approaches to sciatic nerve surgery in the gluteal region iclude the **classical approach** (?-skin incision ➔ larger incision) and the **subgluteal approach**.
- By incision along the direction of the muscle fibers rather than transecting them, this method assures better aesthetical and functional results. It presents an atraumatic technique without the need for muscle suturing.
- Traversing through the gluteal musculature, the appearance of subcutaneous fat signals proximity to the sciatic nerve.
- Bony landmarks are reliable guide: the sciatic nerve is located just lateral to the ischial tuberosity.

Tumors of the *lumbar plexus* are usually situated in the anterior thigh, whereas lumbosacral plexus

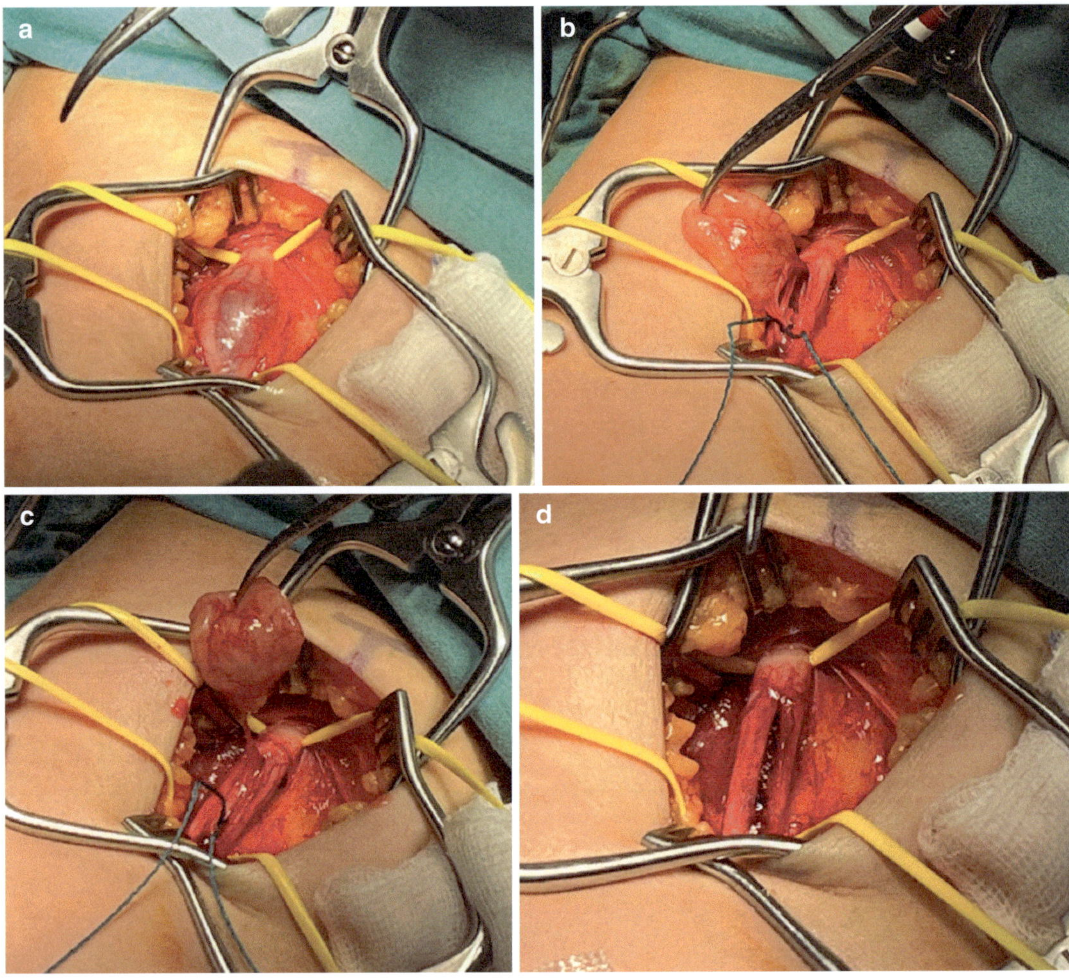

Fig. 8.5 Intraoperative imaging showing a schwannoma of the median nerve at the proximal upper arm (**a**). Careful excision is performed, thereby preserving the fascicles of the median nerve (**b**)

tumors are typically found in the gluteal region and the posterior aspect of the leg.

Neurofibromatosis 1
Case Presentation:

Male patient, 26 years with NF1

History:

The patient had undergone multiple prior surgical resections, including a recent incision of an inguinal tumor, which was histologically confirmed as malignant. He continued to have numerous small cutaneous and subcutaneous tumors, as well as two larger tumors in the lower extremity, all of which were asymptomatic.

The conducted spectrograph though demonstrated elevated signals in the two larger tumors. While not definitively indicative of malignancy, the patient's history of early-onset malignant peripheral nerve tumors prompted oncologists to recommend surgical excision and histological examination.

Intraoperative Findings:

Located along the saphenous nerve, the terminal cutaneous branch of the femoral nerve, the first tumor confirmed intraoperatively as a neurofibroma.

The second tumor was found arising from the superficial peroneal nerve. Access to this lesion

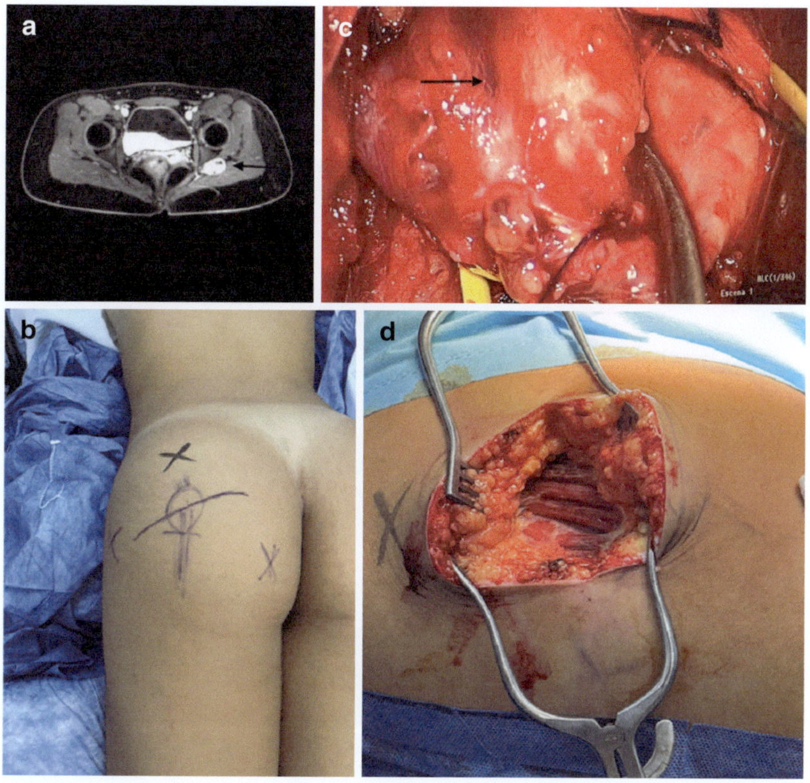

Fig. 8.6 (**a**) Shows a tumor of the left sciatic nerve on the MRI axial plane (arrow). Surgery is performed in prone position and the suspected course of the sciatic nerve is marked according to the anatomical landmarks (**b**). (**c**) microscopically depicts the tumor adherent to the sciatic nerve. Operative field after tumor resection (**d**)

required transection of the anterior talo-fibular ligament, which does not result in functional deficit. Intraoperatively, no individual fascicles were indetifiable entering or exiting the tumor, indicating diffuse nerve involvement consistent with either a neurofibroma or a tumor with potential malignancy. Complete nerve transection was necessary for excision (Fig. 8.7).

Case Presentation:

Male patient with NF1

Clinical Presentation:

He presented with severe pain being his main symptom. The patient had a history of prior neurofibroma resections. Magnetic resonance imaging revealed a tumor mass involving the C8 spinal nerve.

Surgical Plan:

Planned resection of the tumor in collaboration with the orthopedic surgeon for clavicular bone removal was directed.

Intraoperative Findings:

Upon intraoperative stimulation, the C8 spinal nerve demonstrated minimal functional response. The tumor exhibited a plexiform morphology, raising suspicion for malignancy. Opening the epineurium revealed diffuse infiltration of all fascicles, with only a few showing any response to stimulation. Given these findings, the surgical strategy was modified: a single fascicle was excised for biopsy and a decompression was performed to alleviate pain (Fig. 8.8).

Facial Nerve Palsy

Case Presentation—Hypoglossal-to-Facial Nerve Transfer:

Male patient, 30 years

History:

He initially presented with tinnitus. On the MRI, a schwannoma of the facial nerve proximal to the stylomastoid foramen was seen. Surgical resection of the tumor was performed by the otorhinolaryngologist. Postoperatively, the patient developed a complete facial nerve palsy—House-Brackmann grade VI.

Clinical Presentation:

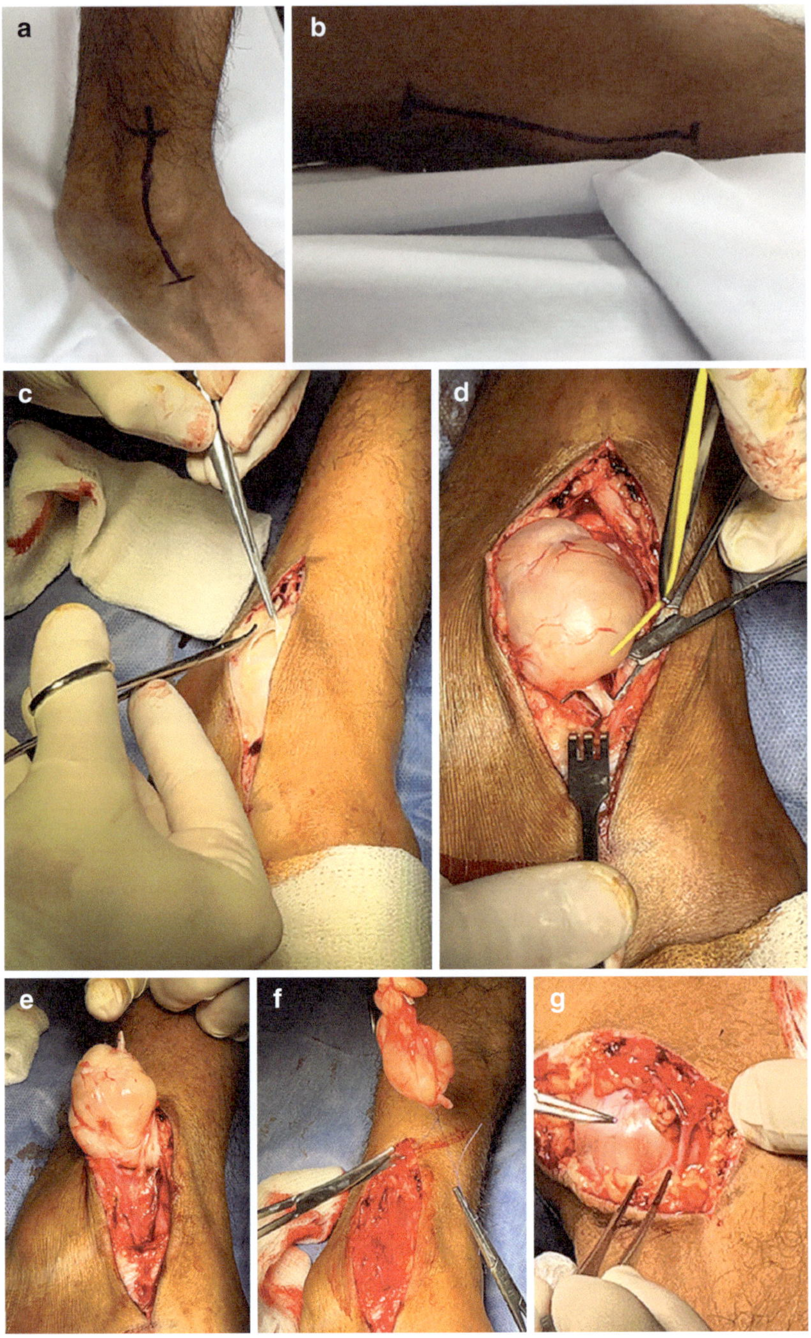

Fig. 8.7 NF 1 patient with 2 large palpable subcutaneous tumors in the lower legs (**a**, **b**). (**c**–**f**) show the steps of surgical resection of the tumor arising from the superficial peroneal nerve. (**g**) depicts the second tumor arising from the saphenous nerve

The patient did not exhibit clinical or electrophysiological evidence of facial nerve regeneration at seven months following tumor resection. A MRI was performed and showed a discontinuity of the facial nerve. Surgical reconstruction via hypoglossal-to-facial nerve transfer was indicated.

Intraoperative Findings:

The bony approach was performed by the otorhinolaryngy team. The facial nerve was

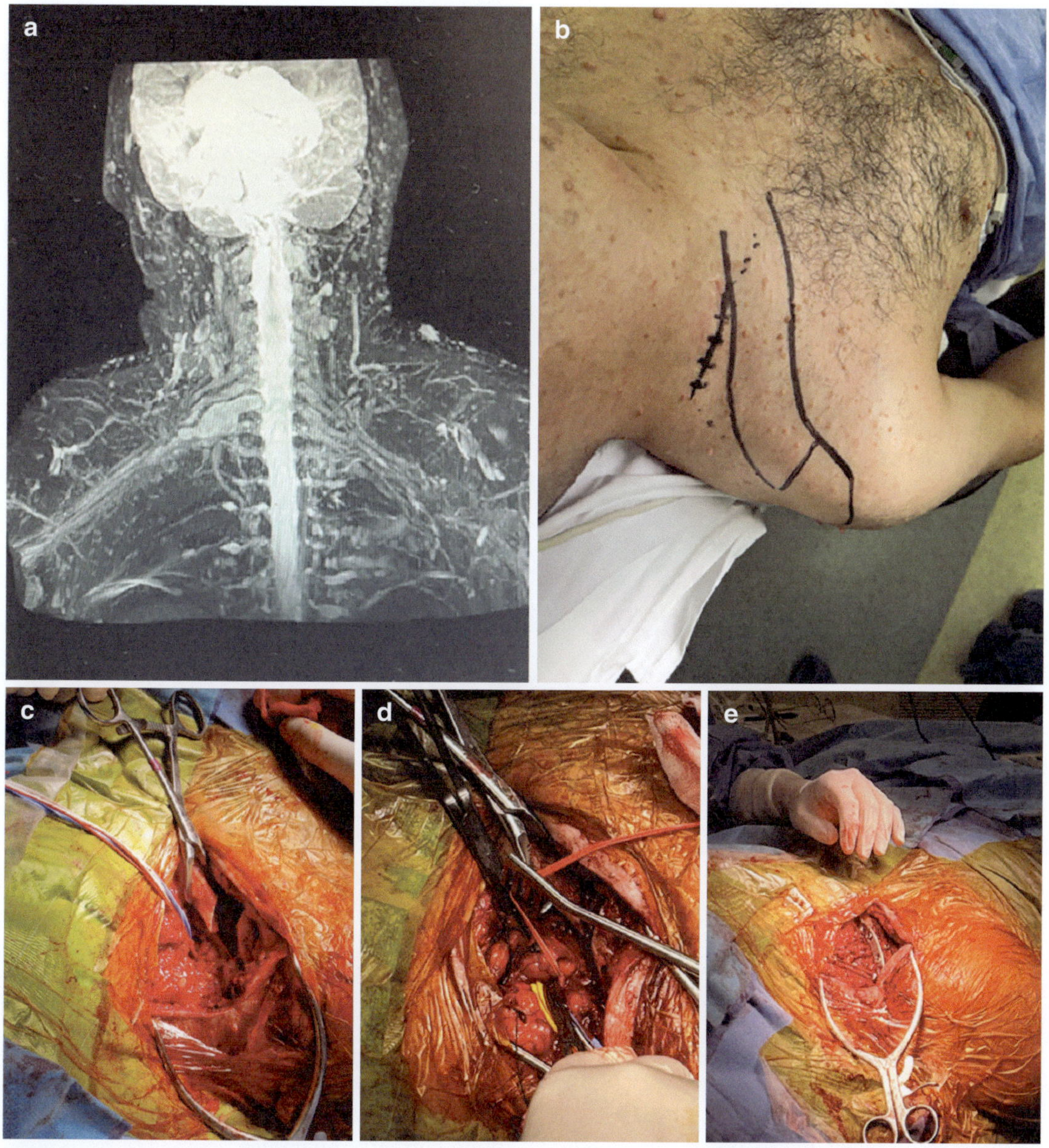

Fig. 8.8 MRI (**a**) of a NF 1 patient reveals numerous tumors with the largest one affecting the right C8 spinal nerve. The incision is determined by anatomical landmarks (**b**). After clavicular bone resection (**c**), an infiltrating mass (**d**) could be identified. (**e**) shows the operative field after reinsertion of the clavicular bone via a plate

transected as proximally as possible, with distal exposure distal to styloid foramen.

The styloid foramen region posed the greatest technical challenge due to the intimate attachment of the nerve to the bony part.

Dissection of the parotid gland was necessary for facial nerve mobilization. The degree of mobilization is limited by the numerous distal branches of the facial nerve.

Only approximately one-third of the hypoglossal nerve was sacrificed to match the diameter of the facial nerve as the hypoglossal nerve is larger. End-to-end coaptation was performed using 10–0 microsutures (Fig. 8.9).

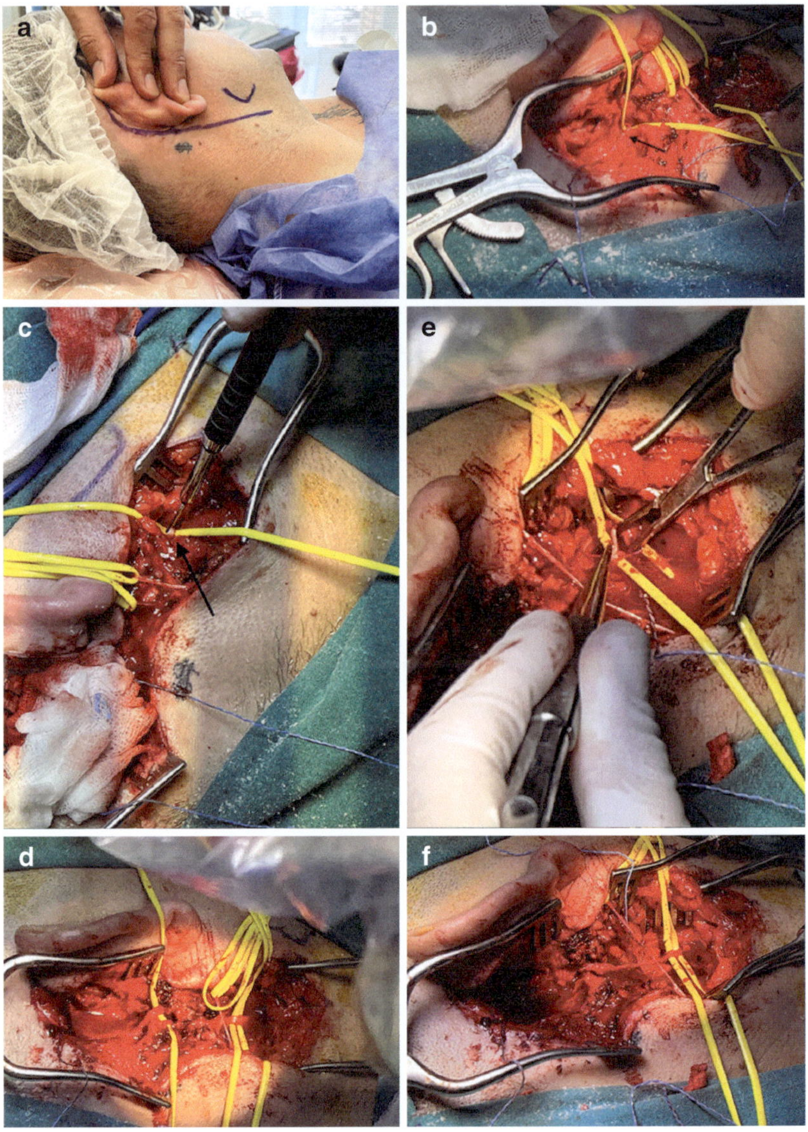

Fig. 8.9 Hypoglossal-to-facial nerve transfer: The planned retroauricular incision is shown in (**a**). First, the facial nerve was dissected (**b**), then, the hypoglossal nerve was identified via stimulation (**c**). Both nerves were put close to each other (**d**) with the hypoglossal being split (**e**) prior to nerve transfer. (**f**) shows the split hypoglossal nerve (donor nerve) sutured to the distal facial nerve stump

In cases of **facial nerve palsy**, the standard approach is to allow for spontaneous recovery, which may take up to 18 months. Immediate surgical intervention is indicated only if the nerve is known to be transected. Outcomes are not negatively affected by waiting for spontaneous recovery. Observational studies suggest that women may experience better functional recovery than men.

The House-Brackmann scale, while commonly used for grading facial nerve function, has limited prognostic utility. Most patients will not achieve better than HB III–IV. No surgery technique currently guarantees complete restoration of facial function.

Full regeneration is constrained by central nervous system limitations. Spontaneous facial expressions, such as smiling, are controlled by the limbic system and are not linked to hypoglossal nerve function. Therefore, voluntary, but not spontaneous facial movements can be restored after hypoglossal-to-facial nerve reconstruction—a fact that emphasizes the limitations of this transfer.

Patients undergoing a hypoglossal-to-facial nerve transfer typically develop hemitongue paralysis which may result in significant deficits regarding speech, mastication, and swallowing. In order to avoid these quite limiting side effects of the hypoglossal-facial nerve transfer, a method called jump graft- can be applied.

Jump grafting describes the interposition of a short nerve graft, that is interposed between the hypoglossal nerve (sutured end-to-side proximally) and the distal facial nerve stump (direct end-to-end suture distally). This technique preserves a greater proportion of hypoglossal function, reducing tongue deficits.

The masseteric nerve can be used for facial nerve reconstruction too. It is usually smaller than the hypoglossal nerve and primarily innervates the lower part of the face, with limited contribution to the upper face. It is thought to allow smiling—a motion of the limbic system—due to potential cross-innervation.

8.3 Trauma

Axillay Nerve

Case Presentation—Triceps Branch to Axillary Nerve Transfer:

Male patient, 34 years

Clinical Presentation:

He presented seven months after a motorcycle accident. On clinical examination, the patient exhibited an isolated axillary nerve palsy with both motor and sensory deficits. Concomitant injuries to the shoulder ligaments and the rotator cuff was evident. Immediate surgical repair for reconstruction of the shoulder ligaments had been performed post-accident; however, the axillary nerve palsy persisted. Due to prior immobilization, it remains unclear whether the nerve injury was a direct consequence of the trauma or an iatrogenic injury during ligament reconstruction.

During functional assessment, active abduction of the shoulder was preserved, likely due to compensatory function of other rotator cuff muscles.

The surgical plan was reconstruction of the axillary nerve via nerve transfer using a motor branch from the triceps muscle (Fig. 8.10).

Preoperative assessment of triceps function prior to surgery is essential to ensure suitability as a donor nerve.

Axillary nerve transfer considerations: The anterior division of the axillary nerve is typically larger and positioned more anteriorly during a posterior surgical approach compared to the posterior division. Functionally, the anterior division is more critical for shoulder function, making it the preferred recipient in axillary nerve reconstruction.

> The posterior division can serve as a donor in nerve transfer procedures, for example in radial nerve injuries.

Three triceps branches of the radial nerve can be considered as potential donors for nerve transfer—the branch to the medial, the branch to the lateral, and one branch to the long head of triceps muscle. Selection should consider functional priorities rather than branch size alone. For example, the long triceps branch may be needed to compensate for arm abduction deficits, making the lateral branch a more suitable donor in such cases.

Radial Nerve

Case Presentation:

Male patient, 53 years

History:

The patient sustained a gunshot-wound seven months ago, resulting in injury to the radial nerve and the anterior interosseous branch of the median nerve.

Clinical Presentation:

The median nerve recovered spontaneously, while there was no regeneration of the radial nerve observed. Sonography revealed discontinuity of the radial nerve with surrounding fibrotic tissue suggesting the presence of a neuroma.

Surgical Plan:

Exploration via the external bicipital canal, resection of the neuroma, and reconstruction by direct coaptation of the nerve was planned.

Intraoperative Findings:

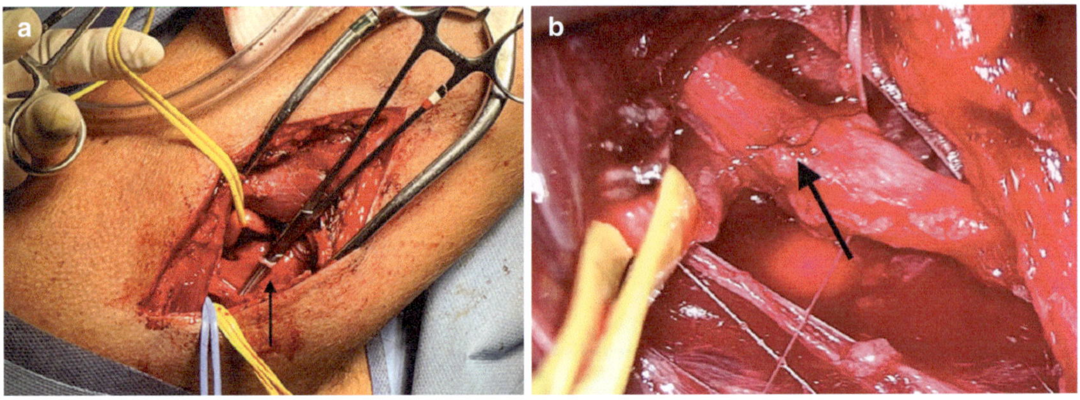

Fig. 8.10 Posterior approach for triceps-to-axillary nerve transfer: The axillary nerve is identified and marked with a yellow loop. One of the triceps branches are revealed in **a** (arrow). (**b**) shows the microscopical view after nerve transfer. A 10–0 microsuture was used for nerve coaptation

The distal radial nerve segment was easily identified. The proximal segment was initially difficult to locate, but careful dissection revealed the neuroma. A Resection of the neuroma created a 5 cm nerve gap—too large for direct coaptation. Reconstruction was performed using rural nerve graft—with the rural nerve being folded four times to reach the diameter of the radial nerve -and fibrin glue was applied to secure the coaptation sites (Fig. 8.11).

The radial nerve generally has a good prognosis for recovery. The best function to recover is hand extension, followed by finger extension and finally thumb function.

For reconstruction of the radial nerve, several transfers are frequently used including:

- Posterior branch of the axillary nerve to the long head of the triceps nerve
- Phrenic or intercostal nerves to the radial nerve or long head of triceps nerve
- Spinal accessory nerve to the radial nerve

In contrast, the ulnar nerve has a poor regenerative ability, High lesions, proximal to the elbow, often result in permanent motor deficits of the hand function especially regarding grasping and finger pinching due to weakness of the first dorsal interossei (FDI) and the adductor pollicis (ADP) muscles.

Injury do the ulnar nerve proximal to the elbow will cause those intrinsic hand muscles to denervate, even if nerve reconstruction surgery is successful. This is because the sprouting axons must travel a long distance to reach their target muscles, which often prevents timely reinnervation even after successful surgery.

To prevent permanent hand deficits, Bertelli et al. performed a distal nerve transfer in which the motor branch of the opponens pollicis muscle is transferred to the terminal division of the deep branch of the ulnar nerve. This provides reinnervation of the FDI and ADP, improving grasp and pinch strength [6].

Tibial Nerve

Case Presentation:

Male patient, 48 years

Clinical Presentation:

He developed excruciating pain in the calf radiating to the foot three months after sustaining a gunshot wound in his right leg. He denied paresthesia, but mild weakness of flexor digitorum brevis muscle was observed on clinical examination. On the sonographic exam, a hematoma around or within the nerve was seen, the nerve itself appeared to be in continuity.

Surgical Plan:

The surgical plan was exploration and neurolysis.

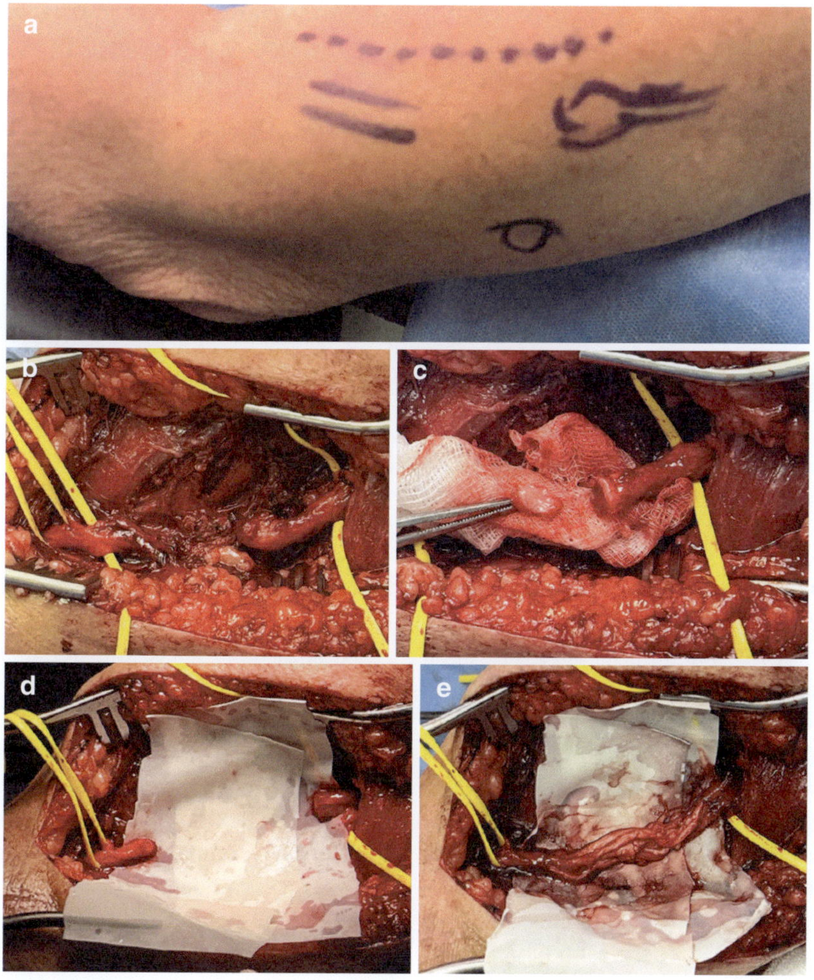

Fig. 8.11 Preoperative marking of the suspected radial nerve (**a**) with the aid of ultrasonography facilitates the planning of the surgery. After neuroma resection (**b**, **c**), the resulting gap was too larger for nerve repair via direct coaptation (**d**). The sural nerve is used as a transplant (**e**)

Intraoperative Findings:

The surgical approach was initiated from healthy tissue to avoid damaging intact structures within the scar tissue; in this case, dissection was performed from distal to proximal.

Upon reaching the affected region, extensive scar tissue and abnormal vascular formations with active bleeding were encountered.

After hemostasis, a neuroma approximately 3 cm in length became visible. Given these findings, the surgical plan was revised to perform a neuroma resection with sural nerve grafting (Fig. 8.12).

> It is critical to preserve any still functional fascicles of the tibial nerve during resection.

The resultant gap was reconstructed using a sural nerve graft. In partial nerve injuries, suturing the graft is often unnecessary—application of fibrin glue is usually sufficient for fixation.

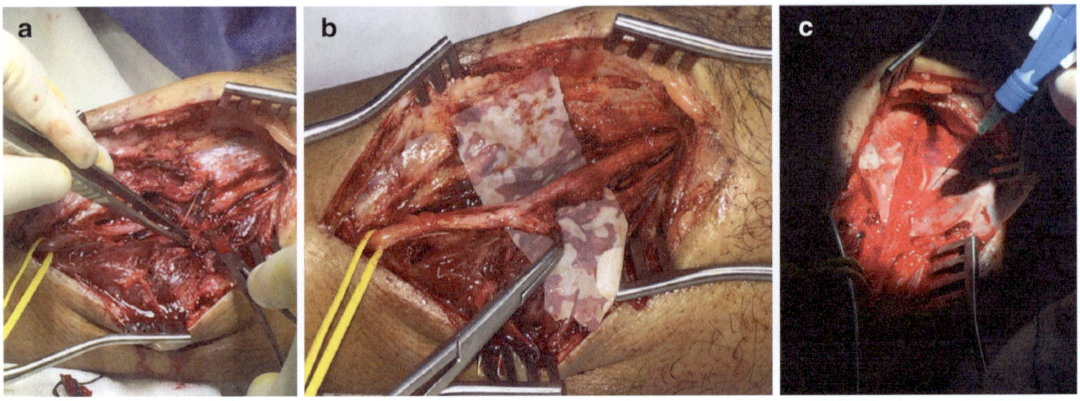

Fig. 8.12 The presence of vessels close to the tibial (**a**) led to extensive bleeding. After hemostasis, a neuroma (**b**) was visible. The neuroma was resected and a sural nerve (**c**) was used to bridge the gap

Sciatic Nerve

In severe sciatic nerve palsies, the sural and the ipsilateral peroneus nerve may be harvested as a graft for reconstruction of the posterior tibial nerve. Although this procedure sacrifices the remaining peroneal nerve function—leading to foot drop—the patient will regain plantar sensation, which is essential for maintaining balance and reducing the risk of complications such as osteomyelitis. Additionally, eversion of the foot will still be possible, and if the strength is sufficient, tendon transfer can later be considered. If not, arthrodesis remains a surgical option.

The **peroneal nerve** has specific anatomical features that contribute to its poor prognosis after injury.

It has a long course down the leg, and is fixed at multiple points—at the fibular head by the peroneus longus muscle and at the ankle joint by the extensor retinaculum of the foot. Along its path, it also runs superficially at the lateral knee, making it highly vulnerable to trauma.

At the sciatic notch and fibular tunnel, as well as at its branching points, the nerve is relatively immobile, which increases its susceptibility to stretch injuries. Moreover, because the peroneal nerve is located laterally within the the sciatic nerve, it is more exposed to external forces.

Its limited vascular supply and an unfavorable ratio of connective tissue to neural tissue further explains its low tolerance to ischemia and compression.

In cases of idiopathic foot drop, it is important to ask about recent weight loss, as this can be an overlooked contributing factor.

A saphenous nerve transfer to the posterior tibial nerve may improve the sensory function in patients with polyneuropathy.

Direct coaptation of the nerve in the lower extremity can sometimes be performed with the knee held in flexion. This technique may enhance regeneration compared with nerve grafting, but it imposes a significant burden on the patient who must endure prolonged immobilization of the leg in a cast with restricted range of motion.

To protect the repair, the epineurium should always be covered to reduce the risk of suture rupture.

Morton Neuroma

Case Presentation:

Male patient, 37 years.

Clinical Presentation:

He reported the sensation of a “stone” on the foot sole while walking, particularly when wearing shoes. On clinical examination, pain was elicited on palpation between digits III and IV of the foot. Mulder sign was positive.

Intraoperative Findings:

A tourniquet was applied to achieve a bloodless operative field.

The intertarsal ligament was opened, and the Mulder maneuver was used intraoperatively to push the neuroma toward the surface. Resection should be performed as proximally as possible to avoid leaving residual compression; the distal aspect is less critical. Care must be taken not to cut the tendon of the extensor digitorum longus muscle. Distal to the neuroma, the nerve characteristically assumes an X-shape due to its bifurcation (Fig. 8.13).

Brachial Plexus Lesion

The primary objective of surgical intervention, are the restoration of shoulder stability and elbow flexion. However, it is indispensable to talk with the patient about the operative strategy as they may prioritize other functions. For example, a patient who is wheelchair-bound may derive greater functional benefit from restoration of wrist extension and grasp strength than elbow flexion.

For surgical exposure, the patient is placed in a supine position with the head rotated laterally toward the contralateral, unaffected side. Placement of a cushion beneath the ipsilateral shoulder facilitates elevation of the neck and improved access of the brachial plexus.

The classical supraclavicular approach provides exposure to the proximal segments of the brachial plexus. The posterior border of the sternocleidomastoid muscle is identified approximately two finger breadths superior to the clavicle. The Birch modification involves medial extension of the incision, whereas the Fiolle-Delmas technique incorporates an additional transverse extension to optimize surgical access (Fig. 8.14).

Nerve transfer options for brachial plexus injury (BPI) with C5 and C6 palsy:

C5 root ➔ Posterior division or triceps nerve

If the C5 root is too weak or injured, think of using axillary nerve instead

Spinal accessory nerve ➔ Suprascapular nerve

Oberlin technique:

Ulnar nerve ➔ Branch of the musculocutaneous nerve to the brachial muscle

Median nerve ➔ Branch of the musculocutaneous nerve to biceps muscle

The median nerve generally provides greater motor function compared to the ulnar nerve.

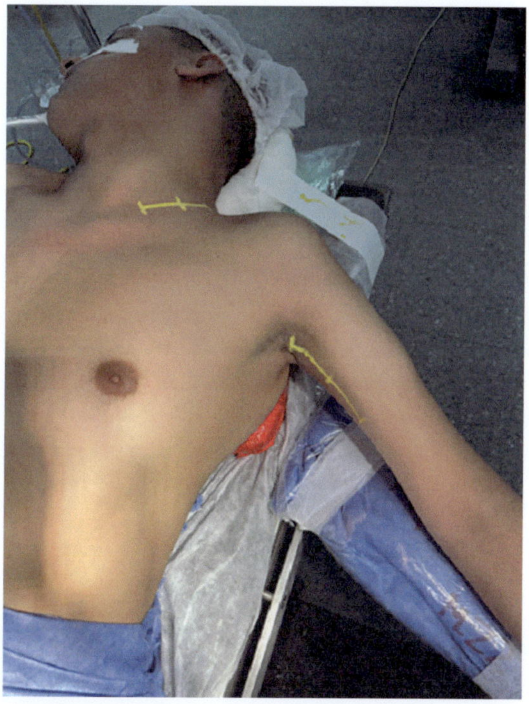

Fig. 8.14 Classical positioning of the patient during brachial plexus surgery. The yellow markings show the supraclavicular approach and the surgical approach for Oberlin procedure at the medial aspect of the upper arm. The arm is classically put on a mobile armboard

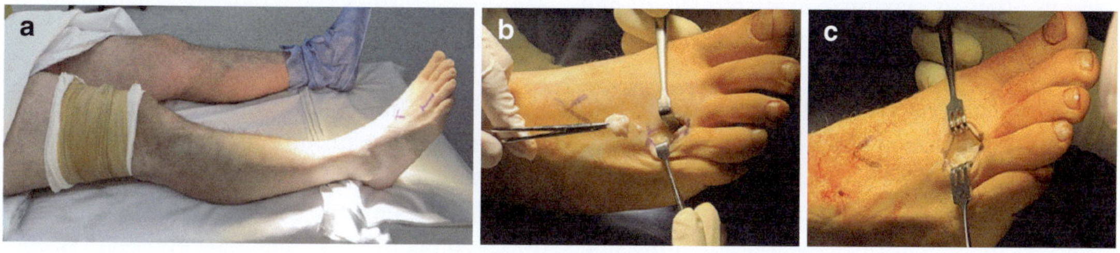

Fig. 8.13 Intraoperative images of Morton neuroma resection: Prior to surgery, a tourniquet was applied for bloodless operative field (**a**). **b** shows the excision of the neuroma. (**c**) demonstrated the postoperative field

However, its distal fascicles are classically more challenging to isolate and dissect, which increases the risk of inadvertent injury of the fascicles responsible for intrinsic hand muscle innervation.

Anatomical Landmarks and Variations During Surgery

- **Transverse cervical artery**: The brachial plexus is located inferior to its vessel and can be reliably identified in relation to it.
- **Omohyoid muscle**: This muscle runs in the same orientation as the brachial plexus and should not be mistaken for neural structures.
- **Exposure beneath the omohyoid**: The first structure encountered is typically the brachial plexus. The superior trunk is identified first, which should then be traced distally to visualize its trifurcation, formed by the suprascapular nerve, the anterior division, and the posterior division.
- **Long thoracic nerve**: This nerve lies proximal to the superior trunk. It is generally not visualized in the classical supraclavicular approach, as it courses too proximally for consistent exposure.
- **Phrenic nerve**: This structure is identified medial to the C5 root and must be preserved to avoid diaphragmatic dysfunction.
- **Infraclavicular approach**: In this exposure, the brachial plexus is located directly beneath the pectoralis minor muscle.

Nerve Grafting and Donor Selection

When performing nerve grafting, the most proximal segment of the recipient nerve and the most distal segment of the donor nerve should be utilized in order to maximize available length and potentially avoid the need for an interpositional graft.

Traditionally, nerve grafts are oriented in reverse to minimize aberrant axonal sprouting.

However, the clinical significance of graft orientation remains debated, with uncertainties regarding the extent of collateral sprouting and the associated axonal loss.

The *intercostal nerves* represent a relatively weak donor source. At least **three intercostal nerves** are typically required to match the caliber of the recipient nerve and achieve satisfactory outcomes. Even with adequate transfer, results remain limited, with functional recovery of elbow flexion observed in only about 20% of patients. Intercostal nerve transfer for elbow flexion is ineffective when combined with an interpositional nerve graft.

The *superficial cervical branch*, encountered during the supraclavicular approach of the brachial plexus, is not an ideal graft option due to its short length, irregular diameter, and multiple branches. Nevertheless, it may be considered in the absence of other viable donor nerves, particularly if a large cervical branch is available.

The *long thoracic nerve* should not be used as a donor nerve, as its sacrifice results in clinically significant morbidity, including painful scapular winging.

Adjunctive therapies:

In selected cases, botulinum toxin injections into the triceps muscle may be employed to temporarily weaken the antagonist, thereby facilitating strengthening and training the biceps muscle in patients with incomplete recovery.

Timing of Reconstruction:

Nerve reconstruction is generally considered ineffective beyond one year after injury, as the denervated muscle undergoes irreversible atrophy. An exception exists when residual muscle activity is present (e.g., contraction without functional movement), including partial innervation. In such cases, reconstruction may still yield meaningful recovery, as the target muscle is not completely denervated.

Muscle Priorities in Upper Brachial Plexus Lesions:

In upper brachial plexus lesion, restoration of external rotation is best achieved by reinnervating the infraspinatus muscle.

Shoulder stability is a prerequisite for functional elbow flexion. Without adequate stabilization, compensatory internal rotation occurs during elbow flexion, limiting function.

Reconstructive Strategies for Shoulder Function

Spinal accessory to suprascapular nerve
Triceps branches to axillary nerve
C5/C6 roots to posterior division of the upper trunk (PDUT)

If the middle or lower trunks are preserved, they should be prioritized as a donor sources for the suprascapular nerve before using the spinal accessory nerve, given the spinal accessory nerve's important contribution to shoulder stability.

Case Presentation:

Male patient, 26 years old

History:

He sustained a motorcycle accident five months prior, resulting in a brachial plexus injury in association with clavicular and tibial bone fracture. The clavicular fracture was managed conservatively, while the tibial fracture required surgical fixation. The initial course was complicated by incomplete foot drop secondary to peroneal nerve injury caused by the tibial fracture.

Clinical Presentation:

Neurologically examination suggested a C5 to C6 injury, with partial C7 lesion, and minimal affection of C8 spinal root.

Recovery of C8 was favorable, with return to triceps strength to M3. While this obviated the need for reconstructive intervention of the triceps, the muscle remained insufficiently strong to serve as a donor for axillary reinnervation.

The peroneal injury improved spontaneously within five months, although weakness of the extensor hallucis muscle persisted.

Surgical Plan:

1. Double Oberlin
2. CN XI to suprascapular nerve
3. C5 root to the posterior division of superior trunk
4. Neurolysis of peroneal nerve with concurrent harvest of the sural graft

Intraoperative Findings:

Supraclavicular exploration and peroneal nerve decompression with sural nerve graft harvest were performed concomitantly by a selected surgical team.

At the level of the superior trunk, significant fibrosis and a neuroma were identified.

The spinal accessory nerve was localized via a supraclavicular approach, traced anteriorly to the trapezius muscle.

In the upper arm, the median and the musculocutaneous nerve were identified first, followed by the branches of the musculocutaneous nerve.

> Enlargement of a nerve segment may suggest an impending branching of the nerve.

Direct electrical stimulation of the musculocutaneous nerve elicited slight muscle contraction, consistent with an incomplete C5/6 lesion, in line with preoperative clinical suspicion.

The ulnar nerve was identified in its typical location in the upper arm, beneath or between two accompanying veins (Fig. 8.15).

C5C6 Brachial Plexus Lesions and Surgical Considerations

In isolated C5/C6 brachial plexus injuries, weakness of the muscles innervated by the median nerve does not typically occur, as the motor contribution to the median nerve arises from the lateral cord, which at this level is predominantly sensory.

Consequently, patients will present with hypoesthesia of the palmar aspect of the first three digits without motor impairment.

In the cases of anatomical variation where the musculocutaneous nerve is absent and its motor function is assumed by the median nerve, the patient will present with biceps and brachial palsy but preserved distal function. In such scenarios, an Oberlin transfer is performed by transferring an ulnar fascicle to the brachial branch and a median fascicle to the median nerve, thereby connecting the non-functional biceps fascicles to functioning fascicles of median nerve.

One rationale for choosing the brachial branch over the biceps branch is that the dissection is

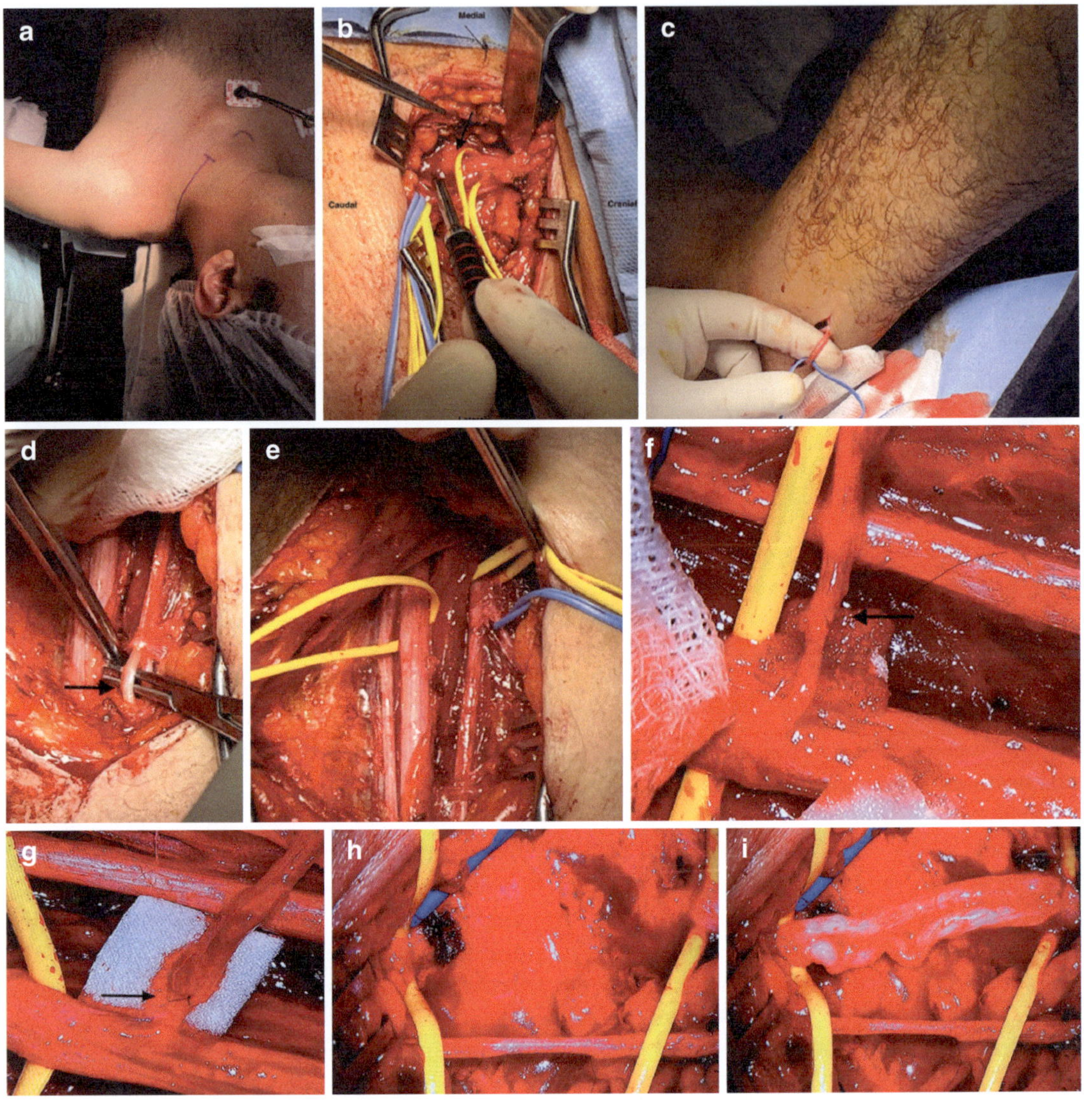

Fig. 8.15 Incision was done via a supraclavicular approach (**a**). After identifying the superior trunk, extensive fibrotic tissue was visible (**b**, arrow). Sural nerve graft harvesting (**c**) was performed it the sam time. (**d**, **e**) the musculocutaneous nerve with its branches was identified, fascicles of the ulnar and median nerve were dissected and prepared to perform a double Oberlin (**f**, **g**). The CN XI was identified to prepare for nerve transfer with the suprascapular nerve. As the gap was too large (**h**), sural nerve graft was used (**i**)

technically easier and provides greater length. The ulnar nerve, however, lies deeper and requires a longer dissection than the median nerve.

When using the ulnar nerve as a donor, the fascicles responsible for wrist flexion should be selected, while preserving those that innervate the intrinsic hand muscles to avoid compromising fine motor function. These fascicles are identified intraoperatively by direct electrical stimulation after opening the epineurium.

The classical Oberlin procedure involves transfer of both median and ulnar fascicles. A single Oberlin transfer may be considered when one donor is not functioning adequately, or when residual function of the biceps or brachial is present and a supercharge transfer is preferred.

During nerve coaptation, tension must be avoided: the nerve should not be too short which would risk traction, nor excessively long, as this unnecessarily increases the regeneration distance for axonal sprouting.

Distally along the musculocutaneous nerve, two branches are typically encountered: the brachialis branch and the cutaneous branch. To differentiate them, the branches must be traced distally—only one will terminate in the brachialis muscle. The cutaneous branch can sometimes be identified by mobilizing it and palpating the overlying skin, though this is not a reliable method.

If an isolated distal branch is found along the musculocutaneous nerve, it is likely to be the brachial branch.

Anatomical Variations:

Approximately 10% of the population lack a musculocutaneous nerve, in which case the median nerve assumes innervation of the biceps and brachialis muscles.

Converesly, the musculocutaneous nerve may give up to seven branches to the biceps muscle.

If multiple branches are present (e.g. three branches), they must be grouped together and coaptated to the fascicle of the median nerve in an Oberlin transfer.

The median nerve normally runs lateral to the artery and gives no branches in the upper arm. However, in some anatomical variants, branches from the median nerve may substitute for musculocutaneous innervation of the biceps and brachial muscles.

Additional considerations:

Wrist extension is mediated by fibers from C8 contributing to C7, rather than from C7 alone.

In C8-T1 lesions surgery may be delayed to 7–9 months post-injury, as the regeneration distance is longer.

In severe traumatic BPI cases, the *suprascapular nerve* may suffer a double crush injury— at the brachial plexus level and additionally at the suprascapular notch. This may explain suboptimal functional outcomes following suprascapular nerve transfers.

A strategy to mitigate this risk is to perform a spinal accessory to suprascapular nerve transfer via a posterior approach. Here, the suprascapular and infraspinatus motor branches are addressed separately. A horizontal incision is made at the level of the scapular spine, with the suprascapular notch located at the midpoint between the acromion and the superior angle of the scapula.

The spinal accessory nerve can typically be identified within the same incision approximately 40% of the distance from the spinal process to the acromion.

Case Presentation:

Female patient, 58-years old

History:

The patient sustained an upper brachial plexus injury following a traffic accident.

Over the subsequent nine months, she experienced spontaneous neurological recovery, regaining triceps muscle strength to M4.

Clinical Presentation:

At the time of presentation, the patient exhibited weakness of the deltoid muscle with muscle atrophy being evident. Additionally, some degree of shoulder subluxation and mild atrophy of the supraspinatus muscle was visible.

Surgical Plan:

Transfer of a triceps branch to axillary nerve to restore deltoid muscle function.

Exploration of brachial plexus, with particular attention to the suprascapular nerve given the persistent shoulder subluxation.

Intraoperative Findings:

A supraclavicular approach was performed. The suprascapular nerve, as well as the anterior and posterior divisions of the superior trunk demonstrated a good response to intraoperative stimulation. Due to the presence of fibrous adhesions, neurolysis was carried out.

Subsequently, a triceps branch to the axillary nerve transfer was performed (Fig. 8.16).

> Because the axillary nerve is relatively immobile, the harvested triceps branch must be of sufficient length to allow tension-free placement and secure coaptation at the level of the axillary nerve.

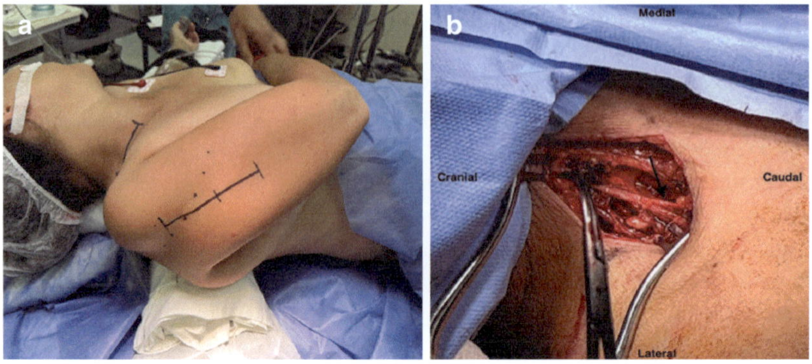

Fig. 8.16 Positioning of the patient for surgery (**a**). The dotted line on the lateral upper arm represents the border of the deltoid muscle. After performing a supraclavicular approach, the anterior and posterior divisions of the superior trunk are depicted by the arrow (**b**)

Case Presentation:

Male patient, 63 years old

Clinical Presentation:

The patient sustained an upper brachial plexus injury following a motorcycle accident approximately six months prior.

Two months earlier, an Oberlin transfer was performed. At the time of evaluation, some biceps contraction was palpable but functional elbow flexion was not yet achieved, consistent with early postoperative recovery. The patient additionally underwent left leg amputation due to infection sequela from the accident and prior surgeries.

Surgical Plan:

Restore shoulder function while avoiding use of the sural nerve as a graft, given the patient's single remaining leg. This precaution minimizes risks of immobilization, thrombosis, paresthesia, infection, or delayed wound healing.

Intraoperative Findings:

Via a suprascapular approach, the superior trunk and the phrenic nerve were identified. Distally, the trifurcation (anterior and posterior divisions, suprascapular nerve) served as the the next anatomical landmark, while the C5 and the C6 roots were visible proximal to the superior trunk. The spinal accessory nerve was also visualized via this approach.

Intraoperatively, all structures could be identified, nevertheless there was extensive fibrous tissue present at the level of the C5 root. Stimulation of the C5 root produced no answer; partial transection was performed to inspect fascicles. Given intact fascicles and a functioning phrenic nerve, the lesion was presumed distal, with no root avulsion.

Whenever considering the **C5 root as a donor** root as a donor, there is a risk of distal lesion that may prevent functional stimulation; unless preoperative MRI provides definite information.

The C5 root was not fully transected to prevent proximal retraction into the tissue thereby losing it.

A transverse cervical nerve (cutaneous/superficial cervical nerve) was harvested and used as a graft to connect the C5 root to the posterior division, thereby avoiding the sural nerve.

The spinal accessory nerve was identified, mobilized, and transected as proximal as possible. Access to the suprascapular nerve was facilitated by resecting connective tissue and partial muscle release, allowing a direct nerve transfer without the need of an intepositional graft (Fig. 8.17).

Obstetric Brachial Plexus Palsy (OBPP)

Case Presentation:

Clinical Presentation:

A 6-months-old infant was presented to the hospital, where a weak C5 and C6 function was observed. Horner syndrome was absent. The

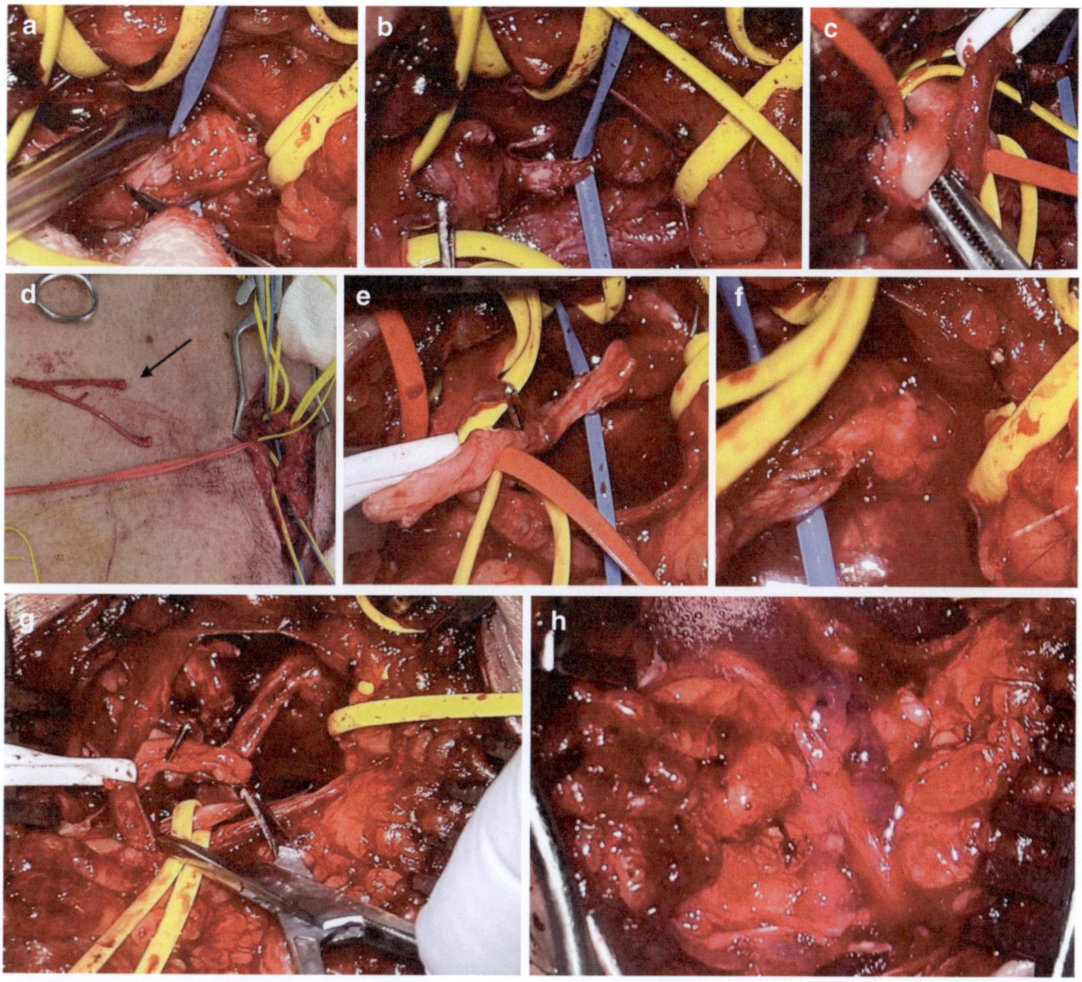

Fig. 8.17 (**a**) Shows the C5 root with a good fascicular structure suggesting a working C5 stump (blue loop). The C5 root was then partially transected (**b**, blue loop)—with the good fascicular structure and a well functioning phrenic nerve (strong answer on stimulation), we could assume that the lesion was more distally and the proximal part of C5 root is working (whenever you are taking the C5 root as a donor, it is a risk because you never know how good it is functioning as stimulation cannot help you). The C5 root was not completely transected to prevent retraction of the nerve. The posterior division (**c**, red loop) of the superior trunk was then prepared for suturing to the C5 root via nerve graft taking the superior cervical nerve (**d–f**). (**g**) shows the suprascapular nerve (yellow loop) which was sutured directly to the spinal accessory nerve to provide shoulder function. Fibrin glue was applied after suturing (**h**)

shoulder deformity was already evident due to weakness of the external rotators.

Surgical Plan:

1. Spinal accessory to suprascapular nerve
2. Repositioning of the glenohumeral joint
3. C7 to C8 spinal root
4. C5 root to the posterior division of the superior trunk

   C5 root to the middle trunk
5. Intercostal nerves to musculocutaneous—addressed at the main trunk level rather than the biceps/brachialis branches due to shorter regeneration distance

Intraoperative Findings:

A suprascapular approach was performed to expose the brachial plexus and identify the spinal accessory nerve. Direct transfer of the supra scapular nerve was feasible without a graft.

Regarding shoulder reconstruction, the subscapular tendon was partially released to reposition the glenohumeral joint and restore external rotation. Postoperatively, the shoulder and arm were immobilized in a thoracobrachial external rotation brace for 1 month.

The sural nerve was then harvested and folded five times to bridge a C7-to-C8 root transfer, addressing C8 root avulsion.

The lateral cutaneous antebrachial nerve was used as a graft to connect the C5 root to the posterior division the superior trunk.

Intercostal nerves were transferred to the musculocutaneous nerve to restore elbow flexion.

Except for the CN XI to the suprascapular nerve transfer, all nerve coaptations were performed using fibrin glue. This was possible due to immobilization in a cast, preventing disruption of the repaired nerves by movement. (Fig. 8.18).

In obstetric brachial plexus palsy (OBPP) the development of shoulder dysplasia must always be considered. Even when nerve reconstruction is successful, a deformed glenohumeral joint will limit shoulder mobility.

Muscle function will adopt abnormally in response to joint dysplasia: the supraspinatus can assume the role of an internal rotator, while the infraspinatus and teres minor muscles may function as abductors. These changes are often indicative for C5/C6 avulsion. Weakness of the external rotators typically result in internal rotation contracture.

To prevent shoulder dysplasia in infants with OBPP, the shoulder should be positioned in external rotation using a cast[7].

It is important to recognize that the triceps muscle receives innervation from both the C7 and C8 spinal roots, which must be considered during reconstruction.

In OBPP, hand function is generally prioritized over elbow and shoulder function; therefore, the median nerve is typically addressed first. Proximal transfers using the C8 root offer the

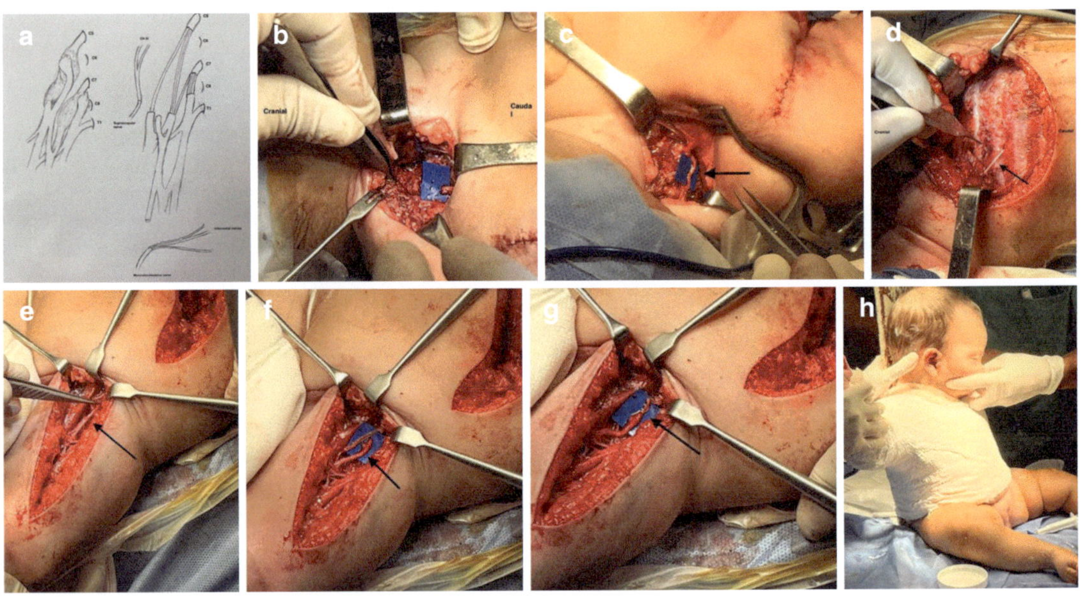

Fig. 8.18 (**a**) Represents the preoperative drawing of the brachial plexus injury (left) and the surgical plan (right). The accessory nerve is transferredventrallytobesuturedtothesuprascapularnerve (**b**, **c**). Next, the intercostal nerves are dissected at the level of the lateral ribs (**d**) and the musculocutaneous nerve is prepared (**e**) to be transferred forthesecondnervetransfer.The intercostal nerves are put to the median upper arm (**f**) and fixed via fibrin glue (**g**). After performing the nerve transfers,theglenohu meraljointisrepositionedandthearmandshoulders are put in a cast (**h**)

advantage of a short regeneration distance but carry the potential risk of axonal misrouting.

A classical nerve transfer procedure for Erb's palsy involves transfer of the spinal accessory nerve to suprascapular nerve, combined with reconstruction of the C5 and C6 spinal nerve stumps—usually with interposition grafts. In cases of total brachial plexus palsy with preganglionic injury, extra-plexal nerve transfers are required.

Shoulder reduction surgery is performed by releasing contracted ligaments of the rotator cuff, particularly those caused by tightness of the subscapularis muscle, to restore proper glenohumeral alignment.

Further Reading

1. Ruettermann M. Challenging the dogma: anterior transposition of the ulnar nerve is indicated in recurrent cubital tunnel syndrome. J Hand Surg Eur Vol. 2021;46(1):45–449. https://doi.org/10.1177/1753193420970022.
2. Byun YS, Lee SU, Park IJ, Im JH, Hong SA. Comparison of in-situ release and submuscular anterior transposition of ulnar nerve for refractory cubital tunnel syndrome, previously treated with subfascial anterior transfer-a retrospective study of 24 cases. Injury. 2023;54(12):111061. https://doi.org/10.1016/j.injury.2023.111061.
3. Nabhan A, Kelm J, Steudel WI, Shariat K, Sova L, Ahlhelm F. Sulcus-ulnaris-Syndrom: Einfache Dekompression oder subkutane Vorverlagerung? [Cubital tunnel syndrome—simple nerve decompression or decompression with subcutaneous anterior transposition?]. Fortschr Neurol Psychiatr. 2007;75(3):168–71. https://doi.org/10.1055/s--2006-955004. German. Epub 2007 Jan 17. PMID: 17230307.
4. Rojas-Gómez MF, Blanco-Dávila R, Tobar Roa V, Gómez González AM, Ortiz Zableh AM, Ortiz Azuero A. Regional anesthesia guided by ultrasound in the pudendal nerve territory. Colomb J Anesthesiol. 2017;45(3):200–9. https://doi.org/10.1016/j.rcae.2017.06.007.
5. Kaur J, Leslie SW, Singh P. Pudendal nerve entrapment syndrome. In: StatPearls. StatPearls Publishing; 2023.
6. Bertelli JA, Soldado F, Rodrígues-Baeza A, Ghizoni MF. Transferring the motor branch of the opponens pollicis to the terminal division of the deep branch of the ulnar nerve for pinch reconstruction. J Hand Surg Am. 2019;44(1):9–17. https://doi.org/10.1016/j.jhsa.2018.09.010.
7. Nixon M, Trail I. Management of shoulder problems following obstetric brachial plexus injury. Shoulder Elbow. 2014;6(1):12–7. https://doi.org/10.1111/sae.12003.